D1252687

OVERUSE INJURIES
of the
MUSCULOSKELETAL
SYSTEM

Marko M. Pečina
Chairman and Professor
Department of Orthopaedic Surgery
School of Medicine
University of Zagreb
Zagreb, Croatia

Ivan Bojanić
Assistant Lecturer
Department of Orthopaedic Surgery
School of Medicine
University of Zagreb
Zagreb, Croatia

CRC Press
Boca Raton   Ann Arbor   London   Tokyo

Library of Congress Cataloging-in-Publication Data

Pećina, Marko.
    Overuse injuries of the musculoskeletal system / by Marko Pećina,
Ivan Bojanić.
      p.   cm.
    Includes bibliographical references and index.
    ISBN 0-8493-4492-1
    1. Overuse injuries. I. Bojanić, Ivan. II. Title.
    [DNLM: 1. Musculoskeletal System--injuries. 2. Atheltic Injuries.
    3. Repetition Strain Injury--diagnosis. 4. Repetition Strain
    Injury--therapy.   WE 175 P365o 1993]
    RD97.6.P43   1993
    617.4'7044--dc20
    DNLM/DLC
    for Library of Congress   93-8061
                                                         CIP

No claim to original U.S. Government works
International Standard Book Number 0-8493-4492-1
Library of Congress Card Number 93-8061
Printed in the United States of America   3 4 5 6 7 8 9 0
Printed on acid-free paper

AAX - 7328

Preface

Related either to athletic activities and recreation or to various professional activities, overuse injuries of the musculoskeletal system are common occurrences in the life of modern humans. Therefore, it is not surprising that overuse injuries are frequently discussed. The mode of this discussion is usually limited to the analysis of different individual painful syndromes, specific localizations of the painful syndrome in the musculoskeletal system, or the specific tissues affected by overuse injuries (tendinitis, stress fractures, etc.). The purpose and scope of this book is to systematically, (and in one place) present today's state of knowledge regarding overuse injuries which affect the musculoskeletal system as a whole. Regardless of the localization and the affected tissue, all clinical entities are presented in the same manner: the name and definition of the syndrome, etiopathogenesis, clinical picture, diagnostic, nonoperative, and operative treatment, and the possibility of prevention.

Besides presenting the newest discoveries reported in the world medical literature, this book also reveals a wealth of individual cases and experiences encompassing pathohistological examinations, x-ray analysis, intraoperative photographs, and the results of both conservative and operative procedures. All patients were treated in the University of Zagreb. I am grateful for the help the University's employees provided during the preparation of this work. A deep debt of gratitude is also due to my family whose patience, love, and support have helped me not only during the writing of this book, but on numerous occasions as well. Apart from the experience of the senior author, the enthusiasm of the younger, already competent co-author was of particular importance during the making of this work.

It goes without saying that the high standard and experience of the publisher, CRC Press, is a significant contribution to the quality of this book for which I am deeply indebted.

Marko M. Pećina
Zagreb

The Authors

Marko M. Pećina, M.D., Ph.D., is Chairman and Professor of Orthopaedic Surgery at the School of Medicine, University of Zagreb. He is also Chief of the Department at Zagreb Teaching Hospital Orthopaedic Clinic.

Dr. Pećina graduated from Zagreb University Medical School in 1964. He was an assistant lecturer at the "Drago Perovic" Anatomic Institute of Zagreb Medical School from 1966 to 1970. He obtained his M.Sc. degree in experimental biology at Zagreb University Faculty of Natural Sciences in 1969 and defended his Ph.D. in medical science at Zagreb University Medical School 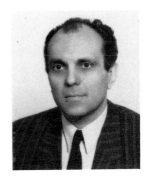 in 1970. Dr. Pećina became an assistant lecturer at Zagreb Medical School Orthopaedic Clinic in 1970. He became senior lecturer in 1978, assistant professor in 1979, associate professor in 1980, and professor in orthopaedics in 1984.

He has visited and worked in many orthopaedic institutions around the world for further professional training (Lyon, Bologna, Basel, London, Milwaukee, New York, Baltimore, Los Angeles, Columbus, and others). He has also participated in numerous symposia and conferences in his country and abroad. He is actively engaged in professional associations, in particular the Croatian Medical Association and Croatian Orthopaedic and Traumatology Society. He is also president of the Croatian Medical Bulletin council and editor-in-chief of the *Croatian Sports Medicine Journal*. Dr. Pećina is a member of the following international societies: International Knee Society, European Spinal Deformities Society, French Society for Orthopaedic Surgery and Traumatology (Société Francaise de Chirurgie Orthopédique et Traumatologigue), European Society of Knee Surgery, Sports Traumatology and Arthroscopy, Italian Club of Knee Surgery (Club Italiano di Chirurgia del Ginocchio), Balkan Medical Union (Union Medicale Balkanique), Collège Européen de Traumatologie du Sport, and the International Association of Olympic Medical Officers. He is a member of the Croatian Olympic Committee and Chairman of the Medical Commission. He is also a member of Société Internationale de Chirurgie Orthopédique et de Traumatologie (SICOT) and is a SICOT national delegate for Croatia and a member of the International Committee. Dr. Pećina is an honorary member of the Hellenic Orthopaedic and Traumatologic Society. He is one of the founders of the European Spinal Deformities Society and was vice-president from 1989 to 1992. Since 1990, he has been a corresponding member of the Editorial Board of International Orthopaedics and the Hip International.

For his professional achievements, Dr. Pećina was awarded numerous tokens of appreciation such as the Balkan Medical Union Award for Scientific Achievement, the Croatian Award of Sports Medicine, and the Croatian Award for Scientific Achievement. He has also received many other diplomas of foreign and domestic associations. He is a regular member of the Croatian Medical Academy and an associated member of the Croatian Academy of Arts and Sciences.

Dr. Pećina is interested in clinical anatomy and applied biomechanics of the locomotor system, scoliosis, knee problems, and sports traumatology. He has published more than 350 expert and scientific papers and several books, including *Tunnel Syndromes* (CRC Press, Boca Raton, 1991).

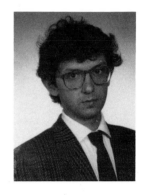

Ivan Bojanić, M.D., is currently in his third year of training as an orthopaedic surgeon. He is also an assistant lecturer at the Department of Orthopaedic Surgery at the School of Medicine, University of Zagreb, Croatia.

Dr. Bojanić obtained his M.D. degree in 1988 from Zagreb University, School of Medicine. He obtained his M.Sc. degree (in biomedicine) in 1991 from Zagreb University, Faculty of Natural Sciences.

Dr. Bojanić is a member of the Croatian Medical Association and Croatian Orthopaedic and Traumatology Society, Croatian Society of Knee Surgery, Sports Traumatology and Arthroscopy. He is the editor of the *Croatian Sports Medicine Journal* and leading doctor of the Croatian track and field national team. He has been participating in international congresses and meetings and thus far has published several articles. Dr. Bojanić's current major research interests are in sports traumatology, arthroscopy, and knee surgery.

Table of Contents

General Part

Chapter

1

Introduction

I. SIGNIFICANCE OF OVERUSE INJURIES

Athletic activities and recreational exercises are the phenomenon of modern civilized societies. The Olympic logo, *"Citius, altius, fortius"*, may serve us better nowadays as "Even faster, even higher, even stronger". If we consider the fact that many sport participants are professionally involved and that sport has become big business and top entertainment in our society, we can understand how sport can be demanding upon an athlete. At the same time, during the last few decades, recreational exercise has become most peoples' everyday lifestyle. About 15% of Americans now jog regularly. This means at least 30 million participants who are in aerobic exercise continue to proliferate, and both swimming and cycling have a growing following with over 75 million participants. However, as exercise continues to proliferate, so do the concomitant injuries. Injuries to the musculoskeletal system that would not normally happen are very frequent due to athletic activities.

Acute mechanical injuries are not a diagnostic and therapeutic problem since they do not differ from injuries happening among the average population. Indeed, various studies indicate that approximately 30 to 50% of all sports injuries are caused by overuse. Many physicians do not make any difference between damage and injury and classify all symptoms under injuries. Injury may be defined as any damage of the tissue that occurred in a well-defined and limited time span. Damage is considered to be the pathological anatomic entity that cannot be proved (evidenced) and, in most cases, the patient did not feel and does not even remember when the damage happened. To sum it up, the main characteristic of an injury is its acuteness, while the damage has chronical character. Damage of the locomotor system is the result of a series of repetitive microtraumas that overwhelm the tissue's ability to repair itself.[34] Therefore, many authors view it as one of the microtraumatic illnesses, but etiologically and pathogenetically, it would be better to term it as an overuse injury.[30]

While overuse of the other major body systems (cardiac, respiratory, renal, nervous, etc.) is relatively easy to test, the overuse of the musculoskeletal system is very hard to prove since there are no morphological and physiological standards with which to compare. The prepathological condition of other major body systems may be objectivized [electrocardiogram (EKG), electromyograph (EMG), electroencephalogram (EEG), etc.], but it is very hard to establish objective standards for overuse injuries of the musculoskeletal system. The common etiology of all of the musculoskeletal overuse injuries is repetitive trauma that overwhelms the tissue's ability to repair itself, including tendons, bursae, cartilage, bone, and especially the musculotendinous unit.

The cause of overuse injuries is much clearer when the biomechanical factors of different sports are analyzed.[7,37] The foot touches the soil between 800 and 2000 times on a 1-mile long run. The ground reactive force at midstance in running is 250 to 300% of body weight. A 70-kg runner at 1175 steps per mile absorbs at least 220 ton of force per mile. Therefore, it is not surprising that even the smallest anatomical or biomechanical abnormalities of the lower extremities, especially if they are submitted to training errors or some other external factors, may lead to overuse injuries of the lower extremities and/or the spine.

To understand the genesis of overuse injuries in the upper extremities, one should only ponder for a couple of seconds on the number of times a javelin thrower throws his spear, a weightlifter lifts his weights, or a handball or waterpolo player takes a shot at the goal. To cite an example, a swimmer will typically make somewhere in the neighborhood of 4000 overhead strokes during one training session. This adds up to more than 800,000 overhead strokes in just one season and simply illustrates why around 60% of the top-class swimmers suffer from overuse injury in the shoulder area.[37]

When talking about overuse injuries, one generally tends to equate it with professional or recreational athletes. However, physicians should be aware of the fact that overuse injuries can also develop in nonathletes and can develop as a result of other human activities,[8,11,14,29] primarily work habits. As an example, we cite the case of an automechanic, who typically works for hours, on a daily basis, with a screwdriver and as a consequence, is at risk for developing lateral (radial) epicondylitis or "tennis elbow". If one takes into account other similarly risk-prone professions such as professional musicians and dancers, dactiolographers, cooks, surgeons, workers on an assembly line, and others, it becomes quite clear that the overuse injury is not just a sports medicine problem, but indeed, a general medical problem. The most important, and at the same time both diagnostically and therapeutically still not completely understood questions are those dealing with overuse in the musculotendinous functional unit, the area where the muscle inserts into the tendon and the tendon inserts into the bone. La Cava[20] refers to this area as the "mioenthesic apparatus". Other authors use the term enthesis, which refers to the area of insertion of the tendon into the bone. This can be carried out either directly or through cartilage, ligament, or membrane (aponeurose). The insertion of the muscle into the tendon is carried out under a more or less sharp angle. This ensures that the direction of the muscle remains relatively constant, despite the fact that the breadth of the muscle is greater than the breadth of the tendon. It is generally believed that at the area of insertion of the muscle fibers into the tendon, there exists an intermediary zone of adhesive tissue of 10 to 100 mm thickness. It is beyond doubt that the musculotendinous unit has some specific characteristics which differentiate it from the muscle, and it is equally beyond doubt that the musculotendinous unit represents a complete and unique functional unit.

The musculotendinous functional unit suffers the greatest strain during muscle contraction. The force of the muscle is relayed to the ends of the musculotendinous unit where the cross area is considerably smaller than the cross area of the muscle. In all cases of longitudinal extension, the maximal forces appear at the ends — in this case, the musculotendinous unit. The elasticity of the musculotendinous unit is smaller than the elasticity of the muscle while its fragility is considerably greater, increasing the risk of its injury. Special proprioceptive bodies are located in the musculotendinous unit which enable it to react in accordance to the state of contraction of the muscle fibers, or in other words to the degree of the mechanical deformation of the muscle.

Since the musculotendinous functional unit has a polymorphic structure, it can be adapted to multifunctional demands of the musculoskeletal system. The musculotendinous unit is also characterized by its susceptibility to injury, which leads to tissue metaplasia (e.g., calcification) in the tendon. One should be aware that the tendon tissue is braditrophic, which explains why it is more often affected by pathological changes due to overuse than other tissues. The changes may affect the musculotendinous area, the tendon itself, its sheath, or the insertion for the bone.[16] They are referred to as miotendinitis, tendinitis, paratenonitis, or just enthesitis, although some authors generally use the term enthesitis for changes on the musculotendinous unit (Figure 1).

When the tendon is overused, the reduction in vascular supply and excessive irritation of nerve ends lead to an aseptic inflammatory reaction which leads to tissue metaplasia, including cartilage, osteoid, and bone metaplasia. The process is chronic and may last for months with frequent reinflammations, causing a condition with constant complaints. To better understand the etiology of the overuse injuries of the musculoskeletal system, it is essential to understand the pathology of the inflammatory process. Regardless of the injury type, the tissue answer is always an inflamma-

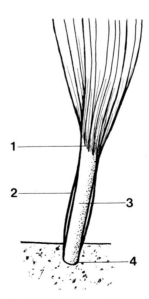

FIGURE 1. Possible localizations of pathological changes in the muscle-tendon union. (1) Miotendinitis; (2) paratendinitis or peritendinitis; (3) tendinitis; (4) enthesitis.

tory response which encompasses a number of changes of the vascular net, blood, and connective tissue. The inflammatory response is a very complex response that includes different cell types, numerous enzymes, and many physiologically active substances. Unfortunately, this response has as yet not been completely elucidated. The cause of the initiation of the inflammatory response is unknown in many cases. One such example is rheumatoid arthritis. On the other hand, the cause may be well known — for instance microorganisms, immunocomplexes or the by-products of the necrotic tissue. This last cause can be directly and causally correlated to the genesis of the overuse injury and the accompanied tissue damage.

Before we elaborate on the etiology and development of the inflammatory response in the overuse injury, it is necessary to elucidate some basic factors concerning this response: vasoactive substances, chemotactic factors, and tissue-damaging agents. Vasoactive substances include prostaglandins, vasoactive amines (histamine, serotonin), anaphylatoxins, and kinins (bradykinin, lysilbradykinin), and it is believed that they cause vasodilation and increased permeability of the blood vessels. The rupture of damaged cells of the tendon releases chemicals which signal other cells to come to the area to aid in cleaning up the damaged tissue. Several different molecules that have chemotactic effect have been isolated. Some of them are of bacterial origin, but others originate from the complement system-activated-by-products. It is discovered that leukotriens and kallikreins also have chemotactic effect. Agents that cause tissue rupture are enzymes hydrolases located inside the lysosomes of the inflamed cells and enzymes located in the extracellular area (e.g., collagenases, elastases, and cathepsin G).

In overuse injuries, the tendon has been loaded repeatedly and the sum of repetitive force leads to microtraumas that initiate the inflammatory response.[10] The initial vasoconstriction is replaced by vasodilation. As a consequence, increase of the intracapillary pressure, permeability of the fine vascular net, and release of the fair amount of transudate in the perivascular area occur. Further permeability increase of the blood vessels causes the accumulation of the fluid containing different cell types and many cell compounds (proteins, white blood cells, thrombocytes). The fluid itself is called *exudate*. Chemotactic chemicals act as signals to draw cells involved with the healing process. Polymorphonuclear leukocytes start degradation of the surrounding tissue by activated hydrolases released from their lysosomes. After a few days, they are replaced by monocytes that soon become macrophages. Other cell types, such as lymphocytes, plasma cells, fibroblast, and mast cells, are also present in the damaged tissue area. Macrophages play the most important role in the inflammatory response. They digest all the by-products of inflammation by process of phagocytosis or endocytosis and thus help in cleaning up the damaged tissue. This event enables the last phase of the response, the healing phase, to take place.

Although the inflammatory response is necessary to initiate healing, it should last only a short time. If the inflammation is prolonged, we must prevent it from becoming chronic. Only under such circumstances should one apply nonsteroidal and steroidal anti-inflammatory drugs. To clarify drug effect, we will describe the role of prostaglandins in the inflammatory response. Prostaglandins are local hormones derived from arachidonic acid. They are metabolized very quickly, but other than that, their biological effects have not been thoroughly investigated yet. In the inflammatory response, they cause local vasodilatation and increased vessel permeability resulting in edema of the inflammated tissue. Together with other mediators of the inflammation, they stimulate pain receptors and are responsible for pain, the first clinical sign of tendinitis. They stimulate osteoclasts and macrophages and, therefore, cause bone resorption as well. Nonsteroidal anti-inflammatory drugs deactivate enzyme cyclooxigenase responsible for the conversion of the arachidonic acid to prostaglandin. Glucocorticoids can also inhibit the biosynthesis of the prostaglandins by locking the enzyme phospholipase.

Generally speaking, healing is the body's response to injury. The process may be divided in phases depending on time needed to activate particular healing mechanisms. Connective tissue healing is divided into two broad stages: proliferative and formative. During the former, which lasts approximately 14 d, cells migrate to the area of the tissue damage and new connective tissue is laid down. This new tissue is remodeled during the next formative stage. The formative stage extends from the end of the proliferative stage until the tissue is as near normal as possible. Chvapil[10] further subdivides connective tissue healing into four stages: (1) cell mobilization (inflammatory response), (2) ground substance proliferation, (3) collagen protein formation, and (4) final organization. Stages 1 to 3 are the proliferative stages of healing, while Stage 4 is formative.

During the stage of cell mobilization, the rupture of damaged cells releases chemotactic substances that initiate the increase in vessel permeability and act as signals to white blood cells, but also help the degradation of damaged tissue. This stage is also called the stage of inflammatory response. It begins when injury occurs, lasts for 48 h, and is important because of the arrival of white blood cells.

Ground substance proliferation does not take place until Day 3 or 4. The existence of an adequate amount of ground substance (which is a gel-like matrix composed of proteins, carbohydrates, and water) is necessary for the aggregation of collagenous proteins into the shape of fibrils.

The stage of collagen protein formation begins at Day 5 following the injury, and is characterized with the transformation of the immature (soluble) collagen into the mature form of the molecule. Collagen transforms as a result of cross-link forming between the tropocollagen molecules. From Day 6 to Day 14, the proportion of cross-linked collagen increases. It is of crucial importance to stop the inflammation before Day 5 because the enzymes prevent formation of cross-links and degrade newly synthesized soluble collagen.

In the final stage, from Day 14 onward, collagen continues to increase and begins to organize into fibrils that reorient themselves in line with the tensile force applied to the tissue. Namely, it is very important to contract the adjacent muscles because the contraction causes the stress of collagen fibrils and generates electric potential due to the piezoelectric effect. The potential itself orients collagen fibrils in line with the tensile force of the muscle contraction. With this event, the process of healing is terminated, and the tendon is capable of withstanding further mechanical loads.

Although conditions concerning tendons and tendon insertions are primarily considered overuse injuries of the musculoskeletal system, some of them are bones,[15,24] muscles, joint cartilage, bursae,[25] and peripheral nerves.[29] One joint that appears to be particularly susceptible to overuse conditions is the patellofemoral joint, where abnormal wear of hyaline cartilage on the retropatellar surface may occur, resulting in anterior knee pain. This condition will be further elaborated in Chapter 7. Chapter 10 is dedicated to the inflammation of the bursae (bursitis), stressing problem of the chronic bursitis caused by repetitive trauma from either friction of the overlying tendon or external pressure applied above the bursae. Nerve tissue is also subject to overuse injury. Sensory, motor, or mixed sensory-motor peripheral nerves may be affected by constant and/or repetitive loading and pressure on nerves, but also by pathomechanics of the special anatomic area such as carpal tunnel, tarsal tunnel, etc.[29] These nerve entrapments of the sports participant are also discussed in Chapter 12.

Pathoanatomical changes that can be seen in overuse injuries of the musculoskeletal system depend on the type of tissue affected and on the localization and clinical stage of the injury. There is a large pathohistological scale from inflammatory response to degenerative changes reported by many authors[10,14,33] and confirmed by intraoperative examination in our own patients. We will briefly describe pathohistological findings concerning different localizations of overuse injuries in our operated patients. The tissue sections were obtained and histologically analyzed courtesy of Nikola Šipuš, from the Institute for Chemical Pathology, University of Zagreb. Tissue samples were obtained from all of the patients who underwent surgery. The samples were taken from the tendon insertion site and from sites of the macroscopic changes in the tendon and its sheath. The tissue samples were fixed in formalin, embedded in paraffin, and stained with hemalaun-eosin. Histological changes of the tendon tissue, bone-tendon interface, and tendon sheath, as well as blood vessels and nerves in the tendon and its sheath, have been analyzed.

The pathohistological sections shown here refer to Achilles tendinitis or patellar tendinitis, which is understandable as these localizations most commonly incite surgical treatment.

The formation of edema and tissue necrosis on certain parts of the tendon are the first noticeable changes that make a tendon different from its normal anatomy (Figures 2 and 3). After a short period of time, inflammatory cells migrate to the damaged area. The most abundant among them are mononuclears (Figure 4). Since the infection is not the issue in this case, among the inflammatory cells, there are very little granulocytes. The first stage of tissue healing, the inflammatory response, is followed by remodeling of the damaged tendon. The remodeling happens through connective tissue proliferation and formation. The proliferation of collagen molecules continues to increase from within the cells of the damaged tendon but soon organizes into collagen fibrils.

The number of blood capillaries also increases, but as the process develops, it decreases back to normal. The scar formed after the tendon is remodeled differs from the normal uninjured tendon in random organization of collagen fibers and greater number of blood capillaries (Figure 5). Changes that affect the bone-tendon interface are characterized by edema development and bleeding and sometimes even by disjunction of the tendon fibers from the bone. Smaller damages of the bone-tendon interface cause edema of all tissue structures, which is then followed by inflamma-

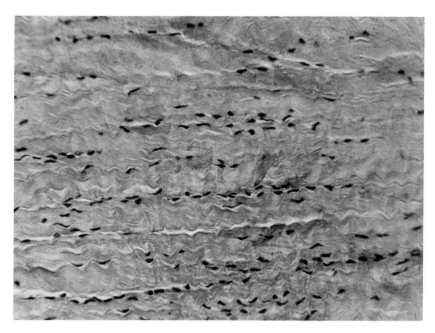

FIGURE 2. Normal tendon (×200).

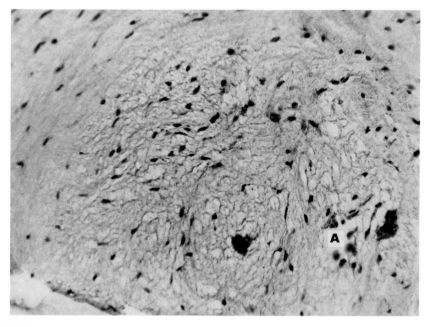

FIGURE 3. Necrotic focus in tendon accompanied by severe edema of the surrounding tissue and initial accumulation of mononuclears (A). (×200).

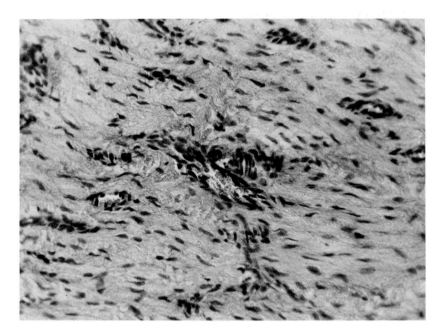

FIGURE 4. Tendon remodeling with proliferation of connective tissue strongly interspersed with blood capillaries. Inflammatory infiltrates of mononuclears are sparce. (×200).

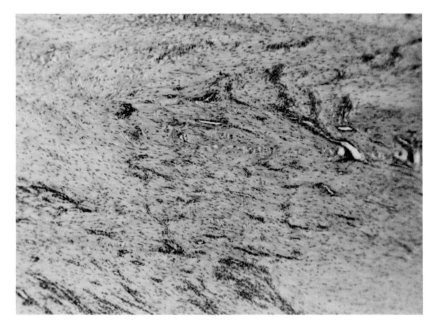

FIGURE 5. Remodeled tendon has irregular structure and contains a greater number of blood capillaries. (×60).

tion. The cells most commonly involved in the inflammatory process are mononuclears and lymphocytes (Figure 6). The connective tissue scar usually degenerates, and the biggest part of the tendon (sometimes even the periost) becomes acellular and full of homogenous hyaline matrix (Figure 7). Those scars are very often spread over surrounding tissue structures, changing the appearance of the surrounding tissue. The first sign of the changes of the tendon sheath is bleeding in the early stages of the injury. Bleeding is soon followed by a secondary inflammation. Since the tendon is poorly provided with blood and lymph, tendon sheath plays an active role in tissue remodeling.

This process is accompanied by a proliferation of macrophages and quite often gigantic cells of the foreign body which fagocite larger particles of the necrotic tendon (Figure 8).

Changes on blood vessels can be divided into changes in the arteries, capillaries, and veins. Inflammatory cells leave the arteries, and capillaries during the inflammatory infiltrates are frequently seen. Although generally younger individuals are involved, the later stages are characterized by a proliferation of endotel accompanied with endarteritic changes which significantly decrease the breadth of the blood vessel. In some cases, this leads to an obliteration of the artery (an example is shown in Figure 9, depicting the area of insertion of the Achilles tendon into the calcaneus). Smaller veins frequently have thrombocytes. In later stages, these thrombocytes are organized (Figure 10) and in some cases recanalized (Figure 11).

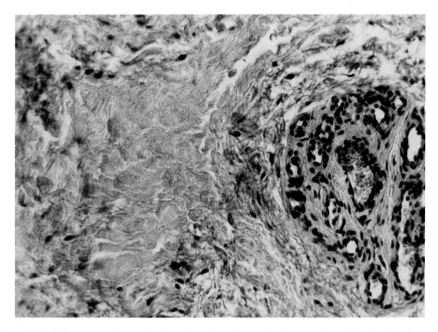

FIGURE 6. Damage to the tendon-bone insertion. Connective tissue edema. Blood capillaries are dilatated and surrounded by inflammatory cells: lymphocytes and mononuclears. (×200).

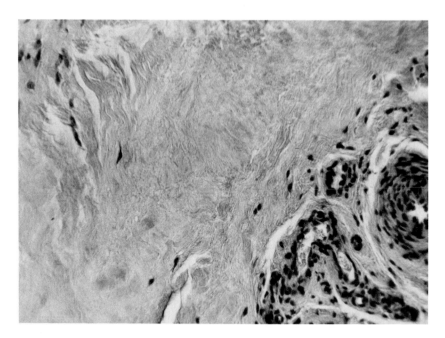

FIGURE 7. Scars on the Achilles tendon insertion site. Strong hyaline degeneration of the tendon's connective tissue makes the connective tissue practically acellular. Mononuclears are rare. (×200).

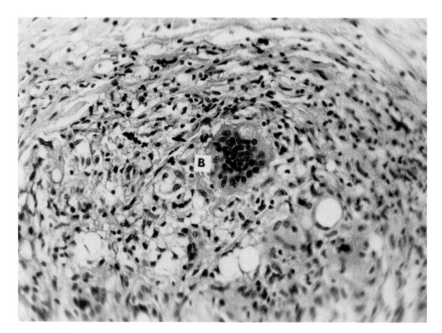

FIGURE 8. Tendon sheath inflammation accompanied by multiplication of granulation tissue rich with macrophages. Rare giant cells of the foreign body are also present, and their cytoplasm contains phagocytic necrotic material (B). (×200).

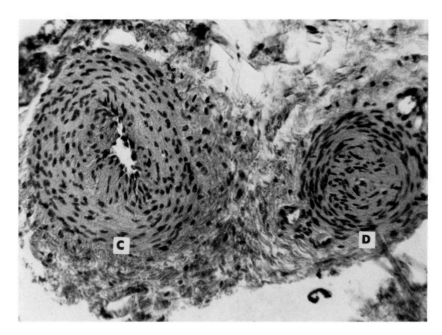

FIGURE 9. Changes affecting arteries close to the scarred tendon insertion site. Severe endarteritis with constriction of the arterial lumen (C) resulting in total obliteration of the artery (D). (×200).

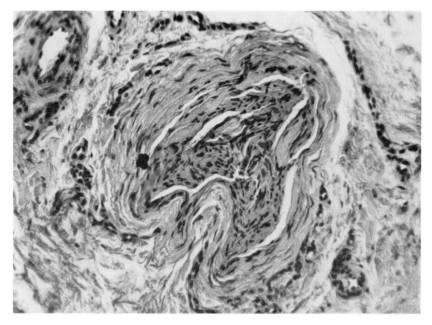

FIGURE 10. Changes in the vein close to the tendon scar. Chronic thrombosis of the vein with thromb organization. (×200).

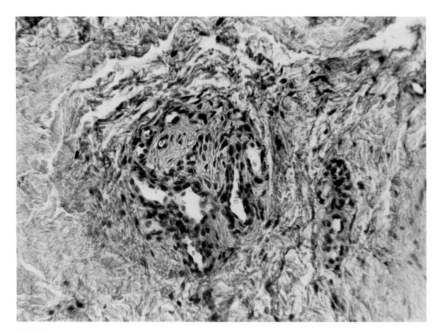

FIGURE 11. Recanalized thromb of a smaller vein localized in the scar on the tendon insertion site. (×200).

Changes in nerves of overuse injuries, up until now, have not been specially analyzed. However, we have found significant changes in the nervous tissue in the area of the injured tendon or in the area of its insertion. To better explain changes affecting nerves, we show a photograph of a normal nerve with a sheath of normal breadth (Figure 12). (According to our opinion, intense pain in the area of the injured tendon, or in the area of its insertion, with frequent morphological insignificant changes is caused by changes on the ends of peripheral nerves.) Our pathohistological analysis has shown the presence of perineuritis accompanied by an increase of breadth of the nerve sheath which later compresses the nerve. These changes are frequently very noticeable (as seen in Figure 13).

Without a complete understanding of the etiopathogenesis of overuse injuries of the musculoskeletal system, there can be no early diagnosis or adequate therapy prescribed. The etiology of these syndromes is multifactorial: In other words, numerous factors contribute to the development of overuse injuries (Table 1).

The clinical picture in the early stages of overuse injuries is characterized by a feeling of tightness. This is generally followed by pain in one part or in the whole musculotendinous unit during its passive or active stretching, during contraction of the affected muscle against resistance, and in lateral stages during normal contraction of the muscle. These symptoms are followed by pain felt during palpation, and sometimes by the presence of swelling in the affected area. The final symptoms include spontaneous pain felt during complete rest, which can in some cases radiate along the length of the whole affected muscle. With regards to the time that the pain appears during athletic activities and to the intensity of the pain, several stages of development are

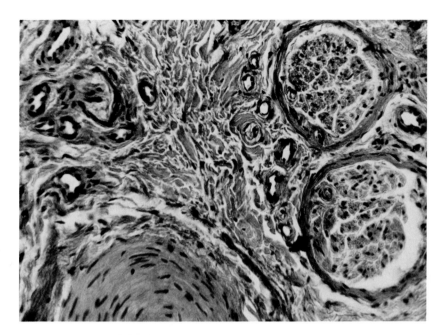

FIGURE 12. Normal nerve with unaffected sheat.

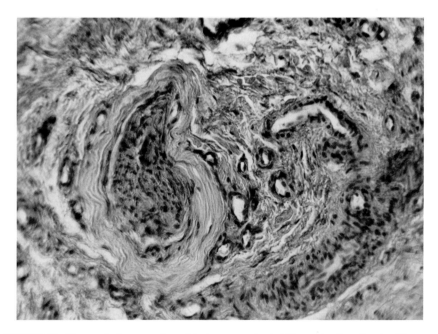

FIGURE 13. Changes in the nerve situated in the scar on the Achilles tendon insertion site. The nerve sheath is thickened and compresses the nerve. (×200).

TABLE 1

Predisposing Factors Leading to Overuse Injuries of the Musculoskeletal System

Internal (intrinsic)	External (extrinsic)
Anatomical Malalignment	Training errors
Leg length discrepancy	Abrupt Changes in intensity, duration,
Excessive femoral anteversion	and/or frequency of training
Knee alignment abnormalities (genu	Poorly trained and unskilled athlete
valgum, varum, or recurvatum)	Surface
Position of the patella (patella	Hard
infera or alta)	Uneven
Excessive Q-angle	Footwear
Excessive external tibial rotation	Inappropriate running shoes
Flat foot	Worn-out running shoes
Cavus foot	
Muscle-tendon imbalance of	
Flexibility	
Strength	
Other	
Growth	
Disturbances of menstrual cycle	

recognized. Based on the correlation between the intensity of the pain, or in other words, the stage of the disease and the remaining athletic capacity, Curwin and Stanish[10] differentiate six stages of development in overuse injuries (Table 2).

II. DIAGNOSIS

The diagnosis of overuse injuries must stem from a careful history as well as a thorough physical examination. To identify the injured structure, it is essential to characterize the pain (e.g., where, when, and how long it lasts) and to ask questions establishing the etiological factors that lay groundwork for the affliction. However, the exclusion of macrotrauma is the key to proper categorization of the injury as one of overuse.

Physical examination is the basic and most important diagnostic method, while all other methods can be regarded as auxilliary methods which are useful only in concert with a detailed physical examination. The characteristics of physical examination with regards to various and specific overuse injuries are discussed in Chapters 2 through 9.

Radiographic examination is rarely of value in establishing the diagnosis of overuse injuries, with the exception of stress fractures (Figure 14). Radiographic examination can be used to detect causative factors that lead to the development of overuse injuries such as malalignment of the extensor system of the knee, static deformation of the lower extremity, and others.

Computerized tomography (CT) is a useful method when diagnosing the presence of an overuse injury and has the added advantage of being able to diagnose changes in muscles and tendons (e.g., in patients with ruptured tendons), as well as those in bone.

TABLE 2
Classification System for the Effect of Pain on Athletic Performance[10]

Level	Description of pain	Level of sports performance
1	No pain	Normal
2	Pain only with extreme exertion	Normal
3	Pain with extreme exertion, 1 to 2 h afterward	Normal or slightly decreased
4	Pain during and after any vigorous activities	Somewhat decreased
5	Pain during activity, forcing termination	Markedly decreased
6	Pain during daily activities	Unable to perform

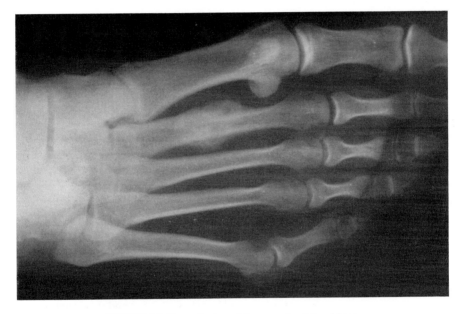

FIGURE 14. Stress fracture of the second metatarsal bone.

Bone scan with technetium-99m diphosphonate is of great help in early diagnosis of stress fractures. In recent times, its diagnostic capabilities have been significantly increased especially with regards to diagnosing changes in tendons and muscles in overuse injuries (Figure 15).

Sonographic examination is, without doubt, the most useful auxillary method used today in diagnosis of overuse injuries. In fact, one could almost say it is an unavoidable method when diagnosing overuse injuries.[12,23] Ultrasonography is very helpful when diagnosing tendinitis (Figure 16), peritendinitis, enthesitis, tendon (Figure 17) and muscle rupture (Figure 18), bursitis, and even stress fractures. The importance of sonographic examination is enhanced by its ability to perform dynamic investigations (e.g., investigation of the muscle during contraction and relaxation, investigation of the tendon during passive and active stretching, and others).

Thermography is an auxillary method which, in recent times has been successfully applied in diagnosing overuse injuries. However, its greatest value is its ability to monitor the course of the disease objectively, both when monitoring the develop-

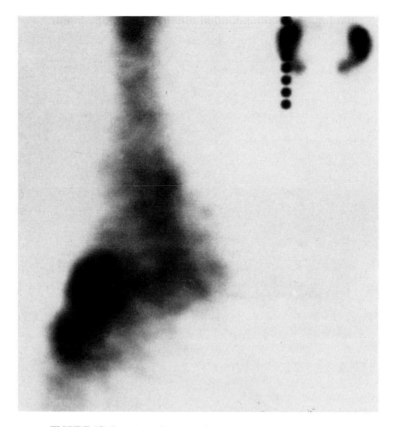

FIGURE 15. Bone scan demonstrating tarsal navicular stress fracture.

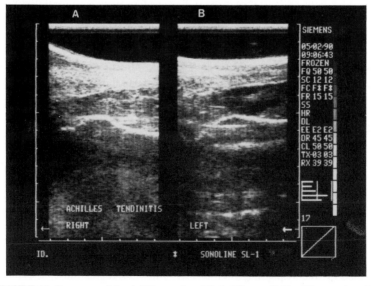

FIGURE 16. Sonogram of the Achilles tendon. (A) Achilles tendinitis; (B) normal tendon.

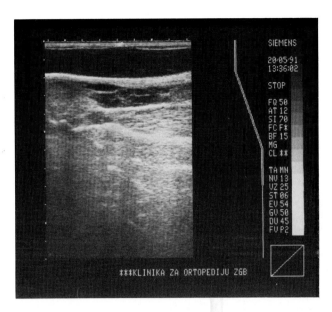

FIGURE 17. Sonogram of the Achilles tendon shows acute rupture of the tendon.

ment of overuse injury *sua sponte,* and when evaluating the effect of prescribed therapy (Figure 19).

Arthroscopy is of significant value in the detection and treatment of injuries to the joint cartilage.[17] It is most commonly applied to the knee joint but is also applied to other larger and smaller joints.

Magnetic resonance imaging (MRI) is the diagnostic method for choice in all pathological changes of the musculoskeletal system and thus is eminently applicable when diagnosing overuse injuries. MRI is able to investigate all of the tissues present in the musculoskeletal system and diagnose any pathological changes in them (Figure 20). In recent times, kinematic analysis has further enhanced the value of this diagnostic method. Despite these advantages, the exact clinical role of MRI has yet to be defined. At present, its clinical application has many limitations, including expense, lack of widespread availability, and technical problems such as limited commercial production of dedicated surface coils.

III. TREATMENT

Treatment of overuse injuries of the musculoskeletal system, in the vast majority of cases is nonoperative. Surgical treatment is rarely required. The basic principle of nonoperative treatment is that it should begin as early as possible — in other words, as soon as the first symptoms appear. The most common error is that the patients do not accord enough attention to the early symptoms and proceed with their everyday athletic or nonathletic activities with unchanged intensity. The basic postulates of nonoperative treatment for overuse injuries are based on the following principles: reducing the pain, controlling the inflammation, facilitating tissue healing, and monitoring further activities.[3,18,26,27,28]

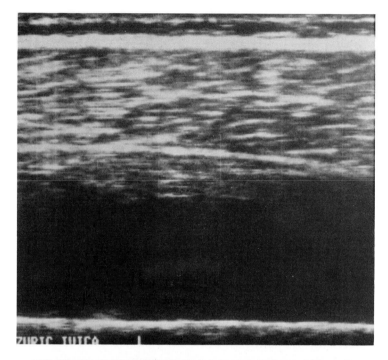

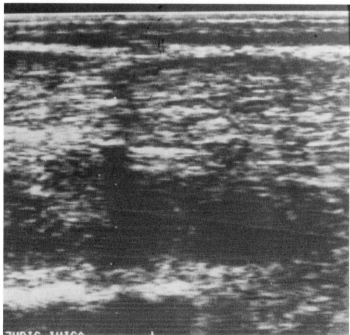

FIGURE 18. Sonogram of the lateral thigh. (A) Hematoma in the region of vastus lateralis muscle; (B) Sonographically controlled function.

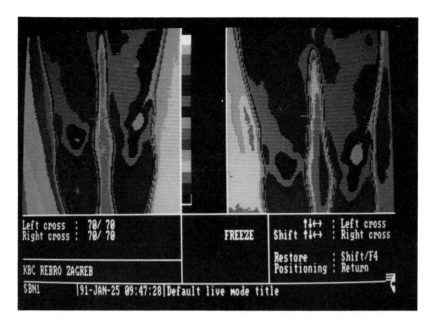

FIGURE 19. Thermography of both knees showing hypothermy in the patellar area of the afflicted knee.

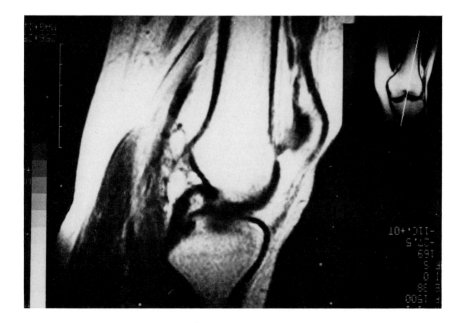

FIGURE 20. Magnetic resonance imaging (MRI) of the knee.

Any nonoperative treatment program which consists of the following must be individually adapted to every patient with regards to both the localization of the pain and to the stage of the disease:[5,9,20,21] a short-term cessation or modification of athletic activities, icing applied to the tender area, application of nonsteroidal anti-inflammatory drugs, stretching exercises for the affected muscles, strengthening exercises for the affected muscle group,[36] correction of the predisposing causative factors (training errors, anatomical deviations that impede the normal biomechanics of running, inadequate athletic footwear, and even the surface on which the athlete habitually trains).

While some authors recommend a total cessation of athletic activities, we believe that in the early stages of disease, complete cessation is not mandatory. The patient, aside from submitting to all other nonoperative methods of treatment, should be encouraged to simply reduce the intensity of his training program, especially those activities that cause pain. In later stages of disease, a complete cessation of athletic activities is mandatory for a period of no less than 3 to 4 weeks. The functional capabilities of the athlete can be kept up during this time by alternative training programs such as swimming or bicycle riding.[26,27]

Icing effectively relieves pain and muscle spasm; it lessens the inflammatory reaction by lowering the level of chemical activity and by vasoconstriction. The principle purpose in applying nonsteroidal anti-inflammatory drugs is to control and regulate the inflammatory process and to monitor its duration in such a manner so it does not last longer than its primary phase, which has a positive effect on tissue healing.

In the treatment of overuse injuries, stretching exercises are also prescribed — principally the so-called passive stretching exercises.[1,2,36] The basic principles of these exercises consist of a precisely defined stance to which the patient must adhere while performing the exercise. He should carry out slow and gradual movements until he feels a stretching sensation; then he should hold that position for a certain period of time.[31] During the performance of passive stretching exercises, the often quoted principle, "no pain, no gain", should be forgotten. The reason for this is the fact that staying in a stretched position that causes pain decreases the length of time the patient can stay in that particular position. It increases the possibility of a reflex muscle contraction and can lead to muscle damage.[19] On the other hand, remaining in the point of "primary" stretching enables the complete relaxation of the targeted muscles, and likewise enables the patient to hold that position for a relatively longer period of time. The athlete who is performing stretching exercises for the first time is advised to hold his position of primary stretching for 15 s. This period of time is gradually increased but should not exceed 30 s. The principal effects of stretching exercises — a decrease of muscle-tendon tension, improvement of vascularization in the musculotendinous functional unit, and an increase in the breadth of movements — reduce the possibility of injury development. Increase of flexibility, which also reduces injury development risk, is another long-term benefit of stretching exercises.

Surgical treatment of overuse injuries of the musculoskeletal system is the final option. In other words, surgical treatment is recommended only after all other nonoperative methods of treatment have failed.[4,6] During surgical procedure, diseased, scarred, and degenerated tissue, calcificates, chronically changed bursae, and other tissue are excised.[30,33] Whenever possible, the surgical treatment should target the causative factors that led to the development of the overuse injury, e.g., removing the tuber of the calcaneus which causes retrocalcanear bursitis or correctly orienting the extensor system of the knee (realignment). In some cases, the aim of the surgical procedure is to increase the vascularization of the injured area. This can be achieved by drilling the bone, by adhesiolysis of the tendon, or by other means. In some cases, surgical treatment is unavoidable, i.e., ruptured tendons, muscle rupture, and depending on the localization, stress fracture. Indications for surgical treatment of various overuse injuries of the musculoskeletal system are discussed in detail in Chapters 2 through 12. However, we would like to stress at this time the importance of postoperative rehabilitation since without an adequately carried out postoperative program of treatment, no surgical intervention, however well carried out, can achieve good results.

According to Curwin and Stanish,[10] the methods of both surgical and nonoperative treatment to be applied should be chosen depending on the stage of healing of the damaged tissue of the musculoskeletal system (Table 3).

Unfortunately, at present, there does not exist one method, either surgical or nonoperative, for any localization of overuse injury that can guarantee 100% good results. For this reason, prevention is of the utmost importance. Unfortunately, this has been made clear only in recent times. To carry out prevention successfully, or in other words to reduce as much as possible the risk of developing overuse injuries, one should be well acquainted with the predisposing factors leading to the development

TABLE 3
Forms of Treatment for Overuse Injuries[10]

Treatment	Used in this stage of healing[a]
Rest	1,2,3
Stop activity	
Cast immobilization	
Taping/support	1,2,3,4
Physical modalities	1,2,3
Ice	
Electric stimulation	
"Deep heat"	
Ultrasound	
Drugs	
Anti-inflammatories (oral)	1,2,3
Steroids (injections)	
Exercise	3,4
Stretching	
Strengthening	
Surgery	1 (rupture) or 4 (chronic)

[a] 1 = cell mobilization (inflammatory response); 2 = ground substance proliferation; 3 = collagen protein formation; 4 = final organization.

of these syndromes. Likewise, one should attempt to assert some influence over them. In prevention, as in the treatment of overuse injuries, the physician should take into account the individual needs of each patient as it is impossible to treat, for instance, a recreational runner with the same therapy one would prescribe for a top-level, professional athlete.[13] Stretching exercises play an important role in the *prevention* of overuse injuries as well. It is also important to note that the prevention of overuse injuries of the musculoskeletal system has been greatly enhanced by numerous investigations carried out during the past 20 years. This research has described many predisposing causative factors of these injuries and has suggested ways of both treating and preventing them.[13,30,35] Perhaps one of the best examples of how these investigations have contributed not only to therapy, but also to decreasing the frequency of some overuse injuries, is Achilles tendinitis. Due to adequate and correct prevention in training (monitoring the training process so that there are no sudden increases in the intensity of training), prevention concerning the surface (avoiding running on steep inclines and on uneven, rough, and hard surfaces), and prevention concerning footwear (wearing adequate athletic footwear), as well as orthotic correction of biomechanical irregularities which cause excessive pronation of the foot during running (pes planovalgus, pes cavus, and others), the incidence of Achilles tendinitis has dropped by more than 50% during the past 10 years. Besides education (to which we hope to contribute with this book), prevention, as well as treatment of overuse injuries of the musculoskeletal system, depends on the close collaboration between the athlete, coach, and physician.

IV. NOMENCLATURE OF THE SYNDROMES

The various terms applied to different overuse injuries have not been recognized by all authors as yet. With regards to the basic pathohistological substrate of overuse injury, whether it is inflammation or a degenerative process, the question arises whether one should use the term tendinitis or tendinopathic change. We believe that the primary cause lies in the inflammation process, which during the course of its chronic stage, leads to degenerative changes. For this reason, we use terms ending with "-itis". When naming various individual syndromes, we also place full attention on the precise localization of the injury. For this reason, we use the term *tendinitis* when the injury is located on the tendon, *peritendinitis,* when the injury is located on the tendon sheath, *miotendinitis,* when the injury is located in the area where the muscle connects with the tendon, and *enthesitis,* when the injury is located in the area of insertion of the tendon to the bone. In most cases, however, we use the term based on the pathoanatomical localization of the injury, or in other words the term which is most commonly known and which is generally used in medical literature. In general terms, overuse injuries have acquired their terms according to the following:

- affected anatomical structure (i.e., epicondylitis humeri radialis, hip external rotators syndrome, bicipital tendinitis, plantar fasciitis, patellar tendinitis, and others)
- athletic activity in which it most frequently occurs (jumper's knee, rower's forehand, pitcher's elbow, swimmer's knee, runner's knee, etc.)

- cause of development (impingement shoulder syndrome, impingement in the wrist or ankle joint, etc.)
- characteristic symptom or clinical picture (trigger finger, low back pain, snapping hip syndrome, anterior knee pain, etc.)
- author who first, or most precisely described the syndrome (Morbus de Quervain, Morbus Hoffa, Morbus Osgood-Schlatter, Morbus Haglund, etc.)

Despite the terms applied, the basic characteristic of all these syndromes is chronic, cumulating microtraumatic injury. Because of this, the most accurate term is the general term, overuse injuries.

REFERENCES

1. **Alter, M. J.** *Science of Stretching.* Champaign: Leisure Press, 1990.
2. **Anderson, B.** *Stretching.* 20th ed. Bolinas: Shelter Publications, 1987.
3. **Andrews, J. R.** Overuse syndromes of the lower extremity. *Clin. Sports Med.,* 1983; 2:137–148.
4. **Benezis, C., Simeray, J., and Simon, L.** (Eds.) *Muscles, Tendons et Sport.* Paris: Masson, 1990.
5. **Brody, D. M.** Running injuries. *Clin. Symp.,* 1987; 39:1–36.
6. **Catonne, Y., and Saillant, G.** *Lesions Traumatiques des Tendons chez le Sportif.* Paris: Masson, 1992.
7. **Ciullo, J. V. and Zarins, B.** Biomechanics of the musculotendinous unit: relation to athletic performance and injury. *Clin. Sports Med.,* 1983; 2:71–86.
8. **Clain, M. R. and Hershman, E. B.** Overuse injuries in children and adolescents. *Phys. Sportsmed.,* 1989; 17:111–123.
9. **Clement, D. B., Taunton, J. E., Smart, G. W.,** et al. A survey of overuse running injuries. *Phys. Sportsmed.,* 1981; 9:47–58.
10. **Curwin, S. and Stanish, W. D.** Tendinitis: *Its Etiology and Treatment.* Lexington: Collamore Press, 1984; 1–67.
11. **Dalton, S. E.** Overuse injuries in adolescent athletes. *Sports Med.,* 1992; 13:58–70.
12. **Fornage, B. D.** *Ultrasonography of Muscles and Tendons.* New York: Springer-Verlag, 1988.
13. **Hess, G. P., Cappiello, W. L., Poole, R. M.,** et al. Prevention and treatment of overuse tendon injuries. *Sports Med.,* 1989; 8:371–384.
14. **Hunter-Griffin, L. Y.** Overuse injuries. *Clin. Sports Med.,* 1987; 6:225–466.
15. **Hulkko, A., and Orava, S.** Stress fractures in athletes. *Int. J. Sports Med.,* 1987; 8:221–226.
16. **Hunter, S. C., and Poole, R. M.** The chronically inflamed tendon. *Clin. Sports Med.,* 1987; 6:371–388.
17. **Johnson, L. L.** *Arthroscopic Surgery: Principles and Practice.* 3rd ed., St. Louis: C. V. Mosby, 1986.

18. **Kannus, P., Jarinen, M., and Niittymaki, S.** Long- or short-acting anesthetic with corticosteroid in local injections of overuse injuries? A prospective, randomized, double blind study. *Int. J. Sports Med.,* 1990; 11:397–400.

19. **Komi, V. P.** (Ed.) *Strength and Power in Sport.* London: Blackwell Scientific Publications, 1992.

20. **La Cava, G.** L'enthesite ou maladie des insertions. *Press Med.,* 1959; 67:9.

21. **Lehman, W. L., Jr.** Overuse syndromes in runners. *AFP,* 1984; 29:157–161.

22. **Lysholm, J. and Wiklaner, J.** Injuries in runners. *Am. J. Sports Med.* 1987; 15:168–171.

23. **Matasović, T.** (Ed.) *Diagnostic Ultrasound of the Locomotor System.* Zagreb: Skolska Knjiga, 1990.

24. **Matheson, G. O., Clement, D. B., McKenzie, D. C.,** et al. Stress fractures in athlete. *Am. J. Sports Med.,* 1987; 15:46–57.

25. **McCarthy, P.** Managing bursitis in the athlete: an overview. *Phys. Sportsmed.,* 1989; 17:115–125.

26. **McKeag, D. B. and Dolan, C.** Overuse syndrome of the lower extremity. *Phys. Sportsmed.,* 1989; 17:108–123.

27. **Micheli, L. J.** Lower extremity overuse injuries. *Acta Med. Scand.* (Suppl.) 1986; 711:171–177.

28. **O'Connor, F. G., Sobel, J. R., and Nirschl, R. P.** Five-step treatment for overuse injuries. *Phys. Sportsmed.,* 1992; 20:128–142.

29. **O'Neill, D. B., and Micheli, L. J.** Overuse injuries in the young athletes. *Clin. Sports Med.,* 1988; 7:591–610.

30. **Pećina, M.** *Sindromi Prenaprezanja Sustava za Kretanje.* Zagreb: Globus, 1992.

31. **Pećina, M.** *Vježbe istezanja — Stretching.* Zagreb: Globus, 1992.

32. **Pećina, M., Bojanić, I., and Markiewitz, A. D.** Nerve entrapment syndromes in athletes. *Clin. J. Sports Med.,* 1993; 3:36–43.

33. **Perugia, L., Postacchini, F., and Ippolito, E.** *The Tendons: Biology-Pathology-Clinical Aspects.* Milano: Editrice Kurtis, 1986.

34. **Rodineau, J. and Simon, L.** (Eds.) *Microtraumatologie du Sport.* Paris: Masson, 1990.

35. **Schwellnus, M. P., Jordaan, G., and Noakes, T. D.** Prevention of common overuse injuries by the use of shock absorbing insoles. *Am. J. Sports Med.,* 1990; 18:636–641.

36. **Stanish, W. D., Rubinovich, R. M., and Curwin, S.** Eccentric exercise in chronic tendinitis. *Clin. Orthop.,* 1986; 208:65–68.

37. **Taunton, J. E., McKenzie, D. C., and Clement, D. B.** The role of biomechanics in the epidemiology of injuries. *Sports Med.,* 1988; 6:107–120.

Special Part

Upper Extremity

The glenohumeral joint is characterized by having the greatest range of movement in the human body. The joint is able to rotate in every direction in order to reach every part of our body. All the movements performed by the shoulder joint are within the eyesight area, i.e., supervised by one's sight which is very important during work and exercise.

The mobility of the shoulder joint is enabled by the unproportional concave and convex joint bodies and the large volume of the joint capsule. On the other hand, the stability of the joint is ensured by the action of many muscles whose tendons are comprised in the joint capsule itself.

The importance of the arm in human activities is of the utmost value especially during work activities and sports involving the arm in an overhead position (racquet sports, volleyball, waterpolo, swimming, etc.). Since there are numerous tendons and bursae in the glenohumeral area, the incidence of overuse syndromes in such an area is expected.

We will illustrate the point with the words of Uhthoff and Sarkar,[67] "We were aware of this problem when we formulated the following classification, which is based on where the lesion originates. If the lesion arises in the substance of the tendon, the category has been designated intrinsic or primary. On the other hand, if the involvement of the tendon is apparently related to lesion in an adjacent or remote structure, or to systemic diseases, the category is extrinsic or secondary" (Tables 1 and 2).

I. IMPINGEMENT SYNDROME OF THE SHOULDER

Impingement syndrome is an entity[20,23,46,47] that includes a series of damages resulting from the clash of the rotator cuff of the glenohumeral joint (m. supraspinatus, m. infraspinatus, m. subscapularis, m. teres minor), subacromial bursa, and sometimes the long head of the biceps brachii muscle tendon against the frontal part of the acromion, acromioclavicular ligament, coracoid processus, and acromioclavicular joint. The clash happens when the arm is lifted high above the head in an overhead position. The rotator cuff of the shoulder and especially the supraspinatus muscle suffer the most damage during this clash. There are other terms found in literature

TABLE 1
Primary (Intrinsic Origin) Tendinopathies of
Rotator Cuff, Bicipital Tendon, or Both

Apparent causative factor(s)	Clinical syndrome
Trauma	Tendinitis
	Impingement
	Rupture
	Instability
Reactive	Calcifying tendinitis with or without impingement
Degeneration	Instability
	Impingement
	Rupture
Hyperelasticity (Ehlers-Danlos syndrome)	Instability
Idiopathic	Frozen shoulder

TABLE 2
Secondary (Extrinsic Origin) Tendinopathies of
Rotator Cuff, Bicipital Tendon, or Both

Apparent causative factor(s)	Clinical syndrome
Anatomic variations of the bony tissue	Tendinitis
Large coracoid process	Impingement
"Beaking" of the acromion	Rupture
Supratubercular ridge	
Pathologic changes in the bony tissue	Tendinitis
Acromial spur	Impingement
Osteophytes of the acromioclavicular (a-c) joint	Rupture
Systemic diseases	Tendinitis
Metabolic	Frozen shoulder
Endocrine	
Rheumatic	
Remote causes	Tendinitis
Cervical disc	Frozen shoulder
Intrathoracic/intraabdominal disorders	

denoting this entity, e.g., rotator cuff tendinitis, supraspinatus syndrome, subacromial compressive syndrome, pitcher's shoulder, and according to our experience, volleyball shoulder.

Ellenbecker and Dersheid[18] reported that impingement syndrome most often results in athletes as a consequence of the shoulder area overuse. Jobe and Bradley[33] describe the increased incidence of the syndrome in baseball, volleyball, tennis, rugby, athletics, waterpolo, and swimming; this means all sports that require an extended use of the arm in an overhead position, including elite rock climbers.[6] An epidemiological survey was conducted by Lo et al.[41] to collect data relating to the prevalence and frequency of shoulder pain and other related problems among different athletic groups who use vigorous upper arm activities. A questionnaire was administered on site, thus ensuring that the response rate was 100%. Analysis of the results revealed that of the 372 respondents, a total of 163 athletes (43.8%) indicated that they had shoulder problems and 109 (29%) were suffering pain as well. Diffuse pain was indicated by 20 respondents (5.4%), while localized pain during movement was reported in 89 respondents (23.9%). The prevalence of shoulder pain ranked highest among volleyball players (N = 28), followed by swimmers (N = 22), while badminton, basketball, and tennis participants were equally affected (N = 10). Neviaser[51] defines impingement syndrome on rotator cuff muscle as tendinitis caused by prolonged tendon pressure on the coracoacromial arch and the acromioclavicular joint. Butters and Rockwood[9] and Neviaser[51] reported that the impingement syndrome is regularly characterized by subacromial (subdeltoid) bursa damage and damage to the long head of biceps brachii tendon because these structures are connected by the synovial sheath of the shoulder joint. The shoulder joint is an example of a spheric joint, granted, with exceptional mobility and dynamic stability.[18,58,59] The joint consists of a spacy joint capsule, enforced with the glenohumeral ligament and the labrum glenoidale on the front side. The shoulder joint roof is composed of the coracoacromial arch which consists of the coracoid processus and the acromion of the scapula connected by the broad coracoacromial ligament (Figure 1). The subacromial (subdeltoid) bursa is situated beneath the coracoacromial arch. It is one of eight synovial bursae that can be found in this area. Dynamic stability of the joint is determined by the synchronous action of the shoulder muscle. The muscles are divided into three major groups: (1) the costohumeral group (pectoralis major muscle and lattisimus dorsi muscle), (2) the spinoscapular group (trapezius

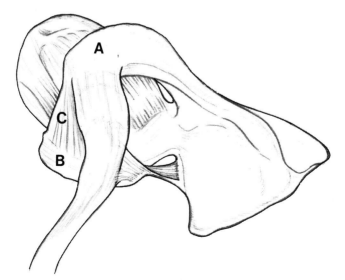

FIGURE 1. The shoulder joint roof is composed of the acromion (A), coracoid process (B), and coracoacromial ligament (C).

muscle, rhomboideus muscle, serratus anterior muscle, and levator scapulae muscle), and (3) the scapulohumeral group (rotator cuff and coracobrahialis muscle).

The rotator cuff of the shoulder joint is built of short muscles: the supraspinatus muscle, infraspinatus muscle, teres minor muscle, and subscapularis muscle. These four muscles set off from the scapula and attach to both tubercules of the humerus. The supraspinatus, infraspinatus, and teres minor muscles attach downwards on the tubercul major, while subscapularis muscle attaches to the tubercul minor. The supraspinatus muscle traverses through the so-called supraspinatus tunnel rimmed with the coracoid processus on the front side, with the acromion and the spina scapulae on the back side, and with the coracoacromial ligament from above. Because of its special anatomic determination, the supraspinatus muscle has an important role in the rotator cuff. It represents the locus minoris resistentiae in the mechanical sense of the rotator cuff.[39,40] It is well known that the musculotendinous units of the rotator cuff act as dynamic stabilizers of the glenohumeral joint, but at the same time prevent the joint capsule from excessive anterior or posterior shift (especially supraspinatus muscle since it is encompassed in the joint capsule from the upper side).

Biomechanical and electromiographic investigations showed the importance of the supraspinatus muscle's preventive role in upper and lower instability.[59] Besides, 1/3 and 1/2 of the shoulder joint strength during external rotation (infraspinatus muscle, teres minor muscle) are due to the rotator cuff muscles, while the subscapularis muscle acts as a strong internal rotator. External rotation plays an important role in abduction of the arm because it prevents the tubercul major from hitting the glenoid and enables arm abduction greater than 90°.[58] Internal rotation of the shoulder joint is important in anteflexion of the arm because of the similar mechanism of avoiding the clash between the humerus head and the coracoacromial ligament. The synchronous action of the teres minor and subscapularis muscles strongly contributes to the fixation of the humerus head (depression action) to the glenoid in any position of arm elevation. The supraspinatus muscle is the fixator of the humeral head in initial abduction that, according to recent findings, does not necessarily start only with supraspinatus muscle contraction. The deltoideus muscle has an equal role in abduction initiation.[28] The role of the long head of the biceps brachii is characterized by assisting the depression and fixation of the humeral head to the glenoid. Its role is stressed in cases of weakness of the first three muscles (infraspinatus muscle, subscapularis muscle, and teres minor muscle).

Recent investigations point to the nutritive role of the rotator cuff. Muscle tension of the rotator cuff of the shoulder mechanically assists the synovial fluid flow through the joint. In this way, the cartilage of the joint surfaces are equally provided with synovial fluid. Finally, the rotator cuff muscles represent a liquid-proof coating of the joint capsule, enabling the loss of synovial fluid due to minor tears of the capsule.

A. Etiopathogenesis

The clash of the humerus head against the coracoacromial arch and the pressure on the surrounding soft tissues result in damage to the rotator cuff tendons; this also leads to an inflammatory reaction characteristic of impingement syndrome. There is an area of relative avascularity on the supraspinatus muscle tendon[8,11,57] near its insertion on the tubercul major of the humerus (Figure 2). A similar region is present on the upper part of the tendon of the long head of biceps brachii. This region is called the *critical zone of the rotator cuff.* Rathburn and McNab[57] suggested that the anatomical position of the rotator cuff tendons plays an important role in the development of the critical zone because it exposes the tendons to constant pressure from the humeral head, squeezing the blood out of the surrounding blood vessels even when the arm is stationary in a position of abduction or neutral rotation.

Investigations carried out on numerous anatomical specimens of the scapula have shown that the development of the impingement syndrome is both correlated and enhanced by an acromion with a lesser inclination and an acromion with a slightly pushed out anterior part or lower area, or by the presence of anterior acromial spurs and inferior acromioclavicular osteophytes.[2] Results obtained by Neer[46,47] indicate that in 95% of the patients suffering from impingement syndrome, damage to the rotator cuff results as a consequence of a similarly or identically developed acromion. In some cases, impingement syndrome can develop as a consequence of the existence of the os acromiale, a special part of the acromion believed to be an ununited ossification center of that acromion. Contrary to the opinion expressed by Neer, Post et al.[55,56] believe that the cause of the impingement syndrome does not necessarily and exclusively have to be related to anatomical deviations. The results of their investigations indicate that the development of the impingement syndrome can also be initiated by weak external rotators of the shoulder joint infraspinatus, and teres minor muscles. An existing weakness of the external rotators of the shoulder joint result in an inadequate fixation of the humeral head in the glenoid fossa in the superior direction. This significantly increases the pressure of the humeral head on

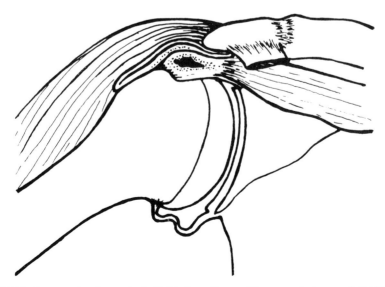

FIGURE 2. Degenerative changes in the "critical zone" area of the supraspinatus muscle tendon.

the tendon blood vessels of the shoulder joint's rotator cuff. This leads to an increasingly greater degeneration of the so-called critical zone accompanied by the progressive development of the impingement syndrome. The development and treatment of impingement syndrome in athletes was described by Jobe et al.[32–35] and Tibone et al.[65] Their results indicate that acute trauma to the shoulder and repeated overhead arm movements, characteristically performed in numerous sports, can increase the speed of progression of the impingement syndrome. Ellenbecker and Derscheid[18] note that concomitant, but unsynchronized, actions of the rotator muscles cause abnormal movements of the upper extremity allowing the clashing of the humeral head against the coracoacromial arch. Jobe and Bradley[33] and Scheib[61] cite their opinion that impingement syndrome develops as a result of the instability of the shoulder joint. According to their opinion, the pathogenetic course of injury to the rotator cuff is comprised of instability of the shoulder joint, subluxation, impingement, and destruction of the rotator cuff. Jobe and Bradley term the preceding course of events as the *shoulder instability complex.* Pieper, Quack, and Krahl[54] describe secondary impingement of the rotator cuff, encountered typically in athletes who participate in "overhead" sports, as caused by the instability of the shoulder joint. Impingement of the rotator cuff can be caused by chronic anterior instability of the shoulder joint. This particular injury is frequently found in athletes who repeatedly engage in overhead arm motions in abduction/external rotation of the arm, in such sports as volleyball, European handball, tennis, badminton, and swimming. Patients who do not respond to conservative treatment such as muscular stabilization are surgically treated.

In brief, we can conclude that there are two principal theories regarding the development of the impingement syndrome: the anatomic and the dynamic theory. Proponents of the anatomic theory believe that impingement syndrome is caused principally by decreased vascularization of some of the tendons of the rotator cuff, while proponents of the dynamic theory place great importance on the relative weakness of those muscles. At the same time it is quite clear that some causative factors can synergistically combine to produce impingement syndrome of the shoulder joint. These include the os acromiale, acute trauma to the shoulder, and excessive repeated strain placed on the upper extremity during some athletic activities. The possible mechanism leading to the development of impingement syndrome of the shoulder is stated in the following. The clash of the humeral head against the acromion causes injury to the surrounding soft tissue, the tendon of the supraspinatus muscle, the long head of the biceps brachii muscle, and the subacromial bursa, which results in inflammatory processes and scarred healing. After a certain period of time, the scar degenerates, frequently resulting in partial or total rupture of the tendon. Depending on the degree of change in the tendons of the shoulder joint rotator cuff, various functions of the rotator cuff are affected. The humeral head is not firmly fixed in the glenoid fossa during arm motions and has a tendency to translate in the superior direction. Such an unstable humeral head causes pain, decreases the range of movements possible in the shoulder joint, causes instability of the shoulder joint, and disrupts the normal flow of the synovial liquid which nourishes the joint cartilage; all this leads to further progression of the injury. The final stages of impingement syndrome are characterized by destruction of the rotator cuff, primarily the supraspinatus muscle and the long head of the biceps brachii muscle (in some cases, morphological changes of the humeral head, also known as arthropathy, caused by injury to the rotators of the shoulder joint).

B. Clinical Picture and Diagnostics

Impingement syndrome is an injury that is characterized by a chronic course. Patients frequently correlate the symptoms of the injury with some acute trauma to the shoulder, but detailed anamnesis usually results in the patient remembering earlier painful sensations in the shoulder joint.

The dominant symptoms of impingement syndrome are tenderness in the shoulder area, crepitations, decreased range of movements in the shoulder joint,[72] and varying loss of strength in the surrounding musculature. The pain may be categorized in intensity depending on arm activities: pain caused while performing strenuous activities of the arm, pain caused by moderate or strong activities, and pain when the arm is stationary.

The condition may appear at any age. Athletes and people with physically hard occupations are at a greater risk to develop these injuries. Neer[46] has developed an elaborate hypothesis on the progression of the impingement syndrome in three stages based on pathoanatomical examinations (Table 3). In Stage 1, edema and inflammation occur. In the beginning of this stage, excessive bowing of the shoulder rotator tendon is noticeable; there is microscopic or partial damage to some of the tendon

TABLE 3
Classification of Impingement Syndrome
According to Neer[45]

Stage 1: Edema and hemorrhage
Typical age | > 25
Differential diagnosis | Subluxation
| A/C arthritis
Clinical course | Reversible
Treatment | Conservative

Stage 2: Fibrosis and tendinitis
Typical age | 25–40
Differential diagnosis | Frozen shoulder
| Calcium deposits
Clinical course | Recurrent pain with activity
Treatment | Consider bursectomy
| C/A ligament division

Stage 3: Bone spurs and tendon rupture
Typical age | < 40
Differential diagnostis | Cervical radiculitis
| neoplasm
Clinical course | Progressive disability
Treatment | Anterior acromioplasty
| Rotator cuff repair

fibers. Bleeding is sometimes present but usually not to a large degree. The age of the patients in this group is usually less than 25 years. The main characteristic of Stage 1 is good prognosis in the sense of reversibility of pathological changes.

Stage 2 lesions are characterized by fibrosis and tendinitis and clearly indicate chronicity. Repetitive episodes of mechanical inflammation of the shoulder rotator tendon, edema, cellular infiltration, and vascular invasion of the tendon are followed by connective tissue reparation and fibrosis of different stages. Nirschl et al.[52] refer to this stage as *angiofibroblastic hyperplasia of the tendons.* The subacromial bursa is also thickened and fibrous. Lesions of this stage are characteristically found in patients between 25 to 40 years of age. The shoulder functions satisfactorily during "easy" activities. However, when performing stronger repetitive movements in an overhead position, such as in throwing sports, the rotator cuff becomes insufficient.

Tears in the tendons of the rotator cuff, tears in the tendon of the long head of the biceps brachii muscle and changes in the bone represent the main characteristics of the Stage 3. Progression of the impingement syndrome is characterized by the appearance of complete, incomplete, or superficial/roughened areas located on the surface of the tendon, which cause bursitis and tears in the tendons of the rotator cuff of the shoulder.[49] Measured at their largest diameter, tears in the tendons of the rotator cuff can be small (less than 1 cm in diameter), average (from 1 to 3 cm in diameter), large (from 3 to 5 cm in diameter), and massive (larger than 5 cm in diameter). Stage 3 is usually found in patients over 40 years of age. Surgical treatment is the only form of therapy for this stage of impingement syndrome.

Lesions in the tendon of the long head of the biceps brachii muscle appear on average in a 1:7 ratio in comparison to lesions in the tendons of the rotator cuff. Lesions in the tendon of the biceps brachii muscle can, however, sometimes represent the first sign of a developing impingement syndrome.[51] Pathological changes in bone tissue, i.e., the collapse of the humeral head, represent the final stage of impingement syndrome. They develop typically only after the presence of long-term destruction of the shoulder rotator tendons and a complete insufficiency of the rotator net. This stage is followed by pathological changes in the whole shoulder joint-cuff tear arthropathy.[32,44,47] The partial or complete destruction of the tendons of the shoulder rotators is sometimes accompanied by nutritive changes in the joint cartilage; this is characterized by the development of hydroxyapatites, active collagenasis, and neutral proteases. This clinical entity is known as *Milwaukee shoulder.*[1] Clinical signs characteristic for impingement syndrome include general tenderness in the anterior part of the acromion or in the humeral greater tubercule area, a painful arch during abduction of the upper extremity above 90°, and a positive impingement sign and hypotrophy of the rotator cuff muscles. The impingement test and the presence of the impingement sign are used in differential diagnosis to ascertain if the painful symptoms are the result of impingement of the shoulder joint and not the result of other changes in the shoulder (Figures 3 and 4).

A positive impingement sign, according to Neer, is the presence of tenderness in the shoulder area when the physician performs anteflexion on the patient's injured shoulder simultaneously with internal rotation of the upper arm. According to Hawkins,[23] a positive impingement sign consists of pain in the shoulder area when the physician performs a strong internal rotation of the patient's arm in a 90°

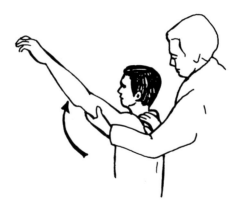

FIGURE 3. Impingement sign performance.

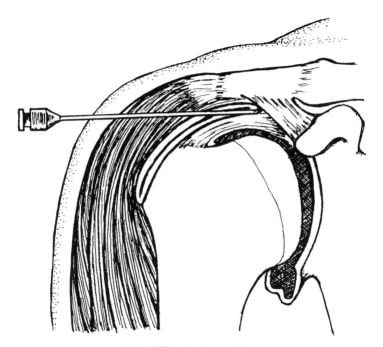

FIGURE 4. Impingement test.

anteflexion position. The impingement test (Figure 4) is used in clinical diagnostics when making differential diagnoses to rule out the possibility of the painful sensations resulting from anterior subluxation of the shoulder joint, acromioclavicular arthritis, cervical radiculitis, "frozen shoulder", traumatic bursitis, calcifying tendinitis, or neoplasmas. A diagnosis of impingement syndrome is confirmed, if after injection of 10 cc of 1.0% xylocain below the anterior edge of the acromion, the patient is able to perform the impingement sign without any pain.

Jobe et al.[32,33] have described a test for the supraspinatus muscle used in differentiating tendon injuries between the supraspinatus muscle and other rotators of the shoulder joint. The test is performed by having the patient stand with his arms held in a position of 90° abduction and horizontal abduction of 30° with full internal rotation. The physician holds the patient's upper arms and resists the patient's efforts to lift his arms in an upward direction (Figure 5). If weakness or pain in the shoulder joint appear, the supraspinatus muscle test is considered to be positive, and the probable localization of the injury to the rotator cuff is the supraspinatus muscle tendon. During the performing of this maneuver, the infraspinatus, subscapularis, and teres minor muscles are completely inactive which can be verified by determining the electrical activity in them.

Lyons and Tomlinson[42] have studied the reported clinical assessment of the presence and extent of a rotator cuff tear in 42 patients in a special shoulder clinic. This preoperative diagnosis was compared with the findings at operation. The clinical tests had a sensitivity of 91% and a specificity of 75%. It is important to exploit clinical examination before resorting to costly and sometimes harmful special investigations.

Radiographic analysis of the shoulder joint includes transaxillar lateral and anteroposterior radiographs during both the internal and external rotation of the humerus. Although not a particularly precise diagnostic method, radiographic analysis sometimes enables the examining physician to confirm the presence of calcium deposits in the tendons of the rotator cuff, sclerotic changes in the greater tubercle of the humerus, a decrease of the subacromial area to less than 6 mm, eburnation of the anterior part of the acromion (Figure 6), and degenerative changes in the acromioclavicular joint.[15,20]

Contrasting arthrography is sometimes employed in the analysis of the continuity of the tendons as well as to verify diagnoses of complete tendon rupture.[38] Subacromial bursography and bursotomography are auxiliary methods used to confirm injury to the joint bursae. Cone et al.[15] consider these methods, as well as fluoroscopy and arthrography, to be useful diagnostic methods for detecting the beginning stages of impingement syndrome and Čičak et al.[17] described ultrasound

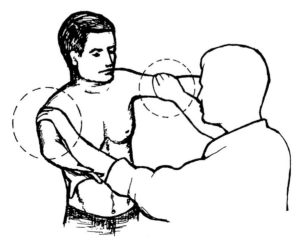

FIGURE 5. Supraspinatus test.

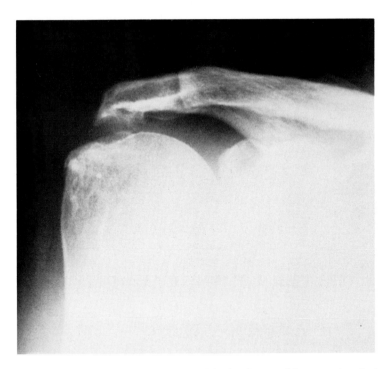

FIGURE 6. Roentgenogram demonstrating subacromial sclerosis, acromial spurs, and cystic changes of the greater tuberosity of the humerus as a result of the impingement process.

guidance of the needle placement for shoulder arthrography. CT is used when analyzing bone pathology of the humeral head and the glenohumeral joint.

Numerous authors[7,14,22,33,36,43,44] have in recent times expressed their belief that ultrasound examination of the rotator cuff is an unavoidable diagnostic method when attempting to determine the presence of partial or total tendon ruptures (Figures 7 and 8) and inflammatory changes in the tendon and tendon sheath.

Wilbourn[73] recommends the use of electromyographic analysis of the muscles of the rotator cuff with the aim of ruling out the possibility of radiculopathy when diagnosing impingement syndrome. Neviaser,[50] on the other hand, points out the exceptional contribution of arthroscopy to both the diagnostics and the treatment of impingement syndrome. Arthroscopy enables a direct view of the current state of the internal structures of the shoulder joint, tendons, burses, cartilage, and tendon and synovial sheaths; at the same time it offers the possibility of a therapeutic intervention.[50,53,62] MRI is a very useful diagnostic method, which enables the detection of even very small lesions in the soft tissues and the neurovascular structures.[16,27,31,66,68]

C. Treatment

Treatment for impingement syndrome, in the most general terms, can be divided into nonoperative and operative treatment. Nonoperative treatment is indicated for the first stage of the disease. Lasting at least several months, it is indicated for patients suffering from Stage 2 of the disease, while surgical treatment is indicated

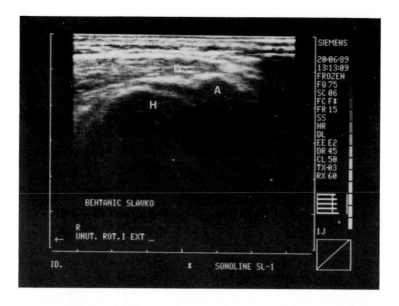

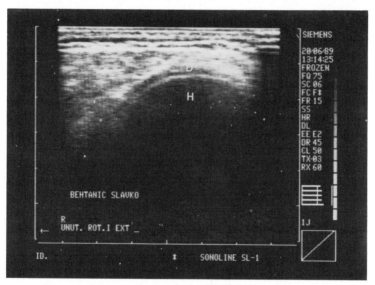

FIGURE 7. Longitudinal (A) and transversal (B) sonograms show a complete tear of the rotator cuff. The cuff lacks apposition of the deltoid muscle (D) to the humeral head (H). (A) Acromion.

only when, and if, conservative treatment fails to produce any significant results. Patients suffering from Stage 3 of the disease must always be treated surgically.

Nonoperative treatment is recommended for patients suffering from Stage 1 and 2 of impingement syndrome. Treatment during the acute, painful stage of the injury consists of rest, physical therapy, electrotherapy, cryotherapy, and application of oral, nonsteroid, anti-inflammatory drugs.[20,22,23,25,58] The local application of corticosteroids is also described as part of the treatment for impingement syndrome. The

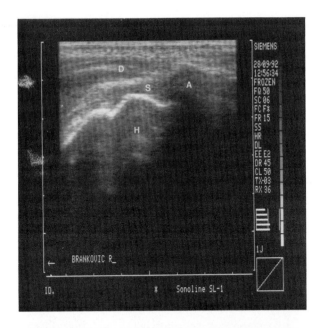

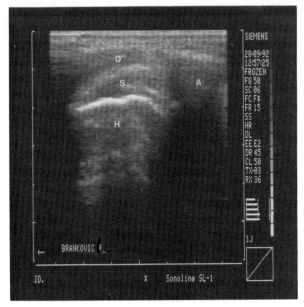

FIGURE 8. Longitudinal sonogram shows focal thinning of the supraspinatus tendon (S). (B) Normal supraspinatus tendon. (H) Humeral head; (A) acromion; (D) deltoid muscle.

corticosteroids are applied onto the inflamed area and not directly on the tissue. The principal effects of corticosteroid therapy include reduction of the edema and the inflammatory reaction. This application carries a certain risk; by repeatedly applying corticosteroids into the same area, their use and application must be tempered with necessary prudence. Friction massage, stretching exercises (Figures 9, 10, and 11) and strengthening exercises for the rotator musculature of the shoulder joint (Figures 12, 13, and 14) are recommended, both as prevention and as part of the treatment, for patients who are not suffering from the acute stage of impingement syndrome.[10,18,29,33]

Operative treatment is indicated for patients suffering from the Stage 3 of the disease.[3,4,12,13,21,24,48,69] Neer[45-47] described an operative technique called *anterior acromioplasty*. The main principle of the procedure consists of remodeling excessively proturburent, large, and downward slanting acromions. Apart from the acromion, inspection of the tendons of the shoulder rotators, the tendon of the long head of the biceps brachii muscle, the subacromial bursa, and the acromioclavicular joint are also carried out during the operation. This is done because it is quite possible for two or more structures of the shoulder to be damaged or injured at the same time. Osteophytes on the acromioclavicular joint and calcificates on the coracoacromial ligament are always removed. Resection of either the acromioclavicular joint or the coracoacromial ligament is performed if it is judged that these structures represent the immediate cause for the development of impingement syndrome. An inflammatorily changed, fibrous subacromial bursa is always excised. Tenodesis is performed when damage to the long head of the biceps brachii muscle is evident.

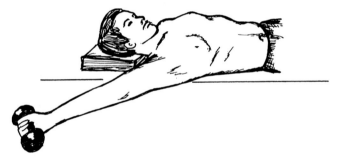

FIGURE 9. Rotator cuff extension. The patient lies on his back with his shoulder in a position of 135° and elbow is in a position of 45°. The weight passively stretches the rotator cuff in the direction of the external rotation.

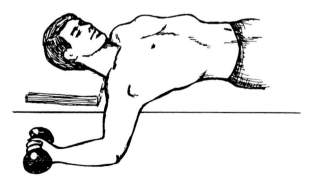

FIGURE 10. Rotator cuff extension. The patient lies on his back with his shoulder and elbow in a position of 90°. The weight passively stretches the rotator cuff in the direction of external rotation.

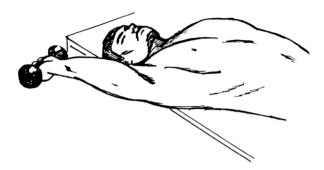

FIGURE 11. Rotator cuff extension. The patient lies on his back with his shoulder in a position of 170° and his elbow at 45°. The weight passively stretches the rotator cuff in the direction of external rotation.

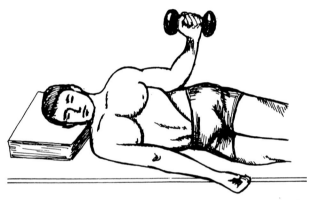

FIGURE 12. Strengthening of the infraspinatus and teres minor muscles. The patient lies on one side and his elbow lies on his thorax in a position of 90°. The weight is slowly lifted in the external rotation direction and slowly lowered in the internal rotation direction.

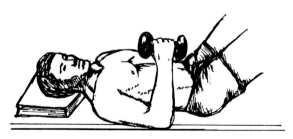

FIGURE 13. Strengthening of the subscapularis muscle. The patient lies on his back, with his elbow along his thorax in a position of 90°. The weight is lowered in a external rotation direction and then lifted in the internal rotation direction.

Anterior acromioplasty, subacromial decompression, shaving of incomplete ruptures in rotator cuff tendons, and refixation of the origins of the rotator muscles in cases of complete rupture are frequently performed arthroscopically.[37,50,53,62,63,71]

All authors agree that anterior acromioplasty and revision of the surrounding tissue generally produce satisfying results visible during the short time that the patient is

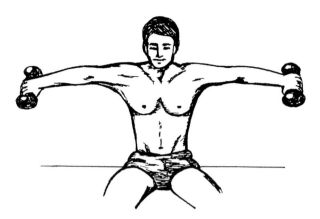

FIGURE 14. Strengthening of the supraspinatus muscle. The patient sits erectly, with his shoulder in a 90° abduction, 30° horizontal abduction, and total interior rotation. The weight is slowly lowered in a 45° arch and then lifted to the strating position.

monitored after the operation.[5,20,22,26,60,64,65] However, recidives of impingement syndrome, after surgical treatment, have been described in patients who have previously participated, at the highest level, in various sports.[26] The long-term success of anterior acromioplasty in athletes significantly depends on scrupulously following the postoperative rehabilitation program. For precisely this reason, Post and Cohen[56] recommend a combination of anterior acromioplasty and stretching and strengthening exercises for the rotator cuff of the shoulder joint. Ellenbecker and Dercheid[18] describe the importance of strengthening the complete musculature of the shoulder joint.

In cases of secondary impingement that has developed as a consequence of instability of the shoulder joint, the primary causative factor must be treated. According to Pieper, Quack, and Krahl[54] and numerous other authors,[19,30,35,70] surgical treatment is indicated for these cases. The treatment consists of anterior reconstruction of the capsule and/or the glenoid labrum, and in addition, if necessary, subacromial decompression and revision of the rotator cuff. Between October 1988 and April 1992, Pieper et al.[54] operated on 66 shoulders in 64 top athletes suffering from chronic anterior or multidirectional instability of the shoulder joint that had led to the development of impingement syndrome of the rotator cuff. In all cases, the athletes themselves were not aware of the instability. Conservative treatment failed to produce any significant results. The success ratio for surgical treatment of the athletes was close to 90%.

II. BICIPITAL TENDINITIS

Bicipital tendinitis is a term used to define overuse of the long head of the biceps brachii muscle. The biceps brachii muscle belongs to the group of anterior, upper arm muscles and is characterized by having two heads — caput longum (long head) and caput breve (short head). The long head of the biceps originates from the supraglenoid tubercle of the scapula, passes over the top of the humeral head, and courses distally, passing through the intertubercular sulcus. The tendon is contained within an invaginated envelope of synovial membrane as it passes through the shoulder joint. The short head originates from the coracoid process of the scapula. The two heads unite approximately in the middle of the upper arm, in the region of the deltoid tuberosity (Figure 15). The biceps brachii muscle ends with two tendons, the stronger and shorter of which attaches itself to the radial tuberosity and, in effect, represents an extension of the caput longum. One tendon plate, the musculus bicipitis brachii aponeurosis, with fibers consisting of extensions from the short head of the biceps brachii, departs from the medial edge of the stronger tendon and proceeds medially into the forearm fascia, which it strengthens. The biceps brachii muscle is a two-joint muscle. The long head of the muscle moves the arm away from the body and rotates it inwardly, while the short head moves the arm toward the body. Synergistic deployment of both heads produces anteflexion of the arm in the shoulder. In the

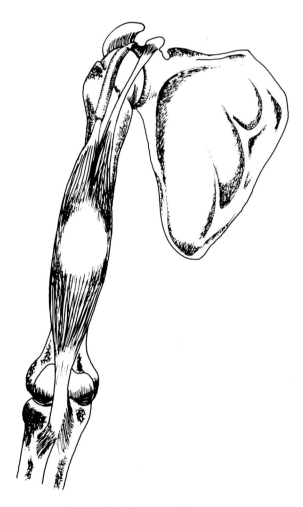

FIGURE 15. Biceps brachii muscle.

elbow joint, the muscle acts as both a flexor and a strong supinator of the forearm. The biceps brachii muscle is inervated by the musculocutaneous nerve.

A. Etiopathogenesis

Bicipital tendinitis is a condition that may occur as an isolated entity, primary tendinitis, or, more frequently, may be seen in conjunction with significant pathology elsewhere in the shoulder, such as impingement syndrome and frontal instability of the shoulder (secondary tendinitis).[82,83,86,90]

The long head of the biceps tendon can be affected at two district sites: inside the joint and inside the bicipital (intertubercular) groove.

In cases of primary tendinitis, the damage to the tendon is localized within the intertubercular groove, characterizing it as a tenosynovitis, an inflammatory process involving the tendon and its sheath. Besides external factors, such as direct trauma or overuse of the arm in an overhead position (smash in volleyball, serve in tennis, or pitching in baseball), development of primary tendinitis may also be due to abnormalities in the soft-tissue parts that surround the tendon (e.g., coracohumeral ligament) and to abnormalities in the intertubercular groove (e.g., in cases with abnormally shallow intertubercular grooves that lead to subluxation of the elbow).

The causes of bicipital tendinitis are definitely age related. Anomalies of the groove and repeated traumas are the most common causes in young individuals, whereas degenerative tendon changes predominate in the older population.

Primary bicipital tendinitis seems to be rare, but it has been reported in volleyball players, swimmers, waterpolo players, tennis players, baseball players, and golfers.[83,86,88]

B. Clinical Picture and Diagnostics

The most consistent complaint when encountering primary bicipital tendinitis is severe pain in the area of the intertubercular groove. The pain increases gradually, usually without any trauma, and is associated with activity; it appears with frequent repetitions of the offending movement and disappears when resting. Typical clinical findings include pain caused by palpating the biceps tendon in its groove, as well as positive Speed's test and Yergason's sign.[83,86,88] In Speed's test, the examiner provides resistance to anteflexion of the arm during concomitant extension in the elbow and full supination of the forearm. In Yergason's test, resistance is provided against supination of the forearm during concomitant flexion of 90° in the elbow. A positive result is indicated when pain appears or intensifies in the intertubercular groove.

Bicipital tendinitis secondary to other pathological conditions in the shoulder appears to represent the more common form of this disorder. Some authors state that it appears in more than 90% of the cases associated with impingement syndrome and anterior instability of the shoulder. When the condition occurs in association with other pathological conditions, it is termed secondary bicipital tendinitis.[83,88] For this reason, all diagnoses of bicipital tendinitis must be accompanied by a thorough and detailed clinical examination, including examinations for the stability of the shoulder and for impingement syndrome.

Besides standard radiographic examinations of the shoulder, diagnosis of bicipital tendinitis requires the taking of special projections, e.g., the Fisk view, which enable the examiner to determine the size of the intertubercular groove.[77,87,89] This is important because short and narrow margins of the intertubercular groove are a well-known predisposition for developing recurrent dislocation of the tendon and consequently bicipital tendinitis.[74,89]

Arthrography of the shoulder is generally used for analysis of the tendon in the intertubercular groove. In recent times, arthroscopy of the shoulder,[76,81,88] for the same purpose, is also frequently performed. An enlarged tendon with characteristic changes (vacuoles) on the tendon sheath indicates bicipital tendinitis.

Ultrasonography of the affected shoulder has also been recently used as an aid in recognizing changes in the biceps tendon (Figure 16). This has the added advantage of enabling examination of the tendon during movement.[79,85] Middleton et al.[85] found that tendinitis is characterized by heterogeneously structured tendon, edema of the tendon, and an enlargement of the tendon sheath.

C. Treatment

Nonoperative treatment of primary bicipital tendinitis entails avoiding offending movements (modified rest), applying nonsteroid anti-inflammatory medications, and performing moderate stretching exercises. Good results are obtained when using a programed therapy consisting of stretching exercises for the shoulder (in abduction,

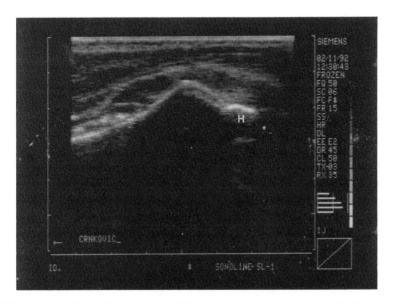

FIGURE 16. Longitudinal (A) and transversal (B) sonograms of the long head of the biceps muscle demonstrating tendinitis in a world champion kayak rider. (H) Humeral head.

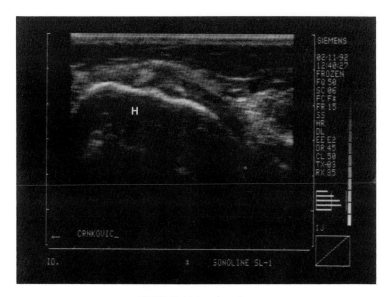

FIGURE 16 (continued).

adduction, and internal and external rotation) before which heat is applied to the injured shoulder. After the stretching exercises, the tender area is massaged with ice. In cases of secondary tendinitis, therapy for the primary disorder must also be carried out.[83,87,88]

Surgical treatment is indicated when the symptoms, despite completing nonsurgical therapy, persist for longer than 6 months. A number of surgical procedures are recommended in medical literature.[91] The best results are obtained by performing tenodesis of the long head of the biceps.[75,78,80,88]

REFERENCES

Impingement Syndrome of the Shoulder

1. **Bateman, J. E.** Neurologic painful conditions affecting the shoulder. *Clin. Orthop.*, 1983; 173:44–55.
2. **Bigliani, L. U., Ticker, J. B., Flatow, E. L., Soslowski, L. J., and Mow, V. C.** The relationship of acromial architecture to rotator cuff disease. *Clin. Sports Med.*, 1991; 10:823–38.
3. **Bigliani, L. U., Cordasco, F. A., McIlveen, S. J., et al.** Operative repair of massive rotator cuff tears: long-term results. *J. Shoulder Elbow Surg.*, 1992; 1:120–130.
4. **Bigliani, L. U., Kimmel, J., McCann, P. D., and Wolfe, I.** Repair of rotator cuff tears in tennis players. *Am. J. Sports Med.*, 1992; 20:112–7.
5. **Bjorkenheim, J. M., Paavolainen, P., Ahovuo, J., et al.** Subacromial impingement decompressed with anterior acromioplasty. *Clin. Orthop.*, 1990; 252:150–5.

6. **Bollen, S. R.** Upper limb injuries in elite rock climbers. *J. R. Coll. Surg. Edinburgh,* 1990; 35 (6 suppl.): 18–20.
7. **Brandt, T. D., Cardone, B. W., Grant, T. H., et al.** Rotator cuff sonography: a reassessment. *Radiology,* 1989; 173:323–327.
8. **Brooks, C. H., Rewell, W. J., and Heatley, F. W.** A quantitative histological study of the vascularity of the rotator cuff tendon. *J. Bone Joint Surg.,* 1992; 74B:151–3.
9. **Butters, K. P. and Rockwood, C. A.** Office evaluation and management of the shoulder impingement syndrome. *Orthop. Clin. N. Am.,* 1988; 194:755–67.
10. **Carson, W. G., Jr.** Rehabilitation of the throwing shoulder. *Clin. Sports Med.,* 1989; 8:657–97.
11. **Chansky, H. A. and Iannotti, J. P.** The vascularity of the rotator cuff. *Clin. Sports Med.,* 1991; 10:807–22.
12. **Codeman, E. A.** Complete rupture of the supraspinatus tendon. Operative treatment with report of two successful cases. *Boston Med. Surg. J.,* 1911; 164:708–710.
13. **Cofield, R. H.** Rotator cuff disease of the shoulder. *J. Bone Joint Surg.,* 1985; 67(A):974–9.
14. **Collins, R. A., Gristina, A. G., Carter, R. E., et al.** Ultrasonography of the shoulder: static and dynamic imaging. *Orthop. Clin. N. Am.* 1987; 18:351–61.
15. **Cone, R. O., III, Resnick, D., and Danzig, L.** Shoulder impingement syndrome. Radiographic evaluation. *Radiology,* 1984; 150:29–33.
16. **Crues, J. V., III and Fareed, D. O.** Magnetic resonance imaging of shoulder impingement. *Top. Magn. Reson. Imaging,* 1991; 3:39–49.
17. **Ciĉak, N., Matasović, T., and Bajraktarević T.** Ultrasound guidance of needle placement for shoulder arthrography, *J. Ultrasound Med.,* 1992; 11:135–137.
18. **Ellenbecker, T. S. and Derscheid, G. L.** Rehabilitation of overuse injuries of the shoulder. *Clin. Sports Med.,* 1989; 8:583–604.
19. **Fu, F. H., Harner, C. D., and Klein, A. H.** Shoulder impingement syndrome. A critical review. *Clin. Orthop.,* 1991; 269:162–73.
20. **Fukuda, H.** Shoulder impingement and rotator cuff disease. *Curr. Orthop.,* 1990; 4:225–32.
21. **Gerber, C.** Latissimus dorsi transfer for the treatment of irreparable tears of the rotator cuff. *Clin. Orthop.,* 1992; 275:152–60.
22. **Habermeyer, P.** Sehnenrupturen in schulterbereich. *Orthopade,* 1989; 18:257–67.
23. **Hawkins, R. J. and Kennedy, J. C.** Impingement syndrome in athletes. *Am. J. Sports Med.,* 1980; 8:151–7.
24. **Hawkins, R. J., Misamore, G. W., and Hobelka, P. E.** Surgery of full thickness rotator cuff tears. *J. Bone Joint Surg.,* 1985; 67A:1349–1355.
25. **Hawkins, R. J. and Abrams, J. S.** Impingement syndrome in the absence of cuff tear (stages 1 and 2). *Orthop. Clin. N. Am.,* 1987; 18:373–83.
26. **Hawkins, R. J., Chris, T., Bokor, D., et al.** Failed anterior acromioplasty. A review of 51 cases. *Clin. Orthop.,* 1989; 243:106–11.
27. **Holder, J., Kursunoglu-Brahme, S., Snyder, S. J., Cervilla, V., Karzel, R. P., Schweitzer, M. E., Flamigan, B. D., and Resnick, D.** Rotator cuff disease: assessment with MR arthrography versus standard MR imaging in 36 patients with arthroscopic confirmation. *Radiology,* 1992; 182:431–6.
28. **Howell, S. M., Imobersteg, A. M., Seger, D. H., et al.** Classification of the role of the supraspinatus muscle in shoulder function. *J. Bone Joint Surg.,* 1986; 68(A):398–404.
29. **Itoi, E. and Tabata, S.** Conservative treatment of rotator cuff tears. *Clin. Orthop.,* 1992; 275:165–73.

30. **Jerosch, J., Castro, W. H., and Sons, H. V.** Das sekundare Impingement-Syndrom beim Sportler. *Sportverletz Sportschaden,* 1990; 4:180–5.

31. **Jerosch, J. and Asshewer, J.** Kernspintomographische Veranderungen der Supraspinatussehne beim Impingement-Syndrom des Sportlers. *Sportverletz Sportschaden,* 1991; 5:12–6.

32. **Jobe, F. W. and Jobe, C. M.** Painful athletic injuries of the shoulder. *Clin. Orthop.,* 1983; 173:117–24.

33. **Jobe, F. W. and Bradley, J. P.** Rotator cuff injuries in baseball. Prevention and rehabilitation. *Sports Med.,* 1988; 6:378–87.

34. **Jobe, F. W.** Throwing injuries in the athlete. In: *Orthopaedic Knowledge Update 3.* Philadelphia: American Academy of Orthopaedic Surgeons, 1990; 293–302.

35. **Jobe, W. J., Tibone, J. E., Jobe, C. M., et al.** The shoulder in sports. In: *The Shoulder.* Rockwood, C. A. and Matsen, F. A., III, Eds., Philadelphia: W.B. Saunders, 1990; 961–990.

36. **Kujat, R.** Impingement syndrome of the shoulder. *Unffalchirurg,* 1986; 89:409–17.

37. **Levy, H. J., Gardner, R. D., and Lemak, L. J.** Arthroscopic subacromial decompression in the treatment of full-thickness rotator cuff tears. *Arthroscopy,* 1991; 7:8–13.

38. **Lindblom, K.** Arthrography and roentgenography in ruptures of the tendon of the shoulder joint. *Acta Radiol.,* 1939; 20:548.

39. **Lindblom, K.** On pathogenesis of ruptures of the tendon aponeurosis of the shoulder joint. *Acta Radiol.,* 1939; 20:563–577.

40. **Lindblom, K. and Palmer, I.** Ruptures of the tendon aponeurosis of the shoulder joint — the so-called supraspinatus ruptures. *Acta Chir. Scand.,* 1939; 82:133–142.

41. **Lo, Y. P., Hsu, Y. C., and Chan, K. M.** Epidemiology of shoulder impingement in upper arm sports events. *Br. J. Sports Med.,* 1990; 24:173–7.

42. **Lyons, A. R. and Tomlinson, J. E.** Clinical diagnosis of tears of the rotator cuff. *J. Bone Joint Surg.,* 1992; 74B:414–5.

43. **Middleton, W. D.** Status of rotator cuff sonography. *Radiology,* 1989; 173:307–309.

44. **Nash, H. L.** Rotator cuff damage: reexamining the causes and treatments. *Phys. Sportmed.,* 1988; 16:128–35.

45. **Neer, C. S.** II. Anterior acromioplasty for the chronic impingement syndrome in the shoulder. *J. Bone Joint Surg.,* 1972; 54(A):41.

46. **Neer, C. S.** Impingement lesions. *Clin. Orthop.,* 1983; 173:70–7.

47. **Neer, C. S., Craig, E. V., and Fukuda, H.** Cuff tear arthropathy. *J. Bone Joint Surg.,* 1983; 65(A):1232–44.

48. **Neviaser, J. S.** Ruptures of the rotator cuff of shoulder. New concepts in the diagnosis and operative treatment of chronic ruptures. *Arch. Surg.,* 1971; 102:483–485.

49. **Neviaser, R. J.** Tears of the rotator cuff. *Orthop. Clin. N. Am.,* 1980; 11(2):295–306.

50. **Neviaser, T. J.** Arthroscopy of the shoulder. *Orthop. Clin. N. Am.,* 1987; 18:361–73.

51. **Neviaser, T. J.** The role of the biceps tendon in the impingement syndrome. *Orthop. Clin. N. Am.,* 1987; 18:383–7.

52. **Nirshl, R. P.** Shoulder tendinitis. In: *AAOS Symposium on Upper Extremity Injuries in Athletes.* Pettrone, F. A. (Ed.). St. Louis: C.V. Mosby 1986; 322–37.

53. **Ogilvie-Harris, D. J. and D'Angelo, G.** Arthroscopic surgery of the shoulder. *Sports Med.,* 1990; 9:120–8.

54. **Pieper, H. G., Quack, G., and Krahl, H.** Secondary impingement of the rotator cuff in overhead sports caused by instability of the shoulder joint. *Croat. Sports Med. J.,* 1992; 7:24–8.

55. **Post, M., Silver, R., and Singh, M.** Rotator cuff tear: diagnosis and treatment. *Clin. Orthop.,* 1983; 173:78–91.

56. **Post, M. and Cohen, J.** Impingement syndrome. Review of late stage 2 and early stage 3 lesions. *Clin. Orthop.*, 1986; 207:126–32.
57. **Rathburn, J. B. and McNab, I.** The microvascular pattern of the rotator cuff. *J. Bone Joint Surg.*, 1970; 52:540–53.
58. **Ribarić, G., Pećina, M., and Bojanić, I.** Impingement sindrom ramena. *Basketball Med. Per.*, 1988; 3:15–23.
59. **Saha, A. K.** Mechanism of shoulder movements and a plea of the recognition of "Zero Position" of glenohumeral joint. *Clin. Orthop.*, 1983; 173:3–10.
60. **Sahlstrand, T.** Operations for impingement of the shoulder. Early results in 52 patients. *Acta Orthop. Scand.*, 1989; 60:45–8.
61. **Scheib, J. S.** Diagnosis and rehabilitation of the shoulder impingement syndrome in the overhand and throwing athlete. *Rheum. Dis. Clin. N. Am.*, 1990; 16:971–88.
62. **Small, N. C.** Complications in arthroscopy: the knee and other joints. *Arthroscopy*, 1986; 2:253–8.
63. **Speen, K. P., Lohnes, J., and Garrett, W. E., Jr.** Arthroscopic subacromial decompression: results in advanced impingement syndrome. *Arthroscopy*, 1991; 7:291–6.
64. **Throling, J., Bjerneld, H., Hallin, G., et al.** Acromiplasty for impingement syndrome. *Acta Orthop. Scand.*, 1985; 56:147–8.
65. **Tibone, J. E., Jobe, F. W., Kerlan, T. G., et al.** Shoulder impingement syndrome in athletes treated by an anterior acromioplasty. *Clin. Orthop.*, 1985; 198:134–40.
66. **Traughber, P. D. and Goodwin, T. E.** Shoulder MRI: arthroscopic correlation with emphasis on partial tears. *J. Comput. Assist. Tomogr.*, 1992; 16:129–33.
67. **Uhthoff, H. K. and Sarkar, K.** Classification and definition of tendinopathies. *Clin. Sports Med.*, 1991; 10:707–720.
68. **Vahlensieck, M., Resendes, M., Lang, P., and Genant, H.** Shoulder MRI: the subacromial/subdeltoid bursa fat stripe in healthy and pathologic conditions. *Eur. J. Radiol.*, 1992; 14:223–7.
69. **Van Holsbeeck, E., Declercq, G., Derijcke, J., Martens, M., Verstreken, J., and Fabry, G.** Shoulder impingement syndrome. *Acta Orthop. Belg.*, 1991; 57:25–9.
70. **Walch, G., Boileau, P., Noel, E., Liotard, J. P., and Dejour, H.** Traitement chirurgical des epaules douloureuses par lesions de la coiffe et du long biceps en fonction des lesions. Reflexions sur le concept de Neer. *Rev. Rheum. Mal. Osteoartic.*, 1991; 58:247–57.
71. **Wasilewski, S. A. and Frankl, U.** Rotator cuff pathology. Arthroscopic assessment and treatment. *Clin. Orthop.*, 1991; 267:65–70.
72. **Watson, M.** The refractory painful arc syndrome. *J. Bone Joint Surg.*, 1978; 60B:544–546.
73. **Wilbourn, A. J.** Electrodiagnostic testing of neurologic injuries in athletes. *Clin. Sports Med.*, 1990; 9:229–47.

Bicipital Tendinitis

74. **Agins, H. J., Chees, J. L., Hoekstra, D. V., and Teitge, R. A.** Rupture of the distal insertion of the biceps brachii tendon. *Clin. Orthop.*, 1988; 234:34–38.
75. **Becker, D. A. and Cofield, R. H.** Tenodesis of the long head of the biceps brachii for chronic bicipital tendinitis. *J. Bone Joint Surg.*, 1989; 71:376–380.
76. **Ciullo, J. V. and Stevens, G. G.** The prevention and treatment of injuries to the shoulder in swimming. *Sports Med.*, 1989; 7:182–204.
77. **Cone, R. O., Danzig, L., Resnick, D., and Goldman, A. B.** The bicipital groove: radiographic, anatomic and pathologic study. *AJR*, 1983; 141:781–788.
78. **Crenshaw, A. H. and Kilgore, W. E.** Surgical of bicipital tendosynovitis. *J. Bone Joint Surg.*, 1966; 48(A):1496–1502.

79. **Čičak, N. and Buljan, M.** Diagnostic ultrasound of the shoulder. In: *Diagnostic Ultrasound of the Locomotor System.* Matasović T. (Ed.). Zagreb: Skolska Knjiga, 1990:155–179.
80. **Dines, D., Warren, R. F., and Inglis, A. E.** Surgical treatment of lesions of the long head of the biceps. *Clin. Orthop.,* 1982; 164:165–169.
81. **Gachter, A. and Seeling, W.** Schulterarthroskopie. *Arthroskopie,* 1988; 1:162–170.
82. **Lupo, S.-C. and Di Biabo, T. M..** La tendinopatia del capo lungo del bicipite brachiale negli atleti participanti pallavolo. *Med. Sport,* 1987; 40:131–140.
83. **Jobe, F. W. and Brodley, J. P.** The diagnosis and nonoperative treatment of shoulder injuries in athletes. *Clin. Sports Med.,* 1989; 8:419–438.
84. **Johnson, L. L.** The shoulder joint: an arthroscopist's perspective of anatomy and pathology. *Clin. Orthop.,* 1987; 223:113–125.
85. **Middleton, W. D., Reinus, W. R., and Totty, W. G.** Ultrasonographic evaluation of the rotator cuff and biceps tendon. *J. Bone Joint Surg.,* 1986; 68(A):440–450.
86. **Naviaser, R. J.** Lesions of the biceps and tendinitis of the shoulder. *Orthop. Clin. N. Am.,* 1980; 11:334–340.
87. **Neviaser, R. J.** Painful shoulder conditions. *Clin. Orthop.,* 1983; 173:63–69.
88. **Post, M. and Benca, P.** Primary tendinitis of the long head of the biceps. *Clin. Orthop.,* 1989; 246:117–125.
89. **Slatis, P. and Aalto, K.** Medial dislocation of the tendon of the long head of the biceps brachii. *Acta Orthop. Scand.,* 1979; 50:73–77.
90. **Uhthoff, H. K. and Sarkar, K.** Classification and definition of tendinopathies. *Clin. Sports Med.,* 1991; 10:707–720.
91. **Walch, G., Boilean, P., Noel, E., Liotard, J. P., and Dejour, H.** Traitement chirurgical des epaules doulouremses par lesions de la coiffe et du long biceps en fonction des lesions. Reflexions sur le concept de Neer. *Rev. Rheum. Mal. Osteoartic.,* 1991; 58:247–257.

Chapter

3

Elbow

I. HUMERAL EPICONDYLITIS

Humeral epicondylitis is an enthesitis which manifests itself at the origin of the forearm extensors on the lateral epicondyle (lateral or radial epicondylitis), or at the origin of the forearm flexors and pronator teres on the medial epicondyle (medial or ulnar epicondylitis).

A. History

The first description of symptoms related to epicondylitis was given in 1873 by the German physician, Runge,[15] who associated this condition with extended use of the arm in writing. In 1882, Morris used the phrase *lawn tennis arm.* One year later, Mayor introduced the term *tennis elbow*[15] in an article in the *British Medical Journal.* In 1896, a German study documented symptoms of lateral epicondylitis in a variety of occupations, including bricklayers, carpenters, plumbers, bakers, shoemakers, and violinists.[5] Bernhard first noted the correlation between tenderness and pain and the excessive use of the forearm extensors.[15] In 1910, Franke introduced the term *humeral epicondylitis.*[12]

Lateral epicondylitis occurs 7 to 10 times more often than medial epicondylitis.[10,11,29,38,40,47,48,52] Humeral epicondylitis is equally common in both sexes, manifests itself usually between the ages of 30 and 50, and occurs 4 times more frequently in the 40s. The dominant arm is most often affected. Bilateral involvement is rare.

Lateral epicondylitis is commonly called *tennis elbow,* while medial epicondylitis has a variety of names: synonimes epitrochleitis, javelin thrower's elbow, and pitcher's elbow. Some authors[7,16] have called both lateral and medial epicondylitis tennis elbow. Nirschl recognizes lateral epicondylitis as *lateral tennis elbow,* medial epicondylitis as *medial tennis elbow,* and triceps tendinitis as *posterior tennis elbow.*

Although humeral epicondylitis is referred to in medical nomenclature by a number of names associated with different sports, in 95% of the cases in clinical practice it is encountered as an occupational hazard in nonathletes, primarily dactilographs, bricklayers, shoemakers, cooks, truck drivers, surgeons, dentists, and in other professions where repeated contractions of the extensor and supinator muscles (in lateral epicondylitis) or flexor and pronator muscles (in medial epicondylitis) are performed. Professions in which repeated contractions are performed against a resisting force are particularly prone to development of humeral epicondylitis. In athletes, who account for 5% of the cases in clinical practice, humeral epicondylitis is most often found in tennis players, javelin throwers, bowlers, fencers, golf players, hockey players, and handball players.

Allander[1] reported an incidence of 1 to 5% of lateral epicondylitis in a population of 15,268 people between 31 and 74 years of age. In a group of women between the ages of 42 to 46 years, he reported an incidence of 10% which is remarkably high when compared to the annual incidence of 1% or less. Luopajaravi et al.[30] reported on a risk-prone population of factory workers and sales assistants with an average age of 39 years. The incidence was 3%. Kivi[27] studied a population of 7,600 manual workers and diagnosed humeral epicondylitis in 88 workers (50 males and 38 females). Lateral epicondylitis was diagnosed in 74 workers (84%), while medial epicondylitis was diagnosed in 14 cases (16%). The mean age of the afflicted workers was 43 years.

A study performed by Gruchow and Palletier[21] analyzed 532 tennis players (278 males and 254 females), between the ages of 20 to 60 years. Their results indicated that age and the amount of daily playing time are correlated to the development of lateral epicondylitis and that the incidence and recurrence of symptoms rises proportionally with age. Lateral epicondylitis was diagnosed in 24.8% of the players under 40 years of age and in 57.4% of the players over 40 years. Further analysis showed that players over 40 years are twice as likely to develop tennis elbow when compared to players under 40 years and that players over 40 years who play more than 2 h/d on average have a 3.5 times greater risk of developing lateral epicondylitis. Their study indicated no significant difference between the incidence and recurrence of symptoms with regards to the weight of the racket and the material from which it is made. Some authors believe that the increased incidence of tennis elbow in players is directly attributable to the materials from which modern rackets are made. With wooden rackets, vibrations that occur when the ball is hit tend to be absorbed, while modern rackets, which are made from metal, graphite, and fiberglass, do not absorb vibrations so effectively. The grip size of the racket can also be one of the causes for development or recurrence of tennis elbow. A grip larger than 4 3/8 in. can lead, especially in older players, to the development of lateral epicondylitis. Some authors emphasize that players with more playing experience have a higher incidence of tennis elbow, a fact they attribute to the greater amount of daily playing time that experienced players have when compared to inexperienced players. Nirschl's[35] study shows that inexperienced tennis players have a higher incidence of tennis elbow because of their improper stroking technique. Priest et al.[39] analyzed the incidence of humeral epicondylitis in a population of tennis players and obtained results similar to those of Gruchow and Palletier[21] with one interesting exception. Their study showed that professional and semi-professional tennis players had a higher incidence of medial epicondylitis, a fact they attributed to the strenuous movements those players performed while serving.

B. Etiopathogenesis

Using the backhand stroke in tennis as an example, we will explain the development of lateral epicondylitis. While performing this stroke, the forearm extensors are contracted to stabilize the wrist and to hold the racket. Repetitive concentric contractions, which occur if the stroke is improperly performed, shorten these muscles as they maintain tension to stabilize the wrist and produce a force that is transmitted via the muscles to their origin on the lateral epicondyle. These repetitive concentric contractions produce chronic overload of the bone-tendon junction which in turn leads to decreased vascularization of the junction and overstimulation of free nerve endings. As a result, there is an aseptic inflammatory reaction.

To illustrate the development of medial epicondylitis, we will describe the mechanics of baseball pitching. The specialized technique used in baseball pitching produces a large valgus stress across the elbow which leads to overstretching of the medial collateral ligament and tension in the bone-tendon junction of the muscles that have their origin on the medial epicondyle. The baseball pitcher, while throwing the ball, extends his arm in the elbow; at the same time, he pronates the forearm and produces a palmar flexion of the wrist just prior to releasing the ball in order to obtain horizontal control of the pitch. Constant repetition of this movement in practice and competition can result in straining the medial collateral ligament or overusing the forearm flexors and pronator teres.

In all cases of lateral epicondylitis, the origin of the extensor carpi radialis brevis muscle is afflicted.[11,24,29,34,36] The origins of the extensor digitorum communis and extensor carpi radialis muscles are affected in 35% of the cases. The extensor carpi ulnaris is rarely involved. In all cases of medial epicondylitis, the origins of the pronator teres and flexor carpi radialis muscles are affected while the origin of the flexor carpi ulnaris muscle is affected in only 10% of the cases[28,34,36] (Figure 1).

Coonrad and Hooper have theorized[10] that macroscopic or microscopic tears in the muscle origin are the likely cause of symptoms. We do not agree with this. In our opinion, the sequence of events is that overuse leads to avascularization of the affected muscle origin which leads to overstimulation of the free nerve ends and results in aseptic inflammation. Further repetition of offending movements causes angiofibroblastic hyperplasia of the origin. Then in the final stage, partial or complete rupture of the tendon occurs. Angiofibroblastic hyperplasia prevents healing, allowing the aseptic inflammation to continue with ultimate damage to the tendon origin. Nirschl states that the degree of angiofibroblastic hyperplasia is correlated to the duration and severity of symptoms.[33–35] The afflicted tendon origin is gray and resembles immature fibrous tissue; it is shiny, is edematose, and easily crumbles. Histological analysis reveals the characteristic invasion of fibroblasts and vascular tissue, the typical picture of angiofibroblastic hyperplasia.

C. Clinical Picture and Diagnostics

The main symptoms consist of pain and tenderness at the lateral epicondyle (in lateral epicondylitis) or at the medial epicondyle (in medial epicondylitis). In most cases, pain is characterized by a gradual onset which, after prolonged repetition of provoking movements, intensifies to the level of severe pain, restricting basically any working activity. A sudden onset of pain is usually associated with one very strenuous movement, i.e., when throwing a heavy object. In lateral epicondylitis, tenderness is produced by palpation on the extensor muscles origin on the lateral epicondyle.

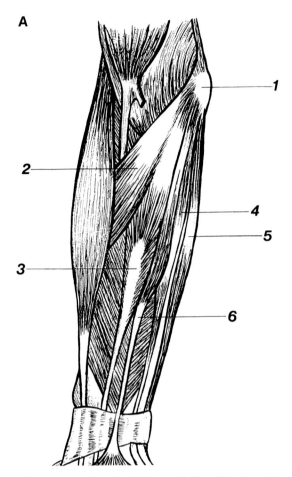

FIGURE 1. Muscle insertion sites from the (A) ulnar and (B) radial epicondylus of the ulna. (A) 1: epicondylus ulnaris (medialis); 2: pronator teres muscle; 3: flexor carpi radialis muscle; 4: flexor digitorum superficialis muscle; 5: flexor carpi ulnaris muscle; 6: palmaris longus muscle.

In some cases, the pain can spread along the radial side of the forearm to the wrist, and in rare cases, even to the third and fourth fingers. The pain can be very intense, i.e., debilitating the patient from turning a key in the lock or even picking up light weights.

According to Warren[48], there are four stages in the development of this injury with regards to the intensity of the symptoms.

1. Faint pain a couple of hours after the provoking activity.
2. Pain at the end of or immediately after the provoking activity.
3. Pain during the provoking activity which intensifies after ceasing that activity.
4. Constant pain which disqualifies any activity.

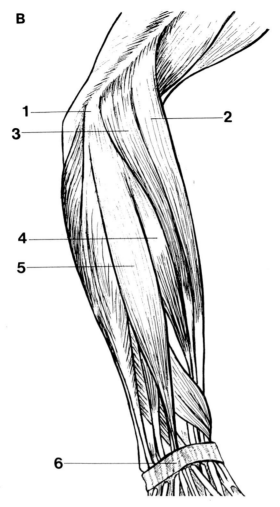

FIGURE 1 (continued). (B) 1: epicondylus radialis (lateralis); 2: brachioradialis muscle; 3: extensor carpi radialis brevis muscle; 4: extensor carpi radialis longus muscle; 5: extensor digitorum communis muscle; 6: retinaculum extensorum.

During physical examination, pain is provoked by palpation on the extensor muscles origin on the lateral epicondyle. The pain will typically intensify if the patient extends the elbow while the examiner palpates the tender area.

The following tests are used to improve localization of the exact area of tenderness and to get a better assessment of the intensity of the pain on the lateral epicondyle.

1. Extending the wrist against resistance while the forearm is in full pronation and extended in the elbow; produces pain at the lateral epicondylar origin. This test was described by Mills[5] in 1928.

2. Extending the middle finger against resistance with the forearm in pronation and the elbow extended; produces pain in the same area. This test was described by Roles and Maudsley[42] (Figure 2).
3. The "chair test". This test employs the use of a small chair with approximately 4 kg in weight and an opening on the sitting surface. The patient pushes his fingers through the opening and attempts to lift the chair with an extended elbow and pronated forearm. The pain will usually appear during the act of lifting. Failing that, the patient should further extend the wrist and if the test is positive, the pain will either appear for the first time or intensify.
4. In Gardner's "stress test",[19] the examiner tries to flex the patient's wrist against the force of the patient's contracted extensor muscles. The elbow is in extension and the forearm in full pronation.

In lateral epicondylitis, flexion and extension are usually complete. However, in some of the chronic cases, hypertrophy of the extensor muscles is visible, and the patient will lack 5 to 15° of wrist extension.[5,8,35,36,52]

Routine anteroposterior and lateral elbow radiographs are usually normal. Calcification of the soft tissues about the lateral epicondyle is occasionally present. Leach and Miller[29] reported an incidence of 22% of cases with calcification in a studied population suffering from lateral epicondylitis.

Thermography of the afflicted elbow can be a very useful aid in diagnosing lateral epicondylitis.[3,28,44] Binder et al.[3] reported that thermography of the afflicted elbow demonstrated in 53 out of 56 patients (95%), with diagnosed lateral epicondylitis, a localized area of greater heat ("hot spot") near the lateral epicondyle with a center that is 1 to 3°C higher than the normal isotherm.

In medial epicondylitis, the area of greatest tenderness is located at the origin of the flexor muscles on the medial humeral epicondyle. In some cases, the pain radiates along the ulnar side of the forearm to the wrist and occasionally even into the fingers. Grip strength is diminished and provokes pain. During physical examination, resisted flexion of the wrist with the elbow extended and the forearm in supination will produce pain in the medial epicondyle area.[5,29,52]

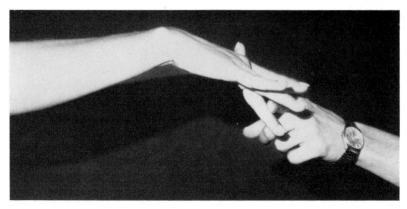

FIGURE 2. Schema of the extension test for the flexed middle finger in the metacarpophalangeal joint against resistance.

Medial epicondylitis in a throwing athlete is differentiated from a chronic medial ligamentous strain by placing the wrist in flexion and the forearm in pronation and then gently applying a valgus stress to the slightly (10 to 20°) flexed elbow. If done gently, this should not be painful if the problem is medial epicondylitis alone. With medial collateral ligament strain or partial rupture, the test will be painful and may demonstrate, in cases of rupture, medial instability of the elbow.

D. Differential Diagnosis

In cases of lateral epicondylitis resistant to nonoperative treatment, differential diagnosis must take into account the radial tunnel syndrome to which some authors refer as *resistant tennis elbow*.[22,42] The radial tunnel whose length is less then 5.0 cm begins proximally at the level of the capitellum of the humerus, which is its posterior wall, and continues to the distal end of the supinator muscle. There are five possible causes of compression in this tunnel: (1) abnormal fibrous band in front of the radial head, (2) a "fan" of radial recurrent vessels, (3) the sharp tendinous origin of the extensor carpi radialis brevis, (4) the arcade of Frohse, and (5) a fibrous band at the distal edge of the supinator muscle. The most common cause of compression is a fibrous arcade of Frohse. Ritts et al.[41] reported that the arcade of Frohse was the cause of 69.4% of the cases of radial tunnel syndrome. Spinnerr's research[37] shows that the arcade of Frohse is absent in fetuses and that only 30% of the mature population have it. Some authors differentiate compression at the arcade of Frohse as a separate syndrome which they call the *supinator muscle syndrome*.[4,9,37]

In radial tunnel syndrome, there may be a spectrum of complaints, including pain, paresthesias, and weakness. A motor deficit is not nearly as common as on a posterior interosseous nerve syndrome. The most common symptom is a dull pain in the posterolateral area of the forearm which sometimes spreads to the dorsal side of the wrist. The pain increases during repeated movements of pronation and extension of the forearm if the wrist is palmarly flexed.

Physical examination must include carefully localizing the point of tenderness. Maneuvers that aggravate or reproduce the patient's symptoms should be carried out, and the most useful test is resisted forearm supination (the elbow is in flexion of 90° and the forearm is in full pronation). This maneuver will worsen or reproduce the symptoms. Extension of the middle finger against resistance with the elbow in complete extension may result in similar symptoms, but not with the same frequency as the resisted forearm supination test.

Although the clinical features of radial tunnel syndrome are quite characteristic, it is often confused with lateral epicondylitis. Werner[50] reported that the radial tunnel syndrome is found with lateral epicondylitis in 5% of the cases, while Beenisch and Wilhelm[4] reported that in 53% of their patients, preoperative tests found supinator muscle syndromes together with lateral epicondylitis.

Differential diagnostics of medial epicondylitis should take into account compressive neuropathy of the median and ulnar nerves in the area of the elbow.

The median nerve is vulnerable to compression as it passes under the lacertus fibrosis or bicipital aponeurosis, through the opening between the heads of the pronator teres muscle, through one of the heads of the pronator teres muscle *(prona-*

tor teres syndrome), and below the fibrous arch of the flexor digitorum superficialis muscle in which case anterior interosseous nerve is affected (*anterior interosseous syndrome* or *Kiloh-Nevin syndrome*).[25,37] Compressive neuropathy of the median nerve in the elbow area is usually characterized by a dull, diffuse pain in the proximal part of the forearm which increases during activity and typically decreases when resting.[25] The area of greatest tenderness is usually located above the point of compression.

The ulnar nerve is vulnerable to compression in the elbow area as it passes through the ulnar groove or between the two heads of the flexor carpi ulnaris muscle *(cubital tunnel syndrome)*.[37] The early stages of ulnar nerve entrapment of the elbow are characterized by paresthesias on the ulnar aspect of the forearm and in the ring and small finger. Sensory changes definitely precede motor changes; however, a careful evaluation of the intrinsic musculature of the hand is essential to detect any weakness. Because of the functional ceasing of the adductor pollicis muscle, Froment's symptom appears. This symptom is characterized by flexion in the interfalangeal joint of the thumb when the patient tries to grip a piece of paper between thumb and forefinger. The same symptoms can be caused by dislocation of the ulnar nerve (luxatio nervi ulnaris) from its groove during elbow flexion. The dislocation can be caused by the shallowness of the groove due to the ripping of the epicondyloolecranon ligament, the valgus position of the elbow, or congenital abnormalities of the humeral epicondyles. During flexion and extension of the elbow, the nerve slips from its groove and slides toward the volar. In most cases, it is squeezed against the medial epicondyle, leading to compression and stretching of the nerve.

Although only Nirschl[34-36] has reported on associated medial epicondylitis with compressive neuropathy of the ulnar nerve (in 60% of his cases), differential diagnosis should always take into account the possibility of ulnar nerve compression whenever a patient localizes the area of greater pain in the vicinity of the ulnar groove. This is especially important in cases with unstable medial collateral ligaments.

E. Treatment

The wide variety of treatments, coupled with the published results, indicate that as yet, no definite type of treatment is universally endorsed.

1. Nonoperative Treatment

Our approach to nonoperative treatment is based on the following principles: relieving pain, controlling the inflammation, and monitoring further activity. Following these principles, we have compiled a program for nonoperative treatment of lateral epicondylitis which we have divided into three phases. The therapy should start as soon as possible; ideally, as soon as the first symptoms appear. One of the most common mistakes is to ignore the early symptoms and continue on as before, repeating offending activities with the same intensity.

a. The First Phase

Eliminating painful activities and resting from work or athletic activities are the most important factors of this phase. While avoiding painful activities, the patient should continue to perform normal, active movements with other parts of the symptomatic extremity to avoid stiffness and other complications. Of oral nonsteroidal anti-inflammatory agents, we generally recommend agents from the oxicamic family (piroxicam) administered in the highest daily doses.

Icing or other types of cryotherapy should be applied 3 times per day for 15 min. This lessens the pain by reducing the conductibility of the sensory nerves. Ice also reduces the inflammatory response by decreasing the level of chemical activity and by vasoconstriction which reduces the swelling. Elevation of the extremity is indicated if an edema of the wrist or fingers is present. In this phase, we also recommend wearing a plastic splint for the wrist ("wrist splint"). A volar splint with the wrist in 20° of extension will usually permit functional use of the hand while preventing overuse of wrist extensors.

b. The Second Phase

The main feature of this phase is stretching exercises. The underlying principle of this phase is based on the fact that by lengthening the tendon during relaxation, we can reduce its stretching during offending movements. Stretching exercises for the extensor muscles of the wrist and fingers should be performed in the following manner: fully extend the elbow and palmarly flex the wrist. While applying pressure with the other hand, increase the palmar flexion as much as possible but stop at the first painful sensation (Figure 3). The patient should remain in the point of maximum nonpainful extension for a period of 15 to 25 s. This exercise is repeated 4 to 5 times a day with two series of ten exercises in each session; the patient should always stop at the first sign of pain. In this phase of therapy, the patient should also perform isotonic exercises, once a day, according to the following plan:

1. Stretching exercises — hold for 15 to 25 s; repeat 10 times
2. Isotonic exercises — three series of 15 repetitions

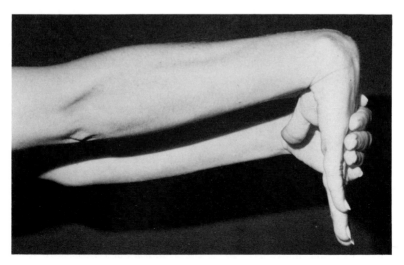

FIGURE 3. Passive stretching of the extensor muscles of the lower arm.

3. Stretching exercises — hold for 15 to 25 s; repeat 10 times
4. Icing — massage the tender area with ice or crushed ice for 10 to 15 min

Isotonic exercises are performed in the following manner: with forearm on a table in a position of full pronation with the wrist hanging over the edge; in this position, perform extension and flexion movements of the wrist. In the beginning phase, the patient should perform the exercise slowly, counting to six after each flexion (the eccentric phase of contraction) and to three after each extension of the wrist (the concentric phase of contraction). When these movements become painless, the patient should gradually increase the speed and resistance. Increasing the speed of the exercises has the effect of increasing the loading on the tendon, while the gradual increasing of outside resistance leads to progressive strain of the tendon, resulting in an increase of its stretching strength. The outside resistance is accomplished by lifting small weights — at first 0.5 kg, and than slowly progressing to 5 kg. The maximum weight should not exceed 10% of the patient's body weight.

As already noted, besides stretching and isotonic exercises, the patient should also perform isometric exercises. A good example is the following: place a rubber band around the gathered fingers and thumb; then perform extension of the fingers against force. The exercise is repeated 3 times a day with 50 repetitions in each series while gradually increasing the tightness of the rubber band. A second useful exercise is to extend the arm in the elbow and abduct the forearm to a horizontal position. An elastic tube or tennis ball is placed in the hand and the patient proceeds to squeeze the object alternately with greater and lesser strength. This exercise is begun in the third week of treatment and is performed 3 times a day with 50 repetitions.

In the first two weeks of therapy, stimulation by high voltage galvanic stimulator is also administered. This produces a piezoelectric effect which promotes tissue healing and enhances localized blood flow. In some patients, it also creates an analgetic effect.

Once all offending movements become painless, the patient can return to his normal daily activities. However, heavy physical work and athletic activities should be avoided. In all activities, the patient should wear a nonelastic elbow brace ("counterforce brace") (Figure 4). This brace plays the role of a secondary muscle attachment site and relieves tension on the attachment at the lateral epicondyle. The brace is applied firmly around the forearm (below the head of the radius) and is tightened enough so that when the patient contracts the wrist extensors, he or she does not obtain a full contraction of the muscles. This phase lasts for 6 to 8 weeks. If the pain recurs or worsens, the intensity of the exercise program is reduced. If the pain persists, the patient is returned to the first phase of treatment.

c. The Third Phase
The patient gradually returns to all activities, but continues to perform stretching exercises and to strengthen the affected muscle groups. A nonelastic elbow brace should be worn during all strenuous activities.

Recurrence of the symptoms is frequent if exercises are not repeated daily to increase the resistance gradually. The patient should be made aware that before any athletic or strenuous activity is undertaken, a long warm-up period of the affected

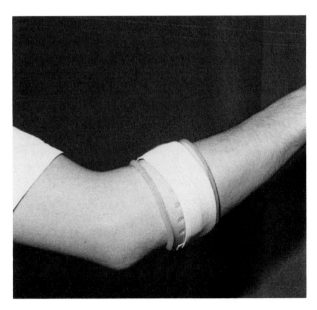

FIGURE 4. Counterforce brace.

muscle group, including stretching exercises, is necessary. Once the activity is finished, stretching exercises and cryotherapy must be performed.

To avoid recidives in cases with professional etiologies, the patient should lighten the weight of his working tools or reduce the frequency of the offending movements. Failing that, rest periods should be increased and the time lengthened to allow relaxation of the muscles; this is to reduce the risk of recurrence. With tennis players, prevention of lateral epicondylitis is accompanied by correcting the improper stroking techniques and way of holding the racket, choosing the optimal shape, material, and weight of the racket, enlarging the grip, and reducing racket string tension.

We believe that local corticosteroid injections should be avoided as long as possible and used only in resistant cases that do not respond to more conservative measures. In these cases, up to three injections deep into the subcutaneous fat tissue can be administered. The injections should not be repeated above the mentioned number because the progressive response to each injection is reduced and the risk of possible complications (subcutaneous atrophy, weakening of the surrounding tissues) increases. Care must be taken not to administer the injection into the tendon because of the increase in pressure in the bradiotroph tissue and because of the possibility of a tendon rupture which is an unwanted side-effect.

2. Surgical Treatment

The symptoms of humeral epicondylitis will prove to be resistant in 5 to 10% of the patients. In those cases, surgical treatment is indicated.[2,6,10,13,14,17,20,26,29,31–36,40,43,45,46,49,51] This treatment is indicated when symptoms persist for longer than 6 months and significantly disable the patient from performing his normal working or athletic activities despite an adequately carried out nonoperative treatment. It is also indicated in cases with frequent recidives and incomplete remissions. A relative indication may be present in athletes for whom the amount of time spent out of competition can be of crucial importance. Different surgical techniques and their modification have been proposed for treating humeral epicondylitis. A review of the literature shows that the most commonly used techniques are modifications of the Hohmann and Bosworth methods. When dealing with lateral epicondylitis, we use the following modification of the Hohmann method. A curvilinear incision is made over the area of the lateral epicondyle. The deep antebrachial fascia is incised, revealing the lateral epicondyle. The tendinous origin of the extensor carpi radialis brevis muscle is part sharply and part bluntly freed from the lateral epicondyle. Using a surgical chisel, the epicondyle is decorticated while the surrounding, less vital structures are excised. A hemostasis is performed after which the wound is closed by layers. Postoperative immobilization is carried out with six layers of sheet cotton and a light circumferential long arm cast with the elbow at 90° and the wrist in functional position. Nirschl[33] reported a 75% success rate using this technique while Stotz et al.[45] reported a 65% success to failure ratio.

Recent knowledge into the etiopathogenesis of humeral epicondylitis has instigated Coonrad and Hooper[40] to develop a new operative method that has been slightly modified by Nirschl and Pettrone.[33] The procedure begins with a lateral 5-cm long incision over the lateral epicondyle. The deep fascia is incised and gently separated, revealing the tendinous origin of the common extensor. Because the origin of the extensor carpi radialis brevis muscle is usually the affected site, the extensor carpi radialis longus muscle is gently lifted to reveal the affected origin. Excision of the affected tendon origin of the extensor carpi radialis brevis muscle is performed, and in some cases, part of the tendon origin of the extensor carpi radialis longus is excised as well. Excision of part of the extensor digitorum communis muscle is very rarely indicated. When necessary, a small opening is made through the synovium for inspection of the radiohumeral joint. Part of the periosteum is removed using an osteotome, or four to five holes are drilled with a small drill down to the spongeous bone. The tendons are than reattached at this site after previously being longitudinally joined. The wound is closed by layers. Post-operative immobilization is carried out with a light circumferential long arm cast with the elbow at 90° and the forearm in a neutral position. Total elevation of the extremity above shoulder level is necessary for 3 d. Mobilization is initiated after 5 to 7 d after which intense rehabilitation is begun. Nirschl and Pettrone[33] reported excellent results using this method without any residual pain contraction or loss of muscle strength in 97.7% of their cases, while Coonrad[11] reported excellent results obtained using this method in all of his patients.

In the last 10 years, percutaneous tenotomy of the extensor muscles in lateral epicondylitis or the flexor muscles in medial epicondylitis has been frequently performed.[2,20,46] The procedure is done in the following manner. The forearm is placed on the operating table in supination while the elbow is in a 90° flexion. The posterior edge of the lateral epicondyle is palpated, and an impression is made 1 cm from the edge towards the middle of the epicondyle on the skin with the thumb. The skin and deeper tissue overlaying the epicondyle are infiltrated with a local anesthetic. Using a No. 11 blade (tenotome), a puncture incision is made through the skin to the bone, and the tendinous origin of the common extensors is freed from the bone. The release is carried down from the proximal to the distal portion of the epicondyle and parallel with the axis of the humerus. The skin is closed with one stitch, and dry sterile dressing is placed on the wound.

A similar procedure is performed on the medial side of the elbow for medial epicondylitis. When releasing the muscles, extreme caution must be taken to prevent damage to the ulnar nerve. To avoid this complication, the index finger of the surgeon's hand is kept in the ulnar groove during the release. Baumgard and Schwartz[2] reported excellent results in 91.4% of the patients on whom a percutaneous tenotomy of the extensor muscles was performed and in 84% of the patients on whom a percutaneous tenotomy of the flexor muscles was performed. Yeger and Turner[46] performed percutaneous tenotomy of the extensor muscles in 109 patients. In 102 of these (93.5%), the results were excellent. The advantages of this operative method, as noted by different authors,[2,20,51] lay in the simplicity of the procedure. The procedure does not require hospitalization, entails very rare postoperative complications, and allows a quick return to normal working activity (on average, 9 d). In athletes and manual workers, however, this procedure is not indicated, in our opinion, since postoperative complications may reduce grip strength.

II. POSTERIOR IMPINGEMENT SYNDROME OF THE ELBOW

Repetitive, sudden, forceful extension of the elbow present in many athletic activities — baseball, handball, tennis and throwing sports — can lead to development of the posterior impingement syndrome of the elbow.[53-58] These movements are characterized by the violent collision of the olecranon against the olecranon fossa. Besides the posterior impingement syndrome of the elbow, these movements can also lead to the development of triceps tendinitis, apophysitis of the olecranon (which can be likened to Osgood-Schatter's disease) and stress fracture of the olecranon (Figure 5). The characteristic symptom of posterior impingement syndrome of the elbow is a sharp pain which manifests itself when the elbow snaps into full extension during activity. The tenderness is localized to the posterior or posterior medial side of the elbow. The patient also complains of reduced mobility, i.e., inability to fully extend the elbow. Crepitations are frequent during movements of the elbow; in some cases, "stiffness" and a diffuse pain accompanied by a swelling of the elbow is also present. During physical examination, pain is discovered over the posterior or posteriomedial area of the olecranon. Pain can also be induced with a strong passive extension of the elbow. The valgus stress test of the elbow will also produce characteristic pain during the last 5 to 10° of elbow extension. In cases of triceps tendinitis, pain will spear during extension against resistance.

Radiographic examination can show what movements provoke collision of the bony parts in the elbow and existence or absence of loose bodies in the elbow. Radiographic examination will also show bony osteophytes on the posteromedial aspect of the olecranon. Cortical thickening of the olecranon fossa, which can be found in both symptomatic and asymptomatic patients, is explained as a physiological adaptation of bone to repetitive stress.

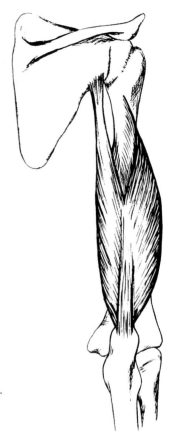

FIGURE 5. Triceps branchii muscle.

Initial treatment consists of reducing stress to the elbow joint (relative rest) and alleviating the pain, swelling, and inflammation. This is accomplished by temporarily ceasing athletic activities, using nonsteroidal anti-inflammatory drugs, and icing the affected area. Taping, with the aim of preventing full extension and valgus of the elbow (an adhesive tape applied to the anterior side of the elbow), can enable the patient to resume athletic activities without pain.

During rehabilitation, exercises which strengthen the elbow flexors (biceps, brachialis, and brachioradialis) should be performed to prevent the maximal extension of the elbow. Stretching exercises of the extensor muscles (triceps) should also be performed. According to Wilson et al.,[58] good results from surgical treatment are short term, and clinical symptoms often recur. Surgical treatment consists of removing the bony osteophytes, performing an osteotomy of the tip of the olecranon, or performing a debridement of the olecranon and olecranon fossa. The latter can be performed arthroscopically.[53–56]

III. MEDIAL TENSION/LATERAL COMPRESSION SYNDROME

Medial tension/lateral compression syndrome is a term used to describe a complex of overuse injuries of the elbow characterized by tenderness, reduced mobility, and the inability to throw a ball without pain. Medial tension/lateral compression syndrome is caused by repetitive valgus stress at the elbow.[59-63] The act of throwing a ball causes a strong valgus stress which leads to stretching of the structures on the medial side of the elbow and at the same time to compression of the lateral side of the joint. Because of this etiology, medial tension/lateral compression syndrome is also known in medical literature due to its high frequency in baseball players, as *pitcher's elbow* in mature athletes and *Little League elbow* in younger athletes (Figure 6).

The syndrome is characterized by extra-articular changes on the medial side of the elbow. In most cases, these changes consist of enthesitis of the wrist flexors and pronator teres on the medial epicondyle of the humerus (medial epicondylitis). Less common are ruptures of these muscles or avulsion fracture of the medial epicondyle. Strain or rupture of the ulnar collateral ligament of the elbow is another frequent symptom. In older athletes, a bony spike on the tip of the ulna (ulnar traction spur) is sometimes found. Some authors believe that compression of the ulnar nerve in this area can also result from the same repetitive stretching movements.

On the lateral side of the elbow, compression causes intra-articular damage. Degenerative changes of the elbow and loose bodies are characteristically found in older athletes while osteochondritis dissecans of the humeral capitulum is typical in younger athletes. Osteochondritis results from repeated valgus stresses incurred while throwing a ball, but also from improper throwing technique.

Radiographic examination is routinely used to diagnose osteochondritis (Figure 7). In the beginning stages, a tomogram can also be indicated. Osteochondritis is seen as an area of greater radiolucency, fragmentation, and deformation of the capitellum.[62] Arthroscopic surgical treatment[59] is the method generally preferred today when dealing with early stages of osteochondritis; the aim is to prevent degenerative

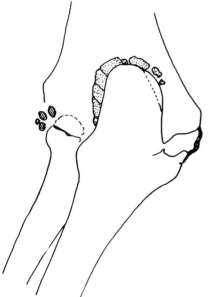

FIGURE 6. Medial tension/laterial compression syndrome of the elbow.

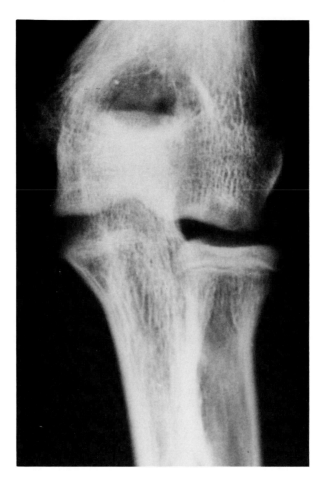

FIGURE 7. Roentgenogram of a top-level gymnast with medial tension/lateral compression syndrome.

changes in the elbow, loose bodies, angular deformation of the radial head, and reduced mobility.

On the posterior side of the elbow, the repetitive collisions of the olecranon against the olecranon fossa produce degenerative changes on the olecranon — in most cases, a bony spur or loose joint bodies. Tenderness of the tip on the medial side of the olecranon is diagnosed during physical examination. A typical symptom of this syndrome, also known as posterior impingement syndrome, is a sharp pain felt during sudden, passive extension in the elbow. Surgical treatment is indicated in most cases.

REFERENCES

Humeral Epicondylitis

1. **Allander, E.** Prevalence, incidence and remission rates of some common rheumatic diseases or syndromes. *Scand. J. Rheumatol.*, 1974; 3:145–153.

2. **Baumgard, S. H. and Schwartz, D. R.** Percutaneous release of the epicondylar muscles for humeral epicondylitis. *Am. J. Sports Med.*, 1982; 10:233–236.

3. **Binder, A., Parr, G., Page Thomas, P., and Hazleman, B.** A clinical and thermographic study of lateral epicondylitis. *Br. J. Rheumatol.*, 1983; 22:77–81.

4. **Beenisch, J. and Wilhelm, K.** Die epicondylitis humeri lateralis. *Fortschr. Med.*, 1985; 103:417–419.

5. **Bojanić, I., Pećina, M., Bilić, R., and Ribarić, G.** Epicondylitis humeri. *Basketball Med. Per.*, 1988; 3:69–81.

6. **Boyd, H. B. and Mc Leod, A. C.** Tennis elbow. *J. Bone Joint Surg.*, 1973; 55(A):1183–1187.

7. **Cabot, A.** Tennis elbow. *Orthop. Rev.*, 1987; 16:69–73.

8. **Chop, W. M., Jr.** Tennis elbow. *Postgrad. Med.*, 1989; 86:301–308.

9. **Coenen, W.** Uber ein diagnostisches zeichen bei der sogenaunten Epicondylitis humeri radialis. *Z. Orthop.*, 1986; 124:323–326.

10. **Coonrad, R. W. and Hooper, R. W.** Tennis elbow: its course, natural history, conservative and surgical management. *J. Bone Joint Surg.*, 1973; 55(A):1177–1182.

11. **Coonrad, R. W.** Tennis elbow. *Instr. Course Lect.*, 1986; 35:94–101.

12. **Cyriax, J. H.** The pathology and treatment of tennis elbow. *J. Bone Joint Surg.*, 1936; 18:921–940.

13. **Čurković B. and Domljan Z.** Radijalni epikondilitis. *Lijec. Vjesn.*, 1982; 104:362–364.

14. **Dobyns, J. H.** Musculotendinous problems at the elbow. In: *Surgery of the Musculoskeletal System.* McCollister, E. C., Ed. New York: Churchill Livingstone, 1983; 211–232.

15. **Emery, S. E. and Gifford, J. F.** 100 years of tennis elbow. *Contemp. Orthop.*, 1986; 12:53–58.

16. **Froimson, A. I.** Tenosynovitis and tennis elbow. In: *Operative Hand Surgery.* Green, D. P., Ed. New York: Churchill Livingstone, 1982; 1507–1521.

17. **Friedlander, H. L., Reid, R. L., and Cape, R. F.** Tennis elbow. *Clin. Orthop.*, 1967; 51:109–116.

18. **Garden, R. S.** Tennis elbow. *J. Bone Joint Surg.*, 1961; 43(B):100–106.

19. **Gardner, R. C.** Tennis elbow: diagnosis, pathology and treatment. *Clin. Orthop.*, 1970; 72:248–253.

20. **Goldberg, G. D., Alroham, E., and Siegel, I.** The surgical treatment of chronic lateral humeral epicondylitis by common extensor release. *Clin. Orthop.*, 1988; 223:208–212.

21. **Gruchow, H. W. and Palletier, B. S.** An epidemiologic study of tennis elbow. *Am. J. Sports Med.*, 1979; 7:234–238.

22. **Heyse-Moore, G. H.** Resistant tennis elbow. *J. Hand Surg.*, 1984; 9:64–66.

23. **Howard, F. M.** Controversies in nerve entrapment syndromes in the forearm and wrist. *Orthop. Clin. N. Am.*, 1986; 17:375–381.

24. **Janda, J. and Koudela, K.** Skelletmuskelbeteiligung bei der enthesopatie des epicondylus lateralis humeri. *Z. Orthop.*, 1988; 126:105–107.

25. **Johnson, R., Spinner, M., and Shrewsbury, M. M.** Median nerve entrapment syndrome in the proximal forearm. *J. Hand Surg.*, 1979; 4:48–51.

26. **Kaplan, E. B.** Treatment of tennis elbow (epicondylitis) by denervation. *J. Bone Joint Surg.*, 1959; 41(A):147–151.

27. **Kivi, P.** The etiology and conservative treatment of humeral epicondylitis. *Scand. J. Rehab. Med.*, 1982; 15:37–41.

28. **Koudela, K. and Novak, B.** Entezopatia epicondyli humeri lateralis: termographic a termometrie loketniho kloubu. *Acta Chir. Orthop. Traumatol. Cech.*, 1985; 52:415–416.

29. **Leach, R. E. and Miller, J. K.** Lateral and medial epicondylitis of the elbow. *Clin. Sports Med.,* 1987; 6:259–272.
30. **Luopajaravi, T., Kuorinka, I., Virolainen, M., and Holmberg, M.** Prevalence of tenosynovitis and other injuries of the upper extremities in repetitive work. *Scand. J. Work Environ. Health,* 1979; 5:48–55.
31. **Neviaser, T. J., Neviaser, R. J., Neviaser, J. S., and Ain, B. R.** Lateral epicondylitis: results outpatient surgery and immediate motion. *Contemp. Orthop.,* 1985; 11:43–46.
32. **Nirschl, R. O.** Tennis elbow. *Orthop. Clin. N. Am.,* 1973; 4:787–800.
33. **Nirschl, R. O. and Pettrone, F. A.** Tennis elbow. *J. Bone Joint Surg.,* 1979; 61(A):832–839.
34. **Nirschl, R. P.** Sports and overuse injuries to the elbow. In: *The Elbow and Its Disorders* Morrey, B. F., Ed. Philadelphia: W. B. Saunders, 1985; 309–341.
35. **Nirschl, R. P.** Tennis elbow (epicondylitis): surgery and rehabilitation of the professional athlete. In: *AAOS Symposium on Upper Extremity Injuries in Athletes.* Pettrone, F. A., Ed. St. Louis: C. V. Mosby, 1986; 244–265.
36. **Nirschl, R. P.** Prevention and treatment of elbow and shoulder injuries in the tennis player. *Clin. Sports Med.,* 1988; 7:289–308.
37. **Pećina, M., Krmpotić-Nemanić, J., and Markiewitz, A. D.** *Tunnel Syndromes.* Boca Raton: CRC Press, 1991.
38. **Penners, W., Schnitzler, M., Kircher, E., and Gottinger, W.** Epicondylitis humeri - Tennis-Ellenbogen. *Forschr. Med.,* 1977; 95:1587–1592.
39. **Priest, J. D., Braden, V., and Gerberich, J. G.** The elbow and tennis. *Phys. Sportsmed.,* 1980; 8:80–88.
40. **Regan, W. D.** Lateral elbow pain in the athlete: a clinical review. *Clin. J. Sports Med.,* 1991; 1:53–58.
41. **Ritts, G. D., Wood, M. B., and Lindscheid, R. L.** Radial tunnel syndrome. *Clin. Orthop.,* 1987; 219:201–205.
42. **Roles, N. C. and Maudsley, R. H.** Radial tunnel syndrome: resistant tennis elbow as a nerve entrapment. *J. Bone Joint Surg.,* 1972; 54(B):499–508.
43. **Routson, G. W. and Gingras, M.** Surgical treatment of tennis elbow. *Orthopaedics,* 1981; 4:769–772.
44. **Shilo, R., Engel, J., Farin, I., and Horochowski, H.** Thermography as a diagnostic aid in tennis elbow. *Handchirurgie,* 1976; 8:101–103.
45. **Stotz, R., Firkowiez, M., and Muller, J.** Beitrag zur operativen therapie der Epicondylitis humeri radialis. *Helv. Chir. Acta,* 1984; 51:189–193.
46. **Vangsness, C. T. and Jobe, F. W.** Surgical treatment of medial epicondylitis. *J. Bone Joint Surg.,* 1991; 73(B):409–411.
47. **Wadswort, T. G.** Tennis elbow: conservative, surgical and manipulative treatment. *Br. Med. J.,* 1987; 294:621–624.
48. **Warren, R. F.** Tennis elbow (epicondylitis): epidemiology and conservative treatment. In: *AAOS Symposium on Upper Extremity Injuries in Athletes.* Pettrone, F. A., Ed. St. Louis: C. V. Mosby, 1986; 233–243.
49. **Wanivenhaus, A., Kickinger, W., and Zweymuller, K.** Die Epicondylitis humeri radialis unter besonderer berucksichtigung der operation nach Wilhelm. *Wien. Klin. Wochenschr.* 1986; 98:338–341.
50. **Werner, C. O.** Lateral elbow pain and posterior interosseous nerve entrapment. *Acta Orthop. Scand.,* 1979; 174(suppl.): 1–110.
51. **Yerger, B. and Turner, T.** Percutaneous extensor tenotomy for chronic tennis elbow. *Orthopaedics,* 1985; 8:1261–1263.

52. **Yocum, L. A.** The diagnosis and nonoperative treatment of elbow problems in the athlete. *Clin. Sports Med.,* 1989; 8:439–451.

Posterior Impingement Syndrome of the Elbow

53. **Carson, W. G., Jr.** Complications of elbow arthroscopy. In: *Arthroscopic Surgery.* Sherman, O. H. and Mankoff, J., Eds. Baltimore: Williams & Wilkins, 1990; 166–179.
54. **Garrick, G. J. and Requa, R. K.** Epidemiology of women's gymnastics injuries. *Am. J. Sports Med.,* 1980; 8:261–264.
55. **Garrick, G. J. and Webb, R. D.** *Sports Injuries: Diagnosis and Management.* Philadelphia: W. B. Saunders, 1990.
56. **Eriksson, E. and Denti, M.** Diagnostic and operative arthroscopy of the shoulder and elbow joint. *Ital. J. Sports Trauma,* 1985; 7:165–188.
57. **Nirschl, R. P.** Prevention and treatment of elbow and shoulder injuries in the tennis player. *Clin. Sports Med.,* 1988; 7:289–308.
58. **Wilson, F. D., Andrews, J. R., Blackburn, T. A., et al.** Valgus extension overload in the pitching elbow. *Am. J. Sports Med.,* 1983; 11:83–88.

Medial Tension/Lateral Compression Syndrome

59. **Andrews, J. R. and Carson, W. G.** Arthroscopy of the elbow. *Arthroscopy,* 1985; 1:97–107.
60. **Barnes, D. A. and Tullos, H. S.** An analysis of 100 symptomatic baseball players. *Am. J. Sports Med.,* 1978; 6:62–67.
61. **Clain, M. R. and Hershman, E. B.** Overuse injuries in children and adolescents. *Phys. Sportsmed.,* 1989; 17:111–123.
62. **Garrick, G. J. and Webb, R. D.** *Sports Injuries: Diagnosis and Management.* Philadelphia: W. B. Saunders 1990.
63. **Ireland, M. L. and Andrews, J. R.** Shoulder and elbow injuries in the young athletes. *Clin. Sports Med.,* 1988; 7:473–494.
64. **Yocum, L. A.** The diagnosis and nonoperative treatment of elbow problems in the athlete. *Clin. Sports Med.,* 1989; 8:439–451.
65. **Wilson, F. D., Andrews, J. R., Blackburn, T. A., et al.** Valgus extension overload in the pitching elbow. *Am. J. Sports Med.,* 1983; 11:83–88.

Forearm and Hand

Since the wrist and hand are well known for a large number of tendons and for their important role in work and sports, overuse injuries are most common in these regions; they are often characterized by tendinitis or tenosynovitis.[2,5,7,18,24] Principal symptoms are pain and tenderness in the affected tendon(s). Pain increases with passive extension of the tendon or with contraction of the appropriate muscle against resistance.[11] The most common overuse injury of the wrist joint is known as *de Quervain's disease* and is characterized by inflammation of the tendons passing through the fibroosseous tunnel of the first dorsal compartment of the wrist at the level of the radial styloid, i.e., m. abductor pollicis longus and m. extensor pollicis brevis. Flexor carpi ulnaris tendinitis is a relatively common overuse wrist injury in athletes, while flexor carpi radialis tendinitis occurs much more rarely. Rowers and weight lifters, to a greater degree than other athletes, often suffer from intersection syndrome, also known as *oarsman's wrist.* Dorsal radiocarpal impingement syndrome is common in gymnasts. In sports medicine, it is often referred to as *gymnast's wrist.* Trigger finger may also be included in overuse wrist syndromes. Long-term sports or working activity may cause the development of nerve entrapment syndromes — carpal tunnel and Guyon's tunnel in particular.

Actually, overuse injuries of the forearm and hand are big problems for people who work with computer keyboards (crippled by computers). The problem, more commonly known as *repetitive stress injuries* (RSI), now strike an estimated 185,000 U.S. office and factory workers a year. The cases account for more than half of U.S. occupational illnesses, compared with about 20% a decade ago.

I. DE QUERVAIN'S DISEASE

De Quervain's disease implies inflammation of the tendons of the abductor pollicis longus muscle and the extensor pollicis brevis muscle as they pass through the first dorsal compartment of the wrist, about 3 cm proximal to the radial styloid (Figure 1). Thickening of tendinous membranes leads to stricture of the lumen of the first carpal canal. Also, thickening of the tendons distally from the narrowed compartment may often be noticed. After passing through the first carpal compartment, the tendons bend under a certain angle, which is somewhat larger in females; this angulation is accentuated by wrist ulnar deviation.[1] Due to this fact, frequent repetitive ulnar abduction of the wrist causes irritation of tendons and their membranes. Naturally, irritation may be caused by altered osseous surface of the radial styloid as

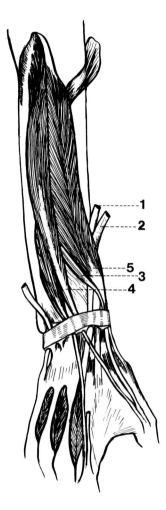

FIGURE 1. Muscles of the first three carpal tunnels. (1) extensor carpi radialis brevis muscle; (2) extensor carpi radialis longus muscle; (3) extensor pollicis brevis muscle; (4) extensor pollicis longus muscle; (5) abductor pollicis longus muscle.

well. In athletes, manual workers, or physical laborers, especially drummers[6] in whom the activity of the thumb is particularly emphasized, tenosynovitis of the first carpal compartment usually takes place. De Quervain's disease develops more often when engaging in racket sports (tennis, squash)[24], but is also seen in athletic throwing disciplines. The condition is more common in females (7 to 9 times) than in males; this is due to greater tendinous angulation and greater range of ulnar wrist abduction in females. In 1895, de Quervain reported about five women with stenosing tendovaginitis. However, in the 13th edition of *Gray's Anatomy* (1893), there is a description of identical changes in the first carpal compartment called *washerwoman's sprain.*[13]

Clinically, pain is dominant with this condition, especially in the area of the radial styloid. Patients also complain of pain upon ulnar deviation and closing of the hand. Pain may radiate to the proximal forearm or distally into the thumb. The pain becomes progressively worse so that the patient eventually ends up with the inability to use his hand. On physical examination, there is localized tenderness and often soft-tissue swelling at the radial styloid. There may be palpable thickening, ganglion cyst formation, and crepitus over the first dorsal compartment. Diagnosis is confirmed on the basis of a positive Finkelstein's test (Figure 2). In this maneuver, the patient's wrist is passive ulnar deviated while the thumb is held adducted in the palm. A positive test is indicated by pain in the region of the radial styloid. The test may also be positive in patients with basal thumb-joint (carpometacarpal, scaphoidotrapeziotrapezoidal, or radioscaphoid joints) arthrosis or intersection syndrome. To minimize false-positive tests, the ulnar deviation stress should be applied to the metacarpal of the index finger. Only rarely can X-ray examination reveal irregularity of osseous surface or thickening of the periosteum in the region of the first carpal compartment. Even if de Quervain's disease is also known as stenosing tendovaginitis, clinical finding of a trigger thumb is extremely rare in this condition.[21] Trigger thumb usually develops as the extensor pollicis brevis tendon passes in a separate fibrous compartment through the first carpal canal. Research has shown evidence of partial or complete septation of the dorsal compartment of the wrist in about 40% of people.[10,12] This fact is important, especially in view of operative treatment of de Quervain's disease.

In the beginning, the treatment is always nonoperative and entails avoidance of aggravating activity, reduction of overall activity, and administration of nonsteroid anti-inflammatory medication. Immobilization of forearm, wrist, and thumb (to the distal interphalangeal skin fold) in a splint (the so-called thumb spica splint) causes symptoms to disappear in more than 70% of patients.[23] Local administration of corticosteroids and anesthetics into the first carpal compartment is also part of nonoperative treatment. This brings dramatic relief, although unfortunately only

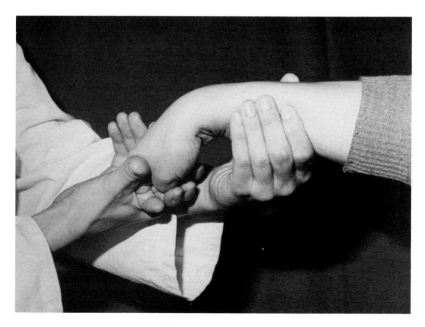

FIGURE 2. Finkelstein's test.

temporary, since it cannot prevent the disease from recurring. Generally, steroid injections should be limited to two or three over a 6-month period; usually, the second and third injection are less effective than the initial one. In an advanced stage of de Quervain's disease, characterized by marked stenosis and thickening of tendinous membranes, successful surgical treatment is the only recourse available.[9] Surgery consists of decompression and release of the first dorsal compartment and also obligatory removal of the altered segments of tendinous membranes. Either a transverse or longitudinal incision may be used. Care should be taken to avoid any undue traction on the radial sensory nerve. The compartment should be released on its dorsal aspect to prevent subluxation of the tendons volarly with the thumb motion. Failure in surgical treatment is usually ascribed to inability to identify the possible anatomic abnormality as the presence of separate fibroosseous canal for each tendon or the presence of multiple tendons of the abductor pollicis longus muscle.[15] During surgery, it happens quite often that only the abductor pollicis longus tendon is decompressed while the extensor pollicis brevis tendon remains intact in its separate compartment; this is the most common cause of repetitive complaints.

II. TENOSYNOVITIS OF OTHER DORSAL COMPARTMENTS

In addition to the first one, tenosynovitis may develop in all other dorsal compartments of the wrist (Figure 3), but most often, this occurs in the sixth one through which the extensor carpi ulnaris tendon passes, and then in the second compartment through which the extensor carpi radialis longus and brevis tendons pass. Tenosynovitis in the second carpal compartment should not be mistaken for oarsman's wrist (intersection syndrome). Tenosynovitis of the fourth and fifth carpal compartment is extremely rare, while tenosynovitis of the third carpal compartment, through which the extensor pollicis longus tendon passes, usually develops as a consequence of changes in the radius following malunion after fractures so that rupture of the extensor pollicis longus tendon often takes place.

As a rule, treatment is nonoperative. Only in the tenosynovitis of the sixth carpal compartment (extensor carpi ulnaris muscle) is surgery required due to thickening of the membranes or formation of calcifications. Sports injuries often cause lesions in the sixth carpal compartment, specifically in terms of the sixth compartment ulnar wall rupture; this usually leads to recurrent subluxation of the extensor carpi ulnaris tendon.[3,14,20] The rupture may occur upon sudden supination, ulnar deviation, and volar flexion. It has been reported in tennis players, golfers, and weight lifters. The patient usually complains of a clicking sensation with forearm rotation, and subluxation of the extensor carpi ulnaris can be visibly palpated and observed. On supination with wrist ulnar deviation, the tendon often displaces with an audible snap when moved in the ulnar and palmar directions. On pronation, it relocates into its normal sulcus. The condition must be differentiated from recurrent subluxation of the distal radioulnar joint. Recurrent subluxation of the extensor carpi ulnaris tendon is treated surgically since reconstruction of the sixth carpal compartment is necessary on the dorsal wrist aspect; it is usually performed by using the extensor retinaculum.

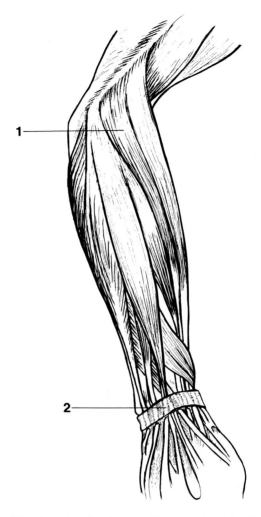

FIGURE 3. Radial and dorsal muscles of the forearm. (1) Lateral epicondyle; (2) extensor retinaculum.

III. INTERSECTION SYNDROME (OARSMAN'S WRIST)

This is an overuse syndrome known by various other terms: peritendinitis crepitans, abductor pollicis longus bursitis, intersection syndrome, squeaker's wrist, oarsman's wrist, and crossover tendinitis. The condition usually develops at the site where the tendons of the extensor pollicis brevis and abductor pollicis longus (muscles of the first dorsal compartment of the wrist) pass across the extensor carpi radialis longus muscle and the extensor carpi radialis brevis muscle (the muscles of the second dorsal compartment of the wrist) (Figures 1 and 3). The typical repetitive wrist motions (extension and radial deviation) cause inflammation of the bursa (according to some authors) normally found there; according to others, this develops as a result of a long-term friction. Athletes who suffer from this disorder more often than others are rowers, canoeists, weight lifters, tennis players, hockey players, and athletic throwers. Painful crepitation with wrist movement as well as weak pinch and diminished grasp are the major symptoms. On physical examination, palpatory tenderness and soft-tissue swelling over the radiodorsal aspect of the distal forearm about 6 to 8 cm proximal to the Lister's tubercle are found.[8] The crepitus, which in some instances may be more like a "squeak", is palpable and audible; this usually occurs during wrist motion and upon palpation of the painful site. Nonoperative treatment consists of avoidance of aggravating activity, immobilization in a splint, and nonsteroid anti-inflammatory medication.[22] Direct steroid injection may be indicated and usually is curative. However, operative exploration and excision of the bursa is rarely required. Surgery should be followed by prolonged protection from the aggravating stresses.

IV. FLEXOR CARPI ULNARIS TENDINITIS

In view of the importance of muscle in wrist motions, flexor carpi ulnaris tendinitis is a relatively frequent condition that affects athletes and others who engage in activities involving repetitive wrist motions. Tenderness and a painful tendon in the wrist joint increase with wrist flexion and ulnar deviation against resistance. The flexor carpi ulnaris tendon ends at the pisiform bone, while the pisohamate and pisometacarpal ligament attach the pisiform bone to the hamate and fifth metacarpal bone. It actually means that the flexor carpi ulnaris tendon ends at the hamate and metacarpal bone, while the pisiform bone, similar to the sesamoid bone, is an integral part of the tendon itself (Figure 4). A synovial sac (bursa) may be found between the tendon and pisiform bone; the pisiform bone also joins with the triquetrum bone. The pisiform bone may become the source of pain, also described as *enthesitis ossis pisiform* by those who consider the flexor carpi ulnaris muscle to be attached to the pisiform bone.[17] However, pain and tenderness in the pisiform bone region may be caused by irritation of the above-mentioned bursa in such a way that it envelops the pisiform bone so that bursitis may be the issue. Also, degenerative changes may take place between the pisiform bone and the triquetrum bone (osteoarthritis). During the wrist flexion, when the examiner moves the pisiform bone laterally, pain will occur. Paley et al.[19] inform about 216 case reports published in world medical literature and conclude that in 44.6% of cases, the patients suffered from enthesitis m. flexor carpi ulnaris or enthesitis of the pisiform bone, while in the remaining cases, the patients had primary or secondary osteoarthritis in the pisotriquetral joint.

Treatment of flexor carpi ulnaris tendinitis consists of avoidance of aggravating motions, i.e., in resting, immobilization of the wrist in a splint, administration of nonsteroid anti-inflammatory drugs, and physical therapy. In the case of pisiform bone enthesitis, bursitis, or arthrosis in the pisotriquestral joint that do not respond to nonoperative treatment procedures, surgery may be contemplated in terms of pisiform bone excision.[4] The pisiform bone is removed subperiosteally, preserving the continuity of the flexor carpi ulnaris tendon; during this procedure, lysis of peritendinous adhesions is also performed if they are present. At times, calcium

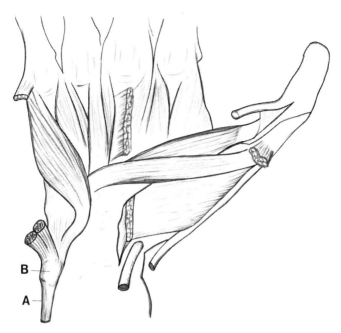

FIGURE 4. The relationship of the ulnar carpal flexor tendon muscle (A) to the pisiform bone (B).

deposits may be found either adhering to or within the tendon, and these should also be removed.

V. FLEXOR CARPI RADIALIS TENDINITIS

Flexor carpi radialis tendinitis occurs much more rarely than tendinitis of the ulnar aspect of the wrist joint; this is mostly because the motion of the wrist joint in its radial aspect is much more limited when compared to the ulnar side. In the case of flexor carpi radialis tendinitis, wrist flexion against resistance and passive extension will cause pain in the affected tendon. The flexor carpi radialis muscle (Figure 5) at about the mid-portion of the forearm continues into the tendon that passes over the carpal root in a separate compartment formed laterally and dorsally by the scaphoid and trapezoid bones, palmarly by the flexor retinaculum, and medially (ulnarly) by the carpi radiatum ligament; this is also a borderline case toward carpal tunnel. The tendon inserts into the palmar surface of the base of the second meta-carpal bone. When passing through its own osseofibrous canal, the tendon is surrounded by the synovial sheath (vagina synovialis). Accordingly, sometimes clinical symptoms of stenosing tenosynovitis of the flexor carpi radialis may develop. These symptoms may require surgical treatment in terms of canal decompression. In the majority of cases, tendinitis and tenosynovitis of the flexor carpi radialis are treated nonoperatively.

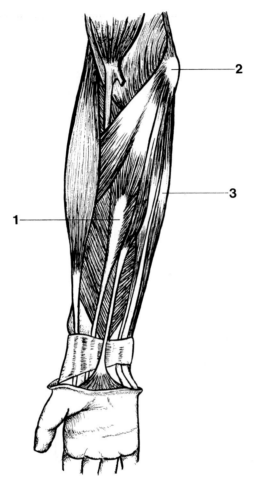

FIGURE 5. The ventral group of forearm muscles. (1) flexor carpi radialis muscle; (2) epicondylus ulnaris (medialis); flexor carpi ulnaris muscle.

VI. DORSAL RADIOCARPAL IMPINGEMENT SYNDROME (GYMNAST'S WRIST)

Repetitive wrist dorsiflexion, especially when performed with an extra load or force as in gymnastics during beam exercises, floor exercises (Figure 6), or jumping, may cause the formation of impingement syndrome in the dorsal aspect of the radiocarpal joint; this is often the reason for pain in the wrist joint in gymnasts.[7,18] Dorsal radiocarpal impingement syndrome is of twofold significance: (1) it causes discomfort and inability to perform exercises, and (2) in its differential diagnosis, it is of utmost importance not to overlook other possible causes of pain in the wrist joint, especially the possibility of fractures of the carpal bones. Pain in the dorsal aspect of the wrist root is the most characteristic sign of the disorder, and its onset is associated with an athletic or working activity. In cases when symptoms persist for

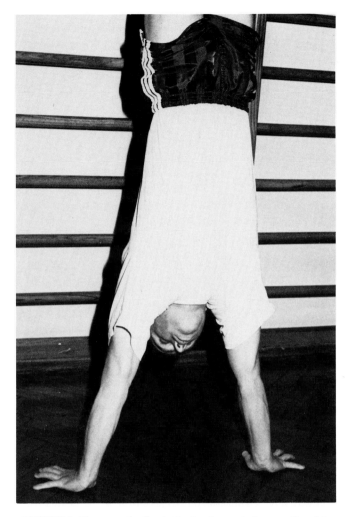

FIGURE 6. The reason leading to the development of gymnast's wrist.

a longer period of time, reduced and painful dorsal flexion of the wrist in regular everyday activities commonly results.

Clinical examination reveals pain and tenderness along the dorsal aspect of the radiocarpal joint, and pain may be elicited by a sudden dorsiflexion of the joint. Painful and limited dorsal flexion of the hand joint is a common finding. Radiology is helpful in differential diagnosis of the impingement syndrome, especially because of the possibility of carpal bone fractures, aseptic necrosis of carpal bones and their stress fractures, injuries of distal radial epiphysis, and subluxation of the lunate bone. Only in exceptional cases will radiogram of the wrist joint in lateral and neutral positions and also at full dorsal flexion show that osseous contact really exists between the radius and carpal bones, causing dorsiflexion block in the wrist joint. Bone scan helps to differentiate stress fracture. It is recommended as an obligatory

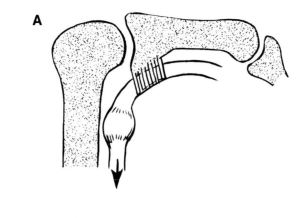

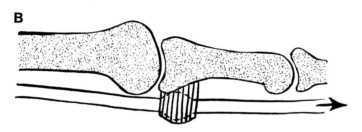

FIGURE 7. Trigger finger. (A) During finger flexion, the thickening of the tendon is situated proximally to the annular ligament. (B) During extension, the entrance is difficult due to the thickening; at certain point (snapping), it enters under the annular ligament.

diagnostic procedure if the symptoms still persist after 2 weeks of treatment for dorsal radiocarpal impingement syndrome. Rest, application of ice, and nonsteroid anti-inflammatory medication are essential for treatment. Relative rest means a limited wrist dorsiflexion that can be achieved by specially designed dorsal immobilization of the wrist using the so-called gym cuff or a special adhesive bandage for the joint.

Rehabilitation is aimed at strengthening the wrist flexor muscles in order to achieve dynamic limitation of the joint dorsiflexion. The extension exercises aimed at achieving a greater range of motion need not always yield the expected results. In the majority of cases, appropriate resting, symptomatic therapy, and physical therapy lead to cessation of the symptoms.

VII. TRIGGER FINGER

When active flexion or extension of the finger is either difficult or impossible, this condition is known as *trigger finger*. If the flexion or extension of the finger is actively performed with difficulty or if when performed passively, a clicking sound may be heard, the finger is behaving as if it were on a trigger, i.e., when the obstacle is conquered the finger snaps. Stenosing tendovaginitis of flexor tendons (most often of the middle finger, then the thumb, and the ring finger), is the pathoanatomic background. Thickening or widening of the flexor tendon has been found at its passing through the tendinous sheath compartment on the palmar aspect of the finger in the region of the metacarpophalangeal joint (Figure 7). However, sometimes the width of the tendon is normal but the compartment is narrow since the sheath is thickened. The lesion occurs more often in women and is common for the right hand. Some authors ascribe this condition to chronic traumatization, thus justifying its classification into overuse syndromes.[24]

Nonoperative treatment consisting of corticosteroid injections into the tendon sheath may be successful, although in a majority of cases, surgery is required.[16] During operation, a longitudinal discission of the tendon sheath is performed in the region of the metacarpophalangeal joint.

REFERENCES

1. **Arons, M. S.** De Quervain's release in working women: a report of failures, complications, and associated diagnosis. *J. Hand Surg.,* 1987; 12A:540–544.
2. **Batt, M. E.** A survey of golf injuries in amateur golfers. *Br. J. Sports Med.,* 1992; 26:63–65.
3. **Burkhart, S. S., Wood, M. B., and Linschied, R. L.** Posttraumatic recurrent subluxation of the extensor carpi ulnaris tendon. *J. Hand Surg.,* 1982; 7:1–3.
4. **Carrol, R. E. and Coyle, M. P.,** Dysfunction of the pisotriquetral joint: treatment by excision of the pisiform. *J. Hand Surg.,* 1985; 10A:703–707.
5. **Dobyns, J. H.** Short-shrift problems: a grab bag of athletic injuries. In: *AAOS Symposium on Upper Extremity Injuries in Athletes.* Pettrone, F. A., Ed. St. Louis: C. V. Mosby, 1986; 170–173.
6. **Fry, N. J. H.** Overuse syndrome in musicians: prevention and management. *Lancet,* 1986; 1:728–731.
7. **Garrick, J. G. and Webb, D. R.** *Sports Injuries: Diagnosis and Management.* Philadelphia: W. B. Saunders, 1990.
8. **Grundberg, A. B. and Reagan, D. S.** Pathologic anatomy of the forearm: intersection syndrome, *J. Hand Surg.,* 1985; 10A:299–302.
9. **Harvey, F. J., Harvey, P. M., and Horsley, M. W.** De Quervain's disease: surgical or nonsurgical treatment. *J. Hand Surg.,* 1990; 15A:83–87.
10. **Jackson, W. T., Viegas, S. F., Coon, T. M., Stimpson, K. D., Frogameni, A. D., and Simpson, J. M.** Anatomical variations in the first extensor compartment of the wrist. *J. Bone Joint Surg.,* 1986; 68A:923–926.
11. **Kulund, D. N.** *The Injured Athlete.* 2nd ed. Philadelphia: J. B. Lippincott, 1988.
12. **Lacey, T., Goldstein, L. A., and Tobin, C. E.** Anatomical and clinical study of the variations in the insertions of the abductor pollicis longus tendon, associated with stenosing tendovaginitis. *J. Bone Joint Surg.,* 1951; 33A:347–350.
13. **Loomis, L. K.** Variations of stenosing tenosynovitis at the radial styloid process. *J. Bone Joint Surg.,* 1951; 33A:340–346.

14. **Loty, B., Memier, B., and Mazas, F.** Luxation traumatique isolée du tendon cubital posterieur. *Rev. Chir. Orthop.,* 1986; 72:219–222.

15. **Louis, D. S.** Incomplete release of the first dorsal compartment — a diagnostic test. *J. Hand Surg.,* 1987; 12A:87–88.

16. **Lyu, S. R.** Closed division of the flexor tendon sheath for trigger finger. *J. Bone Joint Surg.,* 1992; 74(B):418–420.

17. **Mikić, Ž, Somer, T., Tubić, M., and Ercegan, G.** Entezitis piriformne kosti. *Med. Pregl.,* 1985; 523–525.

18. **Osterman, L. A., Moskow, L., and Low, D. W.** Soft-tissue injuries of the hand and wrist in racquet sports. *Clin. Sports Med.,* 1988; 7:329–348.

19. **Paley, D., McMurtry, R. Y., and Cruickshank, B.** Pathologic condition of the pisiform and pisotriquetral joint. *J. Hand Surg.,* 1987; 12A:110–119.

20. **Rowland, S. A.** Acute traumatic subluxation of the extensor carpi ulnaris tendon at the wrist. *J. Hand Surg.,* 1986; 11A:809–811.

21. **Viegas, S. F.** Trigger thumb of de Quervain's disease. *J. Hand Surg.,* 1986; 11A:235–237.

22. **Williams, J. G.** Surgical management of traumatic non-infective tenosynovitis of the wrist extensors. *J. Bone Joint Surg.,* 1977; 59B:408–410.

23. **Witt, J., Pess, G., and Gelberman, R. H.** Treatment of de Quervain tenosynovitis. A prospective study of the results of injection of steroids and immobilization in a splint. *J. Bone Joint Surg.,* 1991; 73(A):219–222.

24. **Wood, M. B. and Dobyns, J. H.** Sports-related extraarticular wrist syndromes. *Clin. Orthop.,* 1986; 202:93–102.

The Spine

Chapter 5

Low Back Pain

I. LOW BACK PAIN IN ATHLETES

In the context of this book, among the numerous factors that cause low back pain, emphasis should be placed on chronic overuse of the lumbosacral area, which manifests itself in some occupations and in professional and nonprofessional athletes. For this reason, we are including cases of low back pain resulting from excessive chronic overuse of the lumbosacral area whose clinical picture corresponds to that of overuse syndromes. This includes some forms of spondylolysis and spondylolysthesis, low back pain in gymnasts, low back pain in some cases of scoliosis and kyphosis, and myofibrositis. Low back pain is the ailment of the century in modern, technological, highly advanced societies. Viewed from a statistical point of view, every adult suffers from low back pain at least 3 times in his life. This, of course, also implies that out of three adults, one will suffer 9 times in his lifetime. According to some statistics, between 50 to 80% of the population in developed industrial countries suffer, or have suffered, from low back pain.[19] The diagram of strain placed upon the lumbal vertebrae in various positions of the body clearly indicates that the frequency of low back pain in modern societies results in part from the way of life and work habits practiced in these societies[28,38] (Figure 1). Loss resulting from absence from work and cost of treatment for low back pain is enormous. To illustrate this, we will cite two examples. The first comes from the U.S. where in one calendar year, loss resulting from low back pain treatment and absence from work was approximated at $14 billion. This is the reason why innovative approaches to prevent and treat low back pain in workers are mandatory. The sports medicine approach for aggressive rehabilitation offers a possible solution.[18] The other example comes from the U.K. where in 1 year, the number of working days lost because of low back pain exceeded 13 million. This clearly indicates that low back pain is also a socioeconomic problem.[14,29]

Low back pain is a term used to describe subjective feelings of pain and tenderness felt in the lumbar or, generally speaking, lower spine. As the term implies, the essence of this syndrome lies in the subjective feeling of pain which can be of different intensity suffered by patients in a very individual manner. A variety of terms are used to describe this painful condition. *Lumbago* is an old expression used to describe acute pain in the lumbar spine area. Nowdays the term *painful lumbar syndrome* is preferred and generally used to describe the same condition. The painful

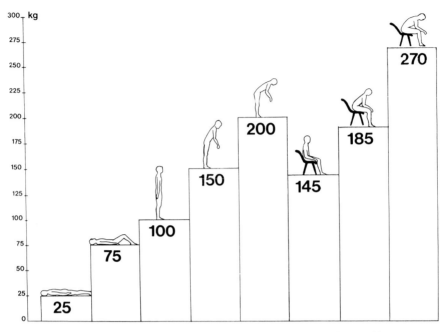

FIGURE 1. Diagram of the strain placed on the lumbar spine in various positions.

lumbar syndrome can be of vertebral origin, meaning the pain manifests itself exclusively in the area in which it originates — in other words, in the lumbar spine area. If painful symptoms manifest themselves in regions far away from the spine, e.g., in the lower extremities, the term *vertebrogenic painful lumbar syndrome* is applied (e.g., lumboischialgia).

When dealing with this condition, one should always have in mind that low back pain is just a syndrome i.e., a number of different symptoms and not a disease in the specific meaning of the word. The pain that is subjectively felt by patients is simply a manifestation of some pathological substrate.[30,31] Very few painful conditions have such a wide variety of possible causative factors as low back pain. The sophisticated methods of modern diagnostics coupled with an increasing amount of knowledge regarding the biomechanics of the spine have enabled researchers to delineate a large, and steadily increasing number of possible causative factors for low back pain.[8] We have composed a table (Table 1) of possible causative factors of low back pain based on our own experience and that of other researchers as reported in the medical literature. Even a cursory examination of Table 1 will reveal that the cause of low back pain is extremely hard to detect; this explains why some patients change a number of physicians before the correct diagnosis is ultimately reached. In everyday clinical practice, the most commonly encountered syndrome is the painful vertebral lumbar syndrome caused by degenerative changes in the lumbar disk and small joints area. From a clinical point of view, back pain can manifest itself in either the acute or chronic stage with the particulars of the clinical picture depending principally on the pathological substrate that led to the development of the syndrome.[6] Treatment, in most cases, (95 to 98%) is nonoperative. It inevitably begins with nonoperative

TABLE 1
Low Back Pain

Congenital and developmental anomalies
    Facet's tropismus
    Transitional vertebra
        Sacralization of the lumbar vertebra
        Lumbalization of the sacral vertebra
    Spina bifida
    Congenital scoliosis and kyphosis
    Scheuermann's disease
    Spondylolysis and spondylolysthesis
Inflammations
    Rheumatic (arthritis rheumatoides, spondylitis ankylosans —
        Bechterew's disease)
    Infections
        Acute (osteomyelitis — spondylitis pyogenes)
        Chronic (osteomyelitis chronica, spondylitis tuberculosa,
        spondylitis mykosa)
Trauma
    Overstrains in lumbar spine
        Acute (injuries)
        Chronic (damages)
    Subluxation of small joints (facet syndrome)
    Infractions and fractures (vertebral body and processuses)
    Subluxations of sacroiliac joints
    Spondylosis and spondylolysthesis
    Posttraumatic kyphosis
Degenerative changes
    Osteochondrosis and spondylosis
    Spondylarthrosis
    Discopathia
    Nerve root entrapment syndrome
    Interspinous arthrosis
    Sacroiliac arthrosis
Tumors
Metabolic disorders
    Osteoporosis
    Osteomalatia
    Paget's disease
    Kummel's disease
Mechanical
    Postural low back pain
    Decrease or increase of lumbar lordosis
    Instability of the spine
    Scoliosis (more than 30°)
    Retropositio of lumbar vertebra
    Muscular changes (myofibrositis, myogelosis, hypertonus)
    Static disorders of the feet
    Abnormal biomechanic of the hip joints (subluxation,
        luxation, contracture)
    Inegality of the legs
    Abnormal biomechanic of the sacroiliac joints
    Venter pnedulus

TABLE 1 (continued)
Low Back Pain

Vascular diseases
Irradiation of the pain from visceral organs
    Gynecological diseases (inflammations, dismenorhoe,
      descensus, prolapse or retroflexion of the uterus)
    Diseases of the gastroentherological system
    Diseases of the urogenital system
    Abscessus subphrenicus
    Diseases of the splenium
Psychogenic

treatment except in cases where an evident pathological substrate that demands surgical treatment is the cause. Examples of the latter include tumors, unstable fractures of the spine, and other similar causes. As part of the nonoperative treatment of painful lumbar syndrome and as an important factor in preventing its development, special emphasis is placed on lifestyle and working habits. For this reason, special "schools" for people suffering from low back pain have been opened to teach people how to live and cope with their disease. While physical therapy, chiefly hydrogymnastics and kinesitherapy, has an outstanding role in nonoperative treatment of low back pain, the physician should always keep in mind that some exercises, especially dynamic exercises, increase the strain on the lumbal vertebrae[38] (Figure 2). Electrophysiological, kinesiological, and biomechanical research have increased our knowledge of kinesitherapy of painful lumbar syndrome. In kinesitherapy, programs with a conspicuous role are reserved for isometric exercises and stretching exercises such as for the hamstrings. The latter are performed with the purpose of affecting lumbar lordosis.[26] Kinesitherapy programs should be individualized with special consideration given to age, sex, bone, ligament, and muscle status of the lumbar spine.[42] The exercises should gradually increase and at all times be adapted to the stage of the disease and to the muscle strength and fitness of the patient.

Low back pain in both professional and nonprofessional athletes corresponds to the general clinical picture of this syndrome and has the same possible causative factors.[5] However, low back pain is unique in professional and nonprofessional athletes in that a clear difference must be made between cases in which a normal and healthy spine is subjected to excessive strain caused by athletic activities resulting in low back pain, and between cases in which endogenous factors such as sacralization or lumbalization of the lower spine causes low back pain in athletes who take part in normal, nonexcessive athletic activities. The worst possible combination is when an athlete suffering from abnormal low back architecture (abnormal endogenous factors) takes part in excessive and high-risk athletic activities (abnormal exogenous factors). Table 2 shows the possible combinations between the condition of the spine and the strain placed on the spine during various athletic activities. Different views are proposed in the current medical literature regarding the risk potential of various sports for developing low back pain and the specific high-risk movements that place excessive strain on the spine.[40] Kujala et al.[25] suggest that high training duration predisposes young athletes to low back pain. The most frequently mentioned high-risk sports for developing low back pain are shown in Table 3. To be successful in

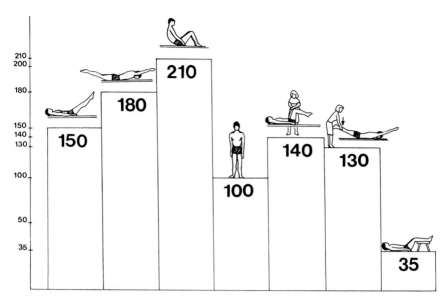

FIGURE 2. Diagram of the strain placed on the lumbar spine during some dynamic exercises.

TABLE 2
Low Back Pain in Athletes

Spine	Strain
Normal	Abnormal (excessive)
Abnormal	Normal
Abnormal	Abnormal (excessive)

TABLE 3
High-Risk Sports for Developing Low Back Pain

	Strain of the spine	
Vertical	**Flexion/extension**	**Rotation**
Horseback riding	Football	Tennis and racquet sports
Gymnastics	Soccer	Golf
Sky diving	Gymnastics	Aerobics
Water skiing	Diving	
Jogging on hard surfaces	Hockey	
	Field hockey	

treating athletes suffering from low back discomfort, the sports medicine specialist must be aware of the psychological impact of low back pain on athletes. Commonly, the injured patient (athlete) wishes to return to activity immediately, with very little respect or knowledge of the biology of healing. In the face of low back pain, the realities of human fragility become obvious, perhaps for the first time. This particular type of injured athlete requires a constant amount of counseling from the sports medicine consultant. The patient must also be made aware of the fact that in some cases, the healing process can be quite long while in other cases complete healing is unobtainable. The patient should be counseled to try to adapt his lifestyle and athletic activities to the limitations imposed on him by the condition of his spine. According to Harvey and Tanner,[12] lumbar spine pain accounts for 5 to 8% of athletic injuries. Although back pain is not the most common injury, it is one of the most challenging for the sports physician to diagnose and treat. A thorough history and physical examination are usually more productive in determining a diagnosis and guiding treatment than imaging techniques. Of the many possible causes of low back pain, we will mention only those that are thought to be or to result from chronic injuries, i.e., from overuse. We will begin with congenital or developmental anomalies, which at first glance, may appear to be contradictory to the above mentioned. However, we would like to reiterate at this point that congenitally abnormal spines (an abnormal endogenous factor) can be damaged by repeated microtraumas and thus result in the classical clinical picture of overuse syndrome.

II. SPONDYLOLYSIS AND SPONDYLOLYSTHESIS

Spondylolysis is a condition that is present in approximately 6% of individuals, but it has been reported in up to 50% of athletes with back pain.[41] This condition is essentially a break in bone continuity resulting from a defect in the junction between the superior and inferior processus articularis; it is most often encountered in the fifth and fourth lumbar vertebra. This junction is known as the *pars interarticularis* or *isthmus* (Figure 3). The defect in the bone is usually fibrocartilaginous in nature. Most authors agree that spondylolysis can be caused by other than congenital factors. Spondylolysis can be caused by trauma and can also result as a consequence of overuse syndrome — from stress fractures. This is especially frequent in female gymnasts. Spondylolysthesis is a condition in which the defect in the vertebral arch causes the slipping of the vertebra in the forward projection. Spondylolysis is, in most cases, asymptomatic and can be detected only by roentgenographic examination. Special slanted oblique projections of the spine are taken, which, in positive cases, show the figure of the "Scottish terrier" with an abnormally extended neck, indicating a defect in the isthmus of the vertebral arch (Figure 4). Some authors believe that spondylolysis can, by itself and without the presence of spondylolysthesis, cause low back pain. Treatment is most often nonoperative. Surgical fixation and bone trans-plantation of the vertebral arch is very rarely indicated.

Spondylolysthesis is a term used to define the slippage of the body of the vertebra above a caudally located vertebra (Figure 5). The slipping, in most cases, is directed in the forward direction, but it can also be directed in the backward projection. The three principal causes of spondylolysthesis are (1) congenital lack of the processus articularis (which is very rare), (2) spondylolysis, and (3) degenerative changes (arthrosis) on the facet joints. Spondylolysthesis caused by degenerative changes on the facet joints (Figure 6) is also called *pseudospondylolysthesis* (false spondylolysthesis) because the slipping of the vertebral body is relatively very slight.[7,15,36] The slipping can appear between any two vertebra, although, in most cases, it is limited to the area between the fourth and fifth lumbar vertebra. Slippage in the backward direction (retrolysthesis) is frequent and is called *retropositio*.[15]

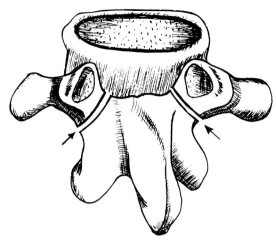

FIGURE 3. Localization of the spondylolitic defect in the vertebral arch (arrows).

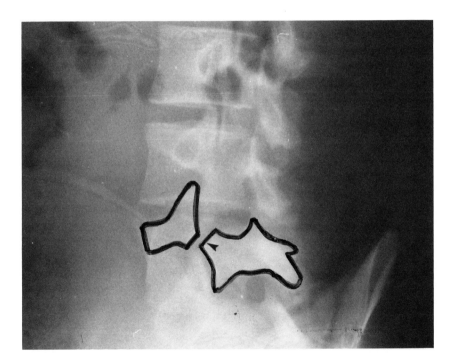

FIGURE 4. Figure of a Scottish terrier.

Neurological side effects are rare in pseudospondylolysthesis. Spondylolysthesis caused by spondylolysis is characterized by the fact that the vertebral body, together with the pedicles (the origins of the vertebral arch from the vertebral body), slip forward together with the processus articularis superiores, which has the effect of displacing the entire spine above that vertebra in the forward direction (Figure 5).

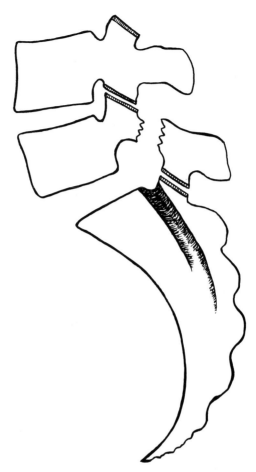

FIGURE 5. Spondylolysthesis of the five lumbar vertebra due to spondylolysis in the arch of the same vertebra.

The lamine and the processus articularis inferiores remain behind in their normal anatomical position. Four grades of spondylolysthesis are recognized by Meyerding, depending on the amount (length) of the forward slipping of the vertebral body. Grade 1 is defined by a 0 to 25% of the posteroanterior vertebral body length of the caudally located vertebra slipping in the forward direction. Grade 2 is defined by 25 to 50%, Grade 3 by 50 to 75%, and Grade 4 by 75% and more vertebral body length forward slippage. In cases when the fifth lumbar vertebra slips over the edge of the sacrum into the pelvis, the term *spondyloptosis* is applied.

The clinical picture of spondylolysthesis caused by an inherited lack of the processus articularis in children and adolescents is characterized by neurological side effects. In pseudospondylolysthesis, the symptoms usually manifest themselves in mature and older patients and are characterized by a painful lower back of vertebral origin. Spondylolysthesis caused by spondylolysis can be both symptomatic and asymptomatic. The symptomatology in this case depends on the amount of vertebral body slippage. The most frequently encountered symptom is low back pain, but in

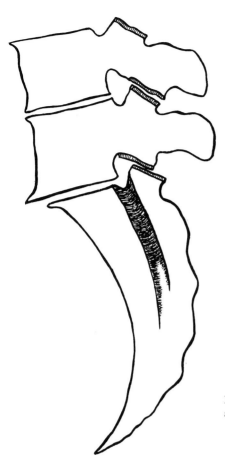

FIGURE 6. Pseudospondylolysthesis due to arthrosis of the small vertebral joints.

some cases, the root of the nerve can also be affected causing lumboischialgia. In clinical diagnostics, the "sign of the step" is characteristic. This sign is best seen by tracing the spinous processus with the tip of the finger in the cranial to caudal direction. At one point (the point of the forward slipping of the affected vertebral body), the finger will encounter a displacement in the form of a step (Figure 5). Depending on the degree of forward slipping, other clinical symptoms can also be seen: the trunk of the patient becomes shorter while the rib arches tend to move closer to the cristae illiacae; in a standing position, the hands reach more distally towards the knees; lumbar lordosis is more pronounced; and the hips are in a flexed position. If painful symptoms are present, they usually appear and/or intensify in a standing or sitting position.

Treatment depends on the gravity of the symptoms, age of the patient, and progression of the spondylolysthesis (if the slipping of the vertebral body continues). In most cases, treatment is conservative and consists of physical therapy, wearing of braces, and adapting the patient's lifestyle and working habits to the limitations placed upon him by the condition of his spine. Conservative treatment should always be attempted before surgery, which is indicated when neurological side effects are apparent or when the patient suffers intense pain. Surgical treatment consists of fusion (spondylodesis) of the affected spinal segments with concomitant bone trans-plantation.

III. MYOFIBROSITIS

Among the mechanical causes of low back pain (caused primarily by continuous exposure to mechanical strain), an important place is reserved for changes in the paravertebral musculature in the form of hypertonus and the appearance of small knots. These changes are known under the general term *fibrositis,*[14] while some authors refer to them as *miogeloses* [as if the muscle has changed from a solid state into a gel state (raw egg vs. hard-boiled egg)]. Histological analysis, however, has failed to prove the presence of fibrositis knots in the muscle. The clinical picture is characterized by the presence of pain in the paravertebral lumbar muscles. This pain is often correlated to the weather, especially changes in weather (a climatic factor). Other, less precisely localized "rheumatic" pains can also be present in other parts of the body.

Physical examination reveals localized tenderness of the affected muscle to palpation. All other clinical or radiological indicators are absent. Movements of the spine are unhindered and a true spasm of the muscles is lacking.

Treatment is empirical and consists of physiotherapy accompanied by massage and exercises, especially stretching exercises.

IV. LOW BACK PAIN IN GYMNASTS

Low back pain, especially in female gymnasts, is a specific sports injury. Most authors today agree that the aggressive factors in gymnastics are the excessive movements in which increased retroflexion is of outstanding importance.[10,11] The excessive flexibility of the spine results from the generalized excessive mobility of the complete locomotor system which is a prerequisite for serious gymnastic training and also the result of the afore-said training. The excessive mobility of, primarily, the lumbar spine is a consequence of the "stretching" of the stabilizing system of the spine. The static and dynamic strain placed on the excessively mobile spine, particu-larly the lumbar area, leads to excessive lumbar curvature, hyperlordosis.[43] At first, this hyperlordosis is limited to relatively infrequent episodes, principally during gymnastic routines, but as time goes on, hyperlordosis becomes habitual (Figure 7). Hyperlordosis represents a biomechanical imbalance in which the center of strain is shifted toward the posterior structures of the vertebrae.[20] The harm of this newly developed situation is best understood when one realizes that the defensive mecha-nism of the lumbar spine to this excessive strain is flexion, shifting the center of the strain to the anterior, more massive structures of the vertebrae. Excessive strain also activates the adaptive mechanism of bone tissue — hypertrophy. The first phase of bone hypertrophy is an increase in osteoclastic activity which prepares the affected area for new hypertrophic bone. During the osteoclastic phase, the bone is exception-ally vulnerable so that intensive training and hyperlordosis are one of the prime biomechanical factors in the development of this ailment. The intensity of training, length, and duration of training and the class of competition are also in direct

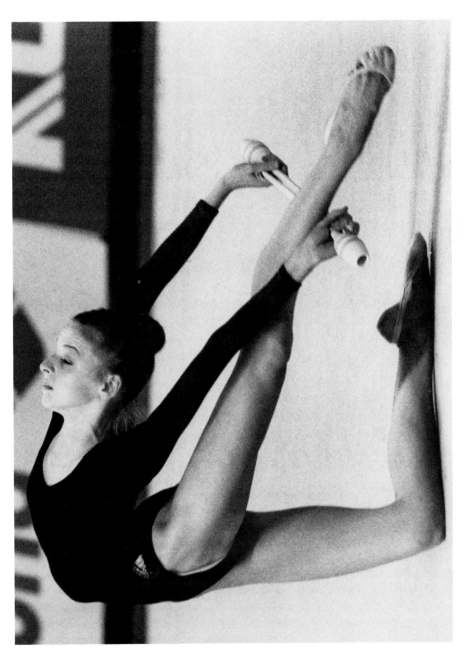

FIGURE 7. (A-C) Characteristic attitudes and hyperlordosis in gymnasts.

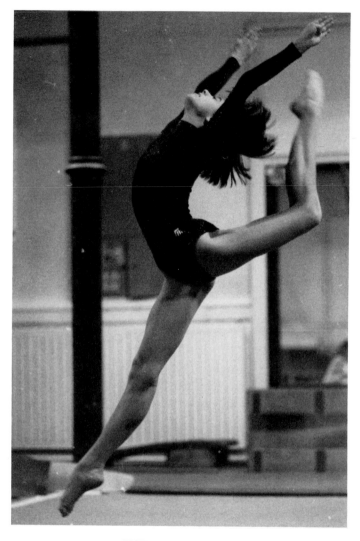

FIGURE 7 (continued).

correlation to the development of this syndrome. The female gymnasts who typically seek counsel from physicians are, in most cases, athletes who have been training for a number of years, who train more than 18 h/week, and who belong to the highest class of competition. The most commonly reported symptom is paravertebral pain, usually unilaterally, in the area of the thoracolumbar junction and the lumbar spine. The dominating symptom is pain. Quite frequently, this is the only symptom present, in spite of extensive diagnostic procedures, and the only sign the physician has that some disorder is present. The principal characteristic of the pain is that it is induced by sporting activities and is progressive. In the beginning phase of the ailment, the pain appears when the gymnast begins her routine, and eases as soon as she stops training. In later stages, the pain persists for a short time after training is finished,

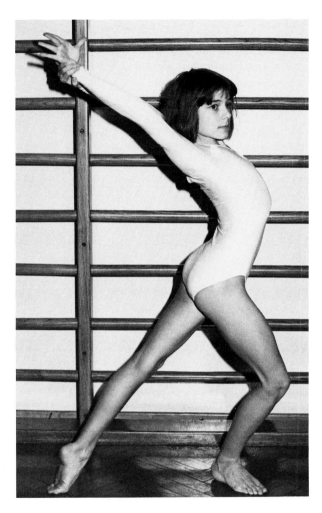

FIGURE 7 (continued).

while the terminal phase is characterized by pain which persists during the whole day. Pain is the only unique and lasting symptom of this disorder. Other symptoms and signs vary, depending on the pathohistological base of the disorder: spondylolysis, protrusion or prolapse of the intervertebral disk, fracture of the vertebra, or spondylogenic pain.[10] Spondylolysis is the most frequent disorder that causes low back pain in female gymnasts.[10,11] The pathological changes are pain in female gymnasts.[10,11] They are usually located on the fourth and fifth lumbar vertebrae. Spondylolysis caused by excessive athletic activity is almost always stable, and very rarely (almost never) progresses into spondylolysthesis of the first degree. This possible development should, however, always be kept in mind during physical examination and diagnostic procedures, especially when the consulted sports medicine specialist encounters a varied and rich symptomatology. The reason for this is that spondylolysis has, with the exception of pain, practically no other symptoms.

Neurological disorders appear only in the terminal phases of spondylolysthesis. In most cases, low back pain induced by gymnastic activity, especially in those activities in which retroflexion is dominant (exercises on the floor, exercises on the beam, landings after jumping over the vault), is the only symptom of spondylolysis. Back muscles, in principle, show no signs of muscle spasm. The mobility of the spine is in order, and the gymnast will typically touch the floor with both her palms while in a standing position with no problem. Because of the generally decreased mobility of people with spine disorders, this exercise will seem to show that every thing is in order. However, the physician should be careful, and try to find out whether this is a case of "relative loss" of mobility. The physician should anamnestically try to find out if there is a subjective feeling of loss of mobility, and then ask the patient to perform a flexion test from the hip from a horizontal position. The gymnast will typically flex her extended foot in the hip for 90°, which is a normal finding in untrained and "not loosened up" patients. Normal flexion for a highly trained, hypermobile female gymnast consists of a 120 to 130° flexion, which represents a relative loss of mobility of 30 to 40° (Figure 8). This relative loss of mobility is caused by the excessive tightness of the knee tendons (hamstrings). The hyperextension test can be used to provoke pain. The test is carried out by having the patient stand on one foot and perform hyperextension (maximal possible retroflexion). The appearance of pain on the ipsilateral side is a strong indicator of spondylolysis.

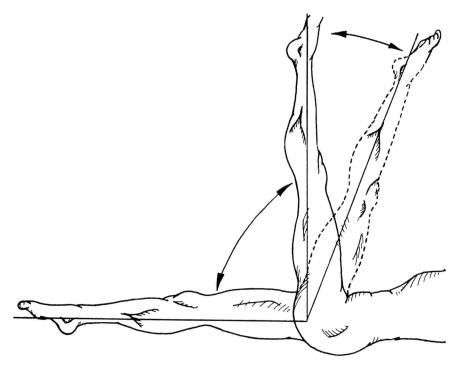

FIGURE 8. Test of hip flexion performed from a lying position. The hip flexion may reach 120 to 130° in trained female gymnast. Untrained individuals and gymnast with decreased mobility achieve hip flexion of only 90°.

Besides this indicator, retroflexion is by itself almost always painful, a fact which is used to provoke pain during extension against pressure from a flexed position. The appearance of pain is a strong indicator of spondylolysis.

A complete radiological examination is exceptionally important and should in fact be a routine examination in gymnasts with low back pain. A complete radiological examination consists of one anteroposterior, one lateral, and two oblique pictures of the spine. The anteroposterior picture registers the so-called "upside down Napoleon hat" phenomenon, a radiographic indicator of well-developed spondylolysthesis of the fifth lumbar vertebra. The effect is caused by the projection of the slipped body of the fifth lumbar vertebra. The lateral radiogram is used to evaluate the stability of the spondylolysis — in other words, to find out if slipping of the vertebral body has occurred.[3]

Radiographic pictures taken from an oblique projection are crucially important as this is the only projection in which the pars interarticularis is clearly visible. The pars interarticularis, as we have already mentioned, is the area in which spondylolysis typically develops (Figure 9). A negative radiological result with persisting low back pain indicates the need for scintigraphic examination (Figure 10). An increased amount of the radioactive isotope coupled with positive anamnestic and clinical findings is a strong indication for a possible diagnosis of spondylolysis. Research has shown that a suspect scintigraphic finding, in a couple of months, turns into radiographically visible spondylolysis. A positive scintigraphic finding, without concomitant anamnestic or clinical confirmation, is not a good enough criterion for positive

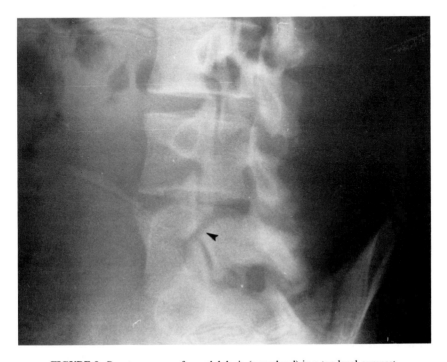

FIGURE 9. Roentgenogram of spondylolysis (arrowhead) in a top-level gymnast.

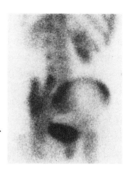

FIGURE 10. Bone scan demonstrating spondylolysis.

diagnosis of spondylolysis or for prescribing therapy. On the other hand, however, negative radiological and scintigraphic findings do not rule out the possibility of spondylolysis as some cases have shown a marked increase in the severity of existing symptoms and the appearance of new, previously not present symptoms. For this reason, pain, as the most persistent and most unique symptom, must be regarded as the fundamental criterion and best orientation for prescribing and evaluating the success of therapy.

Therapy for this overuse syndrome, as for other overuse syndromes, consists of rest for the over-strained tissue. The way in which this is to be accomplished when low back pain is caused by spondylolysis is presently controversial. One group of authors believes that spondylolysis, from the very beginning, should be treated as a fracture, and hence immobilized. To this effect, plastic braces are prescribed with a position of 0° lumbar lordosis. This treatment is prescribed with the aim of lessening the strain on the posterior structures of the vertebra. The brace is worn 23 h/d while the remaining hour is, apart from satisfying the physiological needs of the patient, used for physical therapy: strengthening exercises for the abdominal and pelvic muscles, stretching exercises for the lower extremities, and exercises for correcting lumbar hyperlordosis. The brace is worn for a period of 6 months, or until the initially positive scintigraphic finding turns negative. Mention must be made that an initial negative, "cold" scintigraphic finding, which indicates a decreased reparatory potential of the bone tissue, should not be taken as an absolute counterindication for prescribing the plastic brace. In a number of cases, such a "cold" scintigraphic finding resulted, after application of the plastic brace, into a well-healed case of spondylolysis. Three to four weeks after the initial application of the brace, most patients become asymptomatic. In this period during the hours when the patient is not wearing the brace, (these can be increased to 2 to 3 h) light gymnastic activity is allowed with the exception of exercises performed on the beam and landing practice. The appearance of any symptoms is an absolute counterindication for any activity.

Under the influence of therapy, about one third of the positive scintigraphic findings become negative; this indicates complete bone healing. In such cases, complete sports activities, under full strain, are allowed. Such a result has a favorable long-term prognosis. However, in about 90% of the cases in which complete bone healing is not accomplished within 6 months, pain and any other present symptoms also disappear. This is also considered to be an adequate indicator for complete return to full sports activities. The reasoning behind this is that the stability of spondylolysis, despite induced strain, very rarely turns into spondylolysthesis. Cases in which complete bone healing is not obtained have a less favorable prognosis and a higher risk of reapparition of the symptoms. In this case, the same therapy should be repeated. Quite understandably, some athletes will lack the necessary patience and willpower to go through therapy again. In all probability, they will continue with their gymnastic activities despite the discomfort; as a consequence, the ailment will progress. It will cease to be associated with only athletic activities and will become a permanent fixture in everyday life. In such situations, on rare occasions, spondylolysthesis can develop. As conservative therapy, in this case, is usually not adequate, surgical treatment is indicated. After such treatment, a return to the sports scene is usually possible after 1 year.

Contrary to the before-mentioned group of authors who believe that a brace should be applied immediately, there exists a second group of authors with a different opinion based on the knowledge of the stability of spondylolysthesis. This group believes that there is no need for the application of a brace before physical therapy and rest are utilized. A brace, according to this group of authors, should be applied only if this form of therapy produces no results.

Compression syndrome, or protrusion or prolapse of the intervertebral disk (Figure 11) is a less frequent cause of low back pain in gymnasts. In younger athletes, protrusion or prolapse of the intervertebral disk is not preceded by degenerative changes.[23] The main cause is excessive athletic activity. The clinical picture differs with regard to the one seen in older patients. In most cases, pain is not the dominant symptom. In fact, it is minimal. In the majority of cases, the gymnast, or her trainer, notice a loss of flexibility in the knee tendons (hamstrings), or the beginning of an antalgic position of the spine. Clinical examination reveals a positive Lasegue, irradiation in the area of the sciatic nerve, decreased mobility of the spine in flexion, and when straightening up from a flexed into an upright stance. These maneuvers, as well as flexion in the hip with an extended knee, will typically provoke pain. Neurological side effects as well as clearly seen muscle weakness are extremely rare but possible symptoms.[16] Clinical examination includes a complete radiological examination, computerized tomography, electromyoneurography, myelography, and MRI.

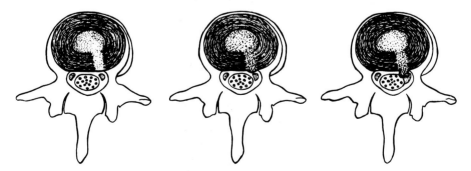

FIGURE 11. The stage of prolapse of the annulus fibrosis and protrusion of the nucleus pulposus in the area of spinal nerve root.

A proven compression syndrome demands treatment according to already established principles. The therapy is based on relieving the affected area by lying in a neutral position. Analgesics, usually aspirin, can also be prescribed as well as cryotherapy and transcutaneous electrostimulation. In younger individuals, a positive response to this treatment is usually seen after about 2 weeks, but this does not by any means indicate that a return to full athletic activities is allowed. Moreover, a general recommendation is that active exercising should cease for a period of 6 to 12 months after a confirmed diagnosis of compression syndrome. During this interval, the patient is advised to wear a somewhat more flexible brace, constructed with 15° lumbar lordosis; this allows the patient to remain mobile, active, and able to attend school. If after 3 weeks of applied conservative therapy, there is no improvement, or if before that time limit, progressive neurological side effects have manifested themselves (such as urinary or anal incontinency), decompression is strongly indicated. The decompression can be carried out either surgically or by injecting chymopapain into the intervertebral disk. Posterolateral fusion of the affected interarticular joints is also recommended in the following cases: if there are radiological indications of the degeneration of the intervertebral disk; if there are radiological or scintigraphic indications of spondylolysis; and if there is anamnestic information of chronic pain in the lumbal spine before the rupture of the disk.

Successful therapy, and by this we imply a full return to sports activities under full strain, is achieved somewhat less frequently than in cases of spondylolysis or fracture. Restitution allowing a complete return to athletic activities is attained in about 50% of the cases.

Spondylogenic pain is the probable diagnosis reached *per exclusionem* after a detailed physical examination has ruled out the possibility of spondylolysis, fracture of the vertebra, and prolapse and protrusion of the disk as other possible causative factors. Symptoms include pain, a hyperlordotic stance, tightness of the hamstrings, lumbodorsal fasciae, and flexors of the hip; in most cases, a relative weakness of the abdominal musculature can also be a symptom. Physical therapy as described in the therapy of spondylosis represents the basic therapeutic treatment in patients with spondylogenic pain. Often, this therapy completely eliminates pain and reduces the curvature of the lumbar lordosis to normal limits. In cases that do not respond to this treatment, the same exercise program is adhered to with the concomitant use of a brace constructed with O° lumbar lordosis with an opened front. The brace is worn for a period of 2 to 3 months. If after this period of time there is no evident improvement, a complete physical examination is indicated again while the physician should also consult with the trainer and parents of the gymnast. It is possible that for some reason, the child is "running" into the disease and that the present symptomatology is the result of a conversive neurosis.

Apart from these causes of low back pain, which are connected with athletic activities, the physician should take into consideration those causes that are not initiated by sports activities. More rare, but differential diagnostically possible causes include osteogenic sarcomas, sacroileitus, and discitis.

The presence of low back pain in gymnasts should be treated as a serious problem.[11] Low back pain syndrome is characterized by its progressive nature. It begins as a slight, barely perceptible pain and continually progresses until the pain and discomfort in the terminal stages of the disease can terminate the sports career of the patient and permanently endanger the health of the gymnast. For this reason, it is mandatory to perform a detailed clinical examination of all gymnasts who experience low back pain for a period of longer than 2 weeks. After treatment and rehabilitation, it is equally important to resume athletic activities gradually and to control the level of strain to which the patient is exposed.

V. SCOLIOSIS AND SPORTS

When attempting to answer the question, *can people with structural scoliosis of the spine take part in athletic activities,* it is essential to recognize some important facts. First of all, one must have a clear conception of what athletic activities mean. In other words, the physician should differentiate between physical education in school and recreational sports, and between the highly competitive professional sports. With regards to scoliosis, the physician should take into account the natural history,[4] degree of deformation, etiology of the scoliosis, and age of the patient.[37] The afore-mentioned facts indicate that there is no general answer to the question posed previously. If such an answer was demanded, it would in all probability have to be affirmative. In other words, patients with structural scoliosis of the spine are allowed to take part in athletic activities. Furthermore, taking an active part in athletic activities is recommended and can in some cases represent a form of therapy in treating scoliosis.[2,9,13,17,33] To underline our opinion on this matter, we would like to cite at this point the opinion of Stagnara who believes that active participation in athletic activities should be incorporated in the therapy recommended for scoliotic patients. Athletic activities should be incorporated in a kinesitherapy program. Without them, therapy would be tedious and boring for the patient.[21] Athletic activities generally improve or stabilize the general state of the organism and have a beneficiary effect on a number of vital functions, especially on the cardiorespiratory system.[1] According to the same author, the criteria that allow a recommendation for taking part in athletic activities depend upon the severity of the scoliosis, and the age and sex of the patient.[39]

Generally speaking, it is better to:

- Recommend a sport that is performed outdoors (or at least partially connected to spending some time out of the house or office) and that places some sort of effort on the cardiorespiratory system (e.g., basketball, volleyball, jogging, etc.).
- Prohibit dangerous sports (skydiving, rugby, judo).
- Exclude athletic activities that demand a high level of specialized technical skills and are connected with physical qualities and considerable strength. These may be beyond the capabilities of the scoliotic patient and may thus discourage him from taking part.
- Choose sports in which the patients can participate for long periods of time, preferrably all of their lives, such as walking, hiking, bicycling, tennis, etc.

Stagnara[39] particularly emphasizes the importance of swimming, which has the advantage of placing the spine in a medium free from strain caused by gravitational forces. It also enables the maintenance of correct posture combined with significant physical activity and respiration and depending on the style of swimming recommended, can force the spine into a position that corrects the deviation. However, we feel it is important to mention at this point that placing the spine in a horizontal position in water does not generate muscle activity in the functional positions of greatest importance to the patient, i.e., when sitting and standing. Furthermore, it is by no means certain that the muscle quality best adapted to the therapeutical idea of extended postural correction is achieved.[39] A special question is the advisability of "asymetric" sporting activities. Stagnara points out that it is impossible to correct a toracal scoliotic deviation by swimming continually with a sidestroke. On the other hand, some athletic activities, due to the constant repetition of asymmetrical movements, can overdevelop one extremity or one side of the body, this cannot be a cause of scoliosis and cannot in all probability worsen the existing scoliosis.[39] Tennis players, even professional tennis players, do not develop structural scoliosis, but simply develop a stronger right or left arm. The beneficiary effects of a sporting activity such as tennis outweigh by far the physician's possible doubts about the harmful side-effects.[35] With regards to physical education in school, we believe that as a general rule, children with structural scoliosis less than 30° should be encouraged to participate actively in all athletic activities, as this is without doubt more beneficial to the child than physical inactivity. The imposed limit of 30° is not arbitrarily determined. Studies have shown that in patients who suffer from scoliosis greater than 30°, the afflicted biomechanics can, by itself, without regard to the etiology of the scoliosis, lead to an increase of the curvature of the spine. When dealing with school-age patients whose scoliosis is greater than 30°, the physician should consider excusing the child from physical education. In collaboration with Professor Ivan Kristofic, who has a special interest in kinesitherapy of scoliosis, we have made a schematic representation and diagram of the differential participation of children in physical education[24,35] with regards to the amount of scoliotic curvature present in the spine of the child (Table 4). An examination of Table 4 will show that we have taken, as the limit for unrestricted participation in physical education, the amount of structural scoliosis not exceeding 20°. The reason why we have chosen the limit of 20, and not 30°, is that we believe not only should the current amount of scoliosis be taken into account, but the physician should also keep in mind the evolutionary character of the disease, i.e., the prognosis. This can be evaluated only by a specially educated orthopedic specialist (who is a specialist in scoliosis), while the practical implementation of the prescribed program is left to the physical education instructor.[22] Precisely because of the discrepancy in the level of expertise between the orthopedic specialist and the physical education instructor, we have taken a lower degree of spinal curvature as the limit for unrestrained physical activity. In view of this, we offer some alternative suggestions, such as partial exception from physical education or exercising under special programs if the set up of these programs is feasible.[24,35] Athletic activities outside of school programs are also recommended with the stipulation that children with scoliosis exceeding 20° should be encouraged to participate in "useful" sports to correct the spine. This is particularly important when one takes into account that nowadays active participation and competition in athletic activities begins at a very early age (as early as 6 or 7 years). Some authors

TABLE 4
Physical Education Program as Related to the Scoliotic Curve

Scoliosis(°)	Physical education
Up to 10	Physical education program without limitation
11 to 20	Physical education program without limitation
	Supervision/regular medical control
21 to 30	Partial exemption from the so-called "lineal program"
	Exemption of jumps over athletic or gymnastic device; some flexibility exercises on the floor — whirling, handstand position, etc.; athletic disk throwing, shot putting, etc.; lifting and carrying
	Capable of participating in a special exercise program, if organized
	Activity of choice: swimming, volleyball, basketball, running, tennis, table tennis, etc.
	Kinesitherapy within a medical center (facultative)
31 to 50	Total exemption from physical education until the end of treatment
	Capable of participating in a special exercise program, provided the program is conducted by instructors graduated in kinesitherapy
	Activity of choice: swimming, volleyball, basketball
	Kinesitherapy within a medical center
More than 51	Permanent exemption from physical education; special exercise programs are not anticipated, although if technically and professionally available, they would be desirable
	Optional activity of choice: swimming, walking
	Kinesitherapy within a medical center

recommend that patients with scoliosis avoid the following sports: throwing (in athletics), fencing, and rowing. This opinion is compatible with the known statistics relative to pathological changes in the vertebrae and professional sports. Pathological changes in vertebrae are encountered in professional athletes with the following distribution: gymnasts (50%), divers (40%), and rowers (50%). There are no precise statistical data on the frequency of pathological changes in wrestlers and weight lifters, but empirical evidence shows that athletes who take part in these sports are also prone to develop scoliotic changes in the spine.

The discussion of scoliosis and sports involves, in our opinion, four points: (1) sports activities and idiopathic scoliosis; (2) sports in the treatment of idiopathic scoliosis; (3) physical education of school children with idiopathic scoliosis; and (4) sports activities in surgically treated patients with idiopathic scoliosis.

In order to deal with the first of these points, we decided to see whether professional athletes with scoliosis of the spine feel any difficulties and constraints in sports activities or in everyday life.

We examined all the students at the School of Physical Education of the University of Zagreb; the total was 541: 353 males and 188 females (aged 19 to 25 years). All were anthropometrically measured and clinically examined by forward bending tests; moreover, all clinically positive cases for scoliosis of the spine were checked by X-ray. All the examinees were also asked to fill out a special question-naire concerning the presence of any spine complaints during their course of studies or engagement in a selected professional sports activity. On clinical examination, scoliosis of the spine was detected in 18.3% of the subjects. After X-ray, 12.05% of the subjects could be said to have scoliosis proper, while only 2.3% of the subjects had scoliosis with a Cobb angle exceeding 10°. The presence of pain or any complaints during sports activities is reviewed in Table 5 for scoliotic subjects and the control group, i.e., subjects presenting no scoliosis of the spine.

As far as the incidence of scoliosis in our subjects is concerned, the results match the incidence established in the general population.[27] It should, however, be noted that our subjects had engaged in sports since their early youth, a fact which also later had a bearing on their choice of the course of study. In terms of the occurrence of pain or difficulties in everyday life or in athletic activities, there were no differences between scoliotic and nonscoliotic subjects. All our scoliotic subjects followed their course of study normally and engaged in professional sports. No one consulted a doctor or discontinued his/her engagement in sports activity, even for a short period of time, because of scoliosis of the spine. This clearly demonstrates that scoliosis was not felt and was not considered by any means as an obstacle to engaging in intensive sports activities. Our study can also provide an indirect answer to the third point raised earlier, i.e., physical education in scoliotic children. It is our view that scoliotic children with an angle of up to 30° feel no constraints as far as physical education in school is concerned. Regarding sports activities in surgically treated patients with idiopathic scoliosis, it is our view that sports activities can be permitted, even up to the highest level, 1 year after surgery. We base this opinion on the fact that we have had examples of surgically treated patients engaging in professional competitive sports such as table tennis (Figure 12), handball, volleyball, etc. Of course, it should be noted that each patient should be considered individually. Therefore, our general answer as to whether individuals with scoliosis of the spine may engage in sports is affirmative, although we are aware of the fact that this matter will require additional extensive research if we are to be strictly accurate and more selective than we are today in answering the question raised, i.e., scoliosis and sports.

Summing up the before mentioned, we feel that is important to stress once again that any physical activity is preferable to physical inactivity for the scoliotic patient.

TABLE 5
Presence of Pain or Complaints in the Spine

Pain/complaints	Scoliosis(%)		Total
	Yes	**No**	
Male			
Yes	21.8	22.1	78
No	78.2	77.9	275
Total	100	100	353
Female			
Yes	37.2	37.2	70
No	62.8	62.8	118
Total	100	100	188

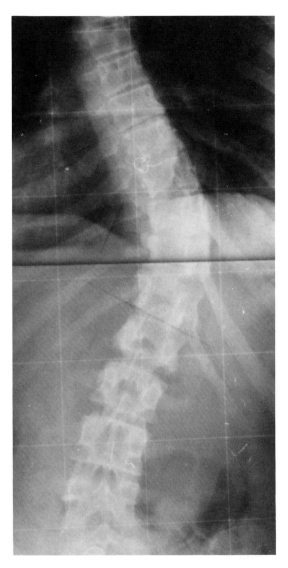

FIGURE 12. Scoliosis in a top-level table tennis player. (A) Preoperative roentgenogram.

VI. JUVENILE (ADOLESCENT) KYPHOSIS — SCHEUERMANN'S DISEASE AND SPORTS

Juvenile (adolescent) kyphosis represents a special clinical entity characterized by an increased, somewhat inferiorly positioned thoracal kyphosis, which in most cases is accompanied by radiologically visible wedge-shaped vertebrae (Figure 13). Nowadays, the criteria for diagnosing Scheuermann's kyphosis are (1) incorrect superior and inferior epiphyseal rings of the vertebral body, (2) decrease of the

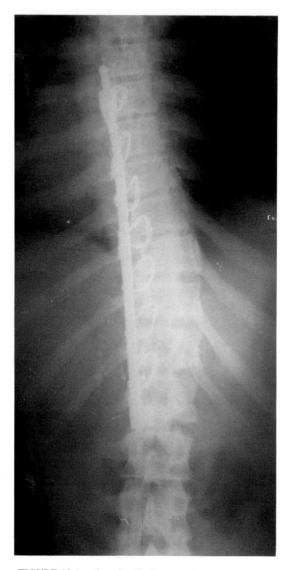

FIGURE 12 (continued). (B) Postoperative roentgenogram.

intervertebral disk space, (3) the presence of one or more vertebra wedged for 5° or more, and (4) an increase of thoracal kyphosis to more than 40°. The etiology of the disease is, as yet, not completely known. The most commonly mentioned cause is thought to be avascular necrosis of the cartilaginous apophyseal rings of the body of the vertebra. This is why this disease is often delegated into the juvenile osteochondrosis group of diseases (epiphysitis and apophysitis). It is quite obvious that the causative factor of this disease is the discrepancy between the strain placed upon and the weight bearing capabilities of the epiphyseal rings of the body of the vertebra. In this context, the question of continued athletic activities presents itself with regard to the manifestation and possible worsening of the adolescent kyphosis of the spine.

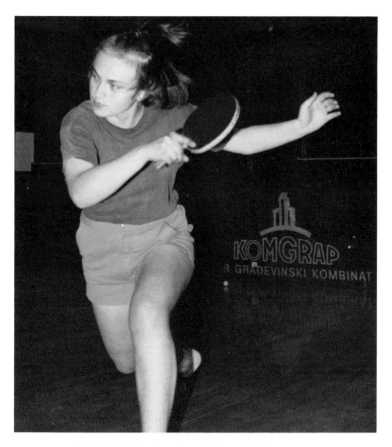

FIGURE 12 (continued). (C) One year after surgery.

When evaluating the ability of patients suffering from Scheuermann's disease to participate in athletic activities, two completely different and controversial viewpoints exist. One holds that the patient should be allowed to continue any and all athletic activities without any constraint, while the other believes that the patient should be forbidden all sports activities.[34] The reason for this difference in opinion is not only in the unclear genesis of this disease, but also in the inability to diagnose precisely the development of the disease. The obvious questions concerning this dilemma are (1) to what degree do athletic activities have a beneficiary effect on the disease? (2) can latent Scheuermann's disease manifest itself in patients who participate in sports? and (3) will the disease show an inclination to worsen in patients who participate in athletic activities (athletic activities as an unfavorable factor)? First we will review all the possible positive effects that participating in sports activities can have on juvenile kyphosis. The positive effects include: "immobilizing" the spine in a functionally correct position caused by a correct stance, strengthening the muscles of the body, decreasing myostatic decompensation, increasing psychological functions such as will and energy, and increasing stamina and general condition, resulting from correct breathing technique and strengthening of the heart and vascular system; this will increase the patient's ability to participate in sports activities. Statistical

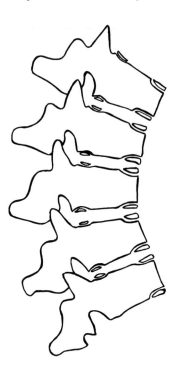

FIGURE 13. Schematic roentgenogram of the thoracal spine affected by Scheuermann's disease.

analysis from the University Hospital in Heidelberg has shown that out of a total sample of 5504 athletes, 437 (7.8%) seek treatment because of pathological changes in the spine. Abstaining from athletic activities was recommended to only one patient. Orthopedic evaluation in professional athletes has shown that out of a total sample of 580 cases from 34 different sports, Scheuermann's disease was found in 18.9% of the cases while an oval back was indicated in 16.8% of the sample. These changes, which frequently appear together, were therefore present in 35.7% of the sample. A recommendation for abstaining from athletic activities was issued in only eight cases. Numerous athletes have often continued training without any discomfort for a number of years despite having certain characteristics of Scheuermann's disease. On the other hand, it is necessary to cite the opinion of Sward.[41] Due to the increased interest in physical fitness and to the fact that athletes start their training at younger ages, the risk for injuries to the growing individual has increased. The spine, as with the rest of the skeleton, is at greater risk of injury during growth, especially during the adolescent growth spurt. Back pain is more common among athletes participating in sports with high demands on the back than other athletes and nonathletes. Disk degeneration, defined as disk height reduction on conventional radiographs and reduced disk signal intensity on MRI, has been found in a higher frequency among wrestlers and gymnasts than nonathletes. Abnormalities of the vertebral bodies including abnormal configuration, Schmorl's nodes, and apophyseal changes are common among athletes. These abnormalities are similar to those found in Scheuermann's disease. Athletes with these types of abnormalities have more back pain than those without.

For this reason, we feel it is imperative to develop a uniform system of classification for patients suffering from juvenile kyphosis, and a uniform set of criteria concerning the advisability of athletic activity in patients with this syndrome.

We believe that kyphotic changes in the spine should be classified into three basic stages:

1. Functional stage — at the end of the first decade of life, characterized by a kyphotic posture, but no radiologically visible changes characteristic of Scheuermann's disease
2. Florid stage — (between the ages of 12 to 14 years) a fully developed clinical picture and characteristic radiological findings
3. Late stage (or the stage following recovery from Scheuermann's disease) — found in patients over 18 years of age; generally referred to as discomforts and pains felt as a consequence of degenerative changes in the spine.

Because of the complexity of the problem, other factors such as the precise localization of the disease, the expected level of strain, and the athletic activity in which the patient is participating, bear considerable weight when reaching the final evaluation.[21] Taking this into account, it is quite logical that a relatively more developed juvenile kyphosis located more distally will have a worse prognosis.

In the following paragraphs, we will mainly concern ourselves with the intensity of the strain and the effect of various athletic activities on different stages of the disease.

In the first stage of the disease, unrestricted individual (partly adapted) athletic activities are allowed. However, physical examinations (at least twice a year) are mandatory. In the event of any pain or discomfort, a consultation with the examining physician is necessary. This is followed by a reduction in the level of strain placed upon the spine and in some cases a complete cessation of athletic activities (Table 6).

With patients in the second stage of the disease, athletic activities are forbidden to those who complain of pain or discomfort, in which case special, targeting medical gymnastics is prescribed. For the remaining patients (those who do not feel any pain or discomfort and who usually make up around 80% of the cases), athletic activities (with certain restrictions) are allowed (Table 7). Table 8 illustrates which athletic activities have a positive effect and which have a negative effect on the course of the disease.[34]

TABLE 6
The Functional Stage of the Kyphosis (Kyphotic Posture)

The level of strain placed upon the spine is unrestricted if the following is adhered to:
Regular physical examination (at least twice a year)
In the event of pain, a reduction in the level of strain

TABLE 7
The Florid Stage of the Disease

In cases where pain or discomfort is felt (20% of the cases)
All athletic activities are forbidden
Specific (targeting) medical gymnastics is carried out

In cases with no pain (80% of the cases)
Reduced activity with regard to bending compression and hyperextension of the spine

TABLE 8
The Effect of the Athletic Activities on the Course of the Disease

Athletic activity	Positive effect on the development of the disease	Negative effect on the development of the disease
Swimming	Backstyle	Butterfly style
	Breaststroke with proper breathing technique	High jumps into water
Bicycling	At the recreational level (with high steering and back support)	At the competitive level
Gymnastics	Exercises that do not bend the spine	Exercises that include bending the spine
Athletics		All jumps (because of bending of the spine); weight lifting
Rowing		Because of bending and general strain on the spine
Games that use a ball: volleyball, basketball, soccer, tennis	Exercises all, for developing the body	

Of the sports with a general positive effect on the course of the disease, special attention should be given to the problem of horseback riding as an integral part of, or as an addition to physical therapy of Scheuermann's disease. Data provided by Harms[34] indicate that horseback riding can be an ideal addition to physical therapy of juvenile kyphosis. When the correct riding technique is employed and the patient is correctly sitting on the horse, the ischial tuberosities of the rider are in direct contact with the saddle while the hips are in a gently flexed position. At the same time, the patient's pelvis is continually and rhythmically turned over, which is the basic aim of medical gymnastics. As a consequence of this, one is forced to adapt oneself automatically (by process of compensation), the thoracal curvature is straightened, and shoulder girdle is placed into a correct position. During the rhythmic movements produced by the walking, trotting, and galloping of the horse, the pelvis is forced to perform alternating movements of bending and straightening which is an ideal way of strengthening the back muscles, loosening up, and relaxing, i.e., unblocking, the spine. For these reasons, we believe that horseback riding is an ideal, and from the patient's point of view almost unconscious, method of performing medical gymnastics. However, the physician should be careful when placing strain (particularly when the strain placed upon the spine is vertical as in horseback riding) on the spine of patients with extreme defects of the spine. These cases are relatively rare, but notwithstanding the practicing physician should bear in mind that excessive vertical strain can negatively affect the already damaged disks. In such cases, horseback riding should be allowed only after an orthopedic brace is correctly put in place. Keeping up with patients who have used horseback riding as part of their therapy for juvenile kyphosis, in varying degrees, has shown that no pain or discomfort has appeared as a result of the worsening of the disease, and also that there has been no increase in the curvature of the spine.

The third stage of the disease, characterized by the state of the patient once he has recovered from the disease, demands a differential evaluation (Table 9). An important fact to keep in mind is that patients belonging to the second group should, by all means, correctly perform their prescribed exercises for strengthening the muscles of the trunk (these exercises are performed solely as a means of increasing the patient's stamina). With patients who belong to the third group, the physician should differentiate between those who suffer daily pain and those who suffer only when exposed to excessive levels of strain. The physician should, likewise, differentiate between patients whose discomforts are caused by muscle insufficiency and those in whom pain is the result of degenerative changes. If the pain is present on a daily basis or if it appears after 30 min or longer periods of standing or walking, the prescribed treatment is shown in Table 9. In cases where the pain is caused by degenerative changes in the spine, the patient is encouraged to participate in athletic activities primarily to strengthen the muscles of the trunk to have a corrective effect on the mobile part of the spine.[21] Such patients are also encouraged to participate in

TABLE 9
The Late Stage of the Disease or the State after Recovery

Evaluation of the general state	Admissible level of strain
A. Immobilization in a correct position, strong muscles of the trunk, absence of pain	Unlimited
B. Immobilization in an incorrect position, strong muscles of the trunk, absence of pain	Limited level of strain (i.e., special training sessions)
C. Immobilization in an incorrect position, weak muscles of the trunk, pain is present	Same level of strain as under B. Medical gymnastics is performed trunk,
Daily pain	Athletic activity with a positive effect on the disease is chosen
Caused by muscle insufficiency	
Caused by secondary degenerative changes	Reduced strain Medical gymnastics
Pain felt when under strain	Same level of strain as under B.

sports that mobilize the spine without exposing it to excessive strain (i.e., sports that involve the handling of a ball).

After reviewing the current state of knowledge, as reported in the medical literature, we feel obliged to report that in the vast majority of cases, patients who suffer from Scheuermann's disease, under medical supervision, can participate in athletic activities.[34] Inherent in this supposition is that the physician is aware of the particular demands that each sport places on the patient. Excessive kyphosing and lordosing (spondylolysis and spondylolysthesis) of the spine should be avoided. Swimming, for instance, is a sport that is often recommended because of its therapeutic and beneficial effects on the patient. However, the physician should be aware that swimming, if performed in the butterfly style, or without the proper breathing technique, can have a negative effect on the further development of the disease. We should also keep in mind that in some athletic activities, particularly at the professional level, pathological changes of the vertebrae are relatively frequent: in gymnastic exercises (50%), high jumps into water (40%), and rowing (50%). For this reason, we advocate orthopedic examinations for adolescents before they take up a particular sport.

In conclusion, we would like to report that patients suffering from Scheuermann's disease can participate in athletic activities. The only mandatory prerequisite is the close collaboration between the athlete, trainer, and sports physician. Other important facts that should be kept in mind are the timely choice of an adequate sport, individual adaptation of the level of strain placed upon the patient, and an interdisciplinary collaboration between all consulted specialists.[34]

REFERENCES

1. **Basmaijan, J. V.** *Therapeutic Exercise*. Baltimore: Williams and Wilkins, 1978.
2. **Cecker, T. J.** Scoliosis in swimmers. *Clin. Sports Med.* 1986; 5:149–157.
3. **Bradford, D. S., Lonstein, J. E., Moe, J., Ogilvie, J. W., and Winter, R. B.** *Moe's Textbook of Scoliosis and Other Spinal Deformities*. 2nd ed. Philadelphia: W. B. Saunders, 1987.
4. **Bunnel, W. P.** The natural history of idiopathic scoliosis. *Clin. Orthop.*, 1988; 229:20–25.
5. **Densiger, R. H.** Biomechanical considerations for clinical application in athletes with low back pain. *Clin. Sports Med.*, 1989; 8:703–715.
6. **Domljan, Z., Curković, B.** Iliolumbalni sindrom. *Lije. Vjesn.*, 1983; 105–107.
7. **Durrigl, P. and Durrigl, T.** Degenerativne afekcije vertebralnog dinamikog segmenta. *Reumatizam,* 1967; 5:165.
8. **Durrigl, T.** Lumbalgije u okviru suvremene medicine rada. *Lije. Vjesn.,* 1961; 83:1079–1082.

9. **Dubravić, S., Pećina, M., Bojanić, I., and Simunjak, B.** Common orthopaedic problems in female athletes. *Croat. Sports Med. J.*, 1991; 6:38–46.

10. **Gašpert, T. and Pećina, M.** Bolni sindromi kralježnice kod gimnasti arki. *Košarkaški Med. Vjesn.*, 1988; 3:63–68.

11. **Goldberg, M. J.** Gymnastic injuries. *Orthop. Clin. N. Am.*, 1980; 11:717–726.

12. **Harvey, J. and Tanner, S.** Low back pain in young athletes. A practical approach. *Sports Med.*, 1991; 12:394–406.

13. **Hopf, C., Felske-Adler, C., and Heine, J.** Empfehlungen zur sportlichen Betatigung von Patienten mit idiopathischen Skoliosen. *Z. Orthop.*, 1991; 129:204–207.

14. **Jajić, I. et al.** *Lumbalni Bolni Sindrom.* Zagreb: Kolska Knjiga, 1984.

15. **Junghanns, H.** *Wirbelsaule und Beruf.* Stuttgart: Hipokrates Verlag, 1980.

16. **Jušić, A.** Klinicka electromioneurografija i neuromuskularne bolesti. JUMENA: Zagreb, 1981.

17. **Jarrouse, Y.** Quel sport pour quel rachis? In: *Muscles, Tendons et Sport.* Benezis, C., Simeray, J., Simon, L., Eds. Paris: Masson, 1990; 73–77.

18. **Keane, G. P. and Saal, J. A.** The sports medicine approach to occupational low back pain. *W. J. Med.*, 1991; 154:525–527.

19. **Kelsey, J. H. and White, A. A.** Epidemiology and impact of low back pain. *Spine*, 1980; 5:133.

20. **Keros, P., et al.** *Functional Anatomy of Locomotor System.* Zagreb: Medicinska Naklada, 1968.

21. **Korbelar, P., Kuera, M., and Sazima, V.** Abweichungen der Wirbelsaule in der sportmedizinischen Praxis. *Sportverletzung Sportschaden*, 1988; 2:69–71.

22. **Kovačić, S., Ed.** *Scoliosis and Kyphosis.* Zagreb: Medicinska Naklada, 1977.

23. **Kramer, J.** Intervertebral disk diseases: causes, diagnosis, treatment and prophylaxis. Stuttgart: G. Thieme, 1982.

24. **Kristofić, I. and Pećina, M.** Ciljana primjena programa preventivnih vježbi u djece sa skoliozom kralježnice. *Acta Med.*, 1982; 8:33–36.

25. **Kujala, U. M., Salminen, J. J., Taimela, S., Oksanen, A., and Jaakkola, L.** Subject characteristics and low back pain in young athletes and nonathletes. *Med. Sci. Sports Exerc.*, 1992; 24:627–632.

26. **Lee, C. K.** Office management of low back pain. *Orthop. Clin. N. Am.*, 1988; 19:797–804.

27. **Lončar-Dušek, M., Pećina, M., Prebeg, Z.** A longitudinal study of growth velocity and development of secondary gender characteristics versus onset of idiopathic scoliosis. *Clin. Orthop.*, 1991; 270:278–282.

28. **Nachemson, A.** Lumbar intradiscal pressure. *Acta Orthop. Scand.*, (suppl.) 1960; 43:1.

29. **Nachemson, A.** Work for all, for those with low back pain as well. *Clin. Orthop.*, 1983; 179:77.

30. **Pećina, M.** Piriformis sindrom u diferencijalnoj dijagnostici bolnih križa. *Acta Orthop. Iugosl.*, 1975; 6:196–200.

31. **Pećina, M.** Contribution of the etiological explanation of the piriformis syndrome. *Acta Anat.* (Basel), 1979; 105:181–187.

32. **Pećina, M., Ed.** *Scoliosis and Kyphosis.* Zagreb: Sveučilična naklada Liber, 1983.

33. **Pećina, M., Dubravčić, S., and Bojanić, I.** Scoliosis and Sport. Proc. Congr. Eur. Spinal Deformities Soc., Lyon, June 1992, Sauramps, Montpellier, 227.

34. **Pećina, M. and Kovač, V.** Morbus Scheuermann i mogućnosti bavljenja sportom. *Sportsko-Med. objave*, 1983; 20:123–129.

35. **Pećina, M. and Krištofić, I.** Tjelesni odgoj u prevenciji i lijeenju skoliotinih držaanja i skolioza. *Fizika kultura,* 1983; 3:93–105.

36. **Schmorl, G. and Junghans, H.** *Die gesunde und die kranke Wirbelsaule in Rontgenbild und Klinik.* Stuttgart: G. Thieme, 1968.

37. **Sires, A.** Rachis de l'enfant et sport: de la prevention a la pratique. In: *Muscles, Tendons et Sport.* Benezis, C., Simeray, J., Simon, L., Eds. Paris: Masson, 1990; 289–295.

38. **Spengler, D. M.** Low back pain: assessment and management. New York: Grune and Stratton, 1982.

39. **Stagnara, P.** *Les Deformations du Rachis.* Paris: Masson, 1985.

40. **Stanish, W.** Low back pain in athletes: an overuse syndrome. *Clin. Sports Med.,* 1987; 6:321–344.

41. **Sward, L.** The thoracolumbar spine in young elite athletes. Current concepts on the effects of physical training. *Sports Med.,* 1992; 13:357–364.

42. **Weiker, G. G.** Evaluation and treatment of common spine and trunk problems. *Clin. Sports Med.,* 1989; 8:399–417.

43. **White, A. A. and Panjabi, M. M.** *Clinical Biomechanics of the Spine.* Philadelphia: J. B. Lippincott, 1978.

The Lower Extremity

6

Hip and Thigh

I. GROIN PAIN

A. Groin Strain

Painful groin syndrome is generally considered to be the most common and most frequent overuse syndrome in some athletic activities, e.g., soccer.[33,34] The term *groin pain,* itself, clearly indicates the site and the principal symptom of the syndrome. However, neither the site nor the pain is precisely defined. When considering the location and anatomic structures affected by overuse, together with the locations and characteristics of pain, the location might be precise, but it could also be the case of diffuse vague pain in the groin region, small pelvis, and upper leg regions. The term *syndrome* is fully justified; indeed, the symptoms are numerous and so are the causes of pain in the groin region. Hence, it is not surprising that modern medical literature abounds with terms defining pain in the groin region: necrotic osteitis pubis, anterior pelvic joint syndrome, traumatic pubic osteitis, Pierson's syndrome, gracillis muscle syndrome, pubic stress symphysitis, pubic symphisis osteoarthropathy, symphysitis, pubic chondritis, and posttraumatic necrosis of the pubic bone.[28,33] These terms and expressions have commonly been used to describe adductor tendinitis, rectus abdominis tendinitis, avulsion injuries of the adductor tendons, postoperative changes without infection in the symphysis region, and a number of arthrotic changes.

To be able to understand the painful groin syndrome, one should have in mind all the muscles that insert in the symphysis region. These muscles attach themselves to the upper and lower branches of the pubic bones: to the very inguinal ligament, to the branch of the ischium, to the small trochanter, and to the iliac crest (Table 1). Also, it should not be forgotten that the groin region is the crossing point of two muscle systems: (1) the trunk muscles, primarily the abdominal ones and (2) the muscles of the lower extremity (Figure 1), the upper leg muscles in the first place, especially the adductor ones (Figure 2). The pelvic region and the hips carry large static and dynamic weight so that both the static and dynamic positions of the pelvis in space ensure equilibrium (balance) of those muscles that are either inserted into or originate from the pelvic bones, especially in the groin region. In general considerations of overuse syndrome development, it is stated that the balance of antagonist muscles and coordination of agonists are essential to the prevention of this syndrome. When we think that the activity and equilibrium of muscles originating from or being inserted into the groin region may also be disturbed because of the changes in the

TABLE 1
Insertion and Origin of Muscles in the Groin Region

Lig. inguinale	M. obliquus abdominis externus
	M. obliquus abdominis internus
Ramus superior	M. rectus abdominis
Ossis pubis	M. obliquus abdominis externus
	M. obliquus abdominis internus
	M. transversus abdominis
	M. pyramidalis
	M. pectineus
	M. adductor longus
	M. adductor brevis
Ramus inferior	M. adductor brevis
Ossis pubis	M. gracillis
	M. cremaster
Ramus ossis ischii	M. adductor magnus
Tuber ossis ischii	M. adductor magnus
	M. semitendinosus
	M. semimembranosus
	M. biceps femoris (caput longum)
Trochanter minor	M. iliopsoas
Spina iliaca anterior superior	M. sartorius
Spina iliaca anterior inferior	M. rectus femoris

lumbar spine or the hip joint, the knee joint, the sacroiliac joints, and the symphysis itself, no wonder the multiple possibilities exist for the development of overuse syndrome affecting certain anatomic structures in the groin region. Besides, it is important to know that the groin region is the site of the inguinal canal located above the inguinal ligament, of lacuna nervorum and vasorum beneath the inguinal ligament, and of the femoral and obturator canals. Of course, these are the openings through which the anatomic structures for the lower extremity pass. Therefore, the groin region is justly referred to as the *Gibraltar of the lower extremity*. All of the above-mentioned information clearly shows that the painful groin syndrome cannot be attributed solely to one particular anatomic structure in the region but rather that the approach to the syndrome, in either prevention, diagnosis or treatment, should be based on the idea of multiple causing factors acting in the development of the syndrome.[33,34] It is precisely the approach we have assumed although we make a difference between the *painful groin syndrome* in a *narrow sense* from the *painful groin syndrome* in a *wider sense,* for which "pain in the groin" seems to be a more appropriate term since it may arise from different pathological conditions in and around the groin region. The painful groin syndrome in a narrow sense primarily implies tendinitis of the adductor muscles — the long adductor muscle and the gracillis muscle in the first place and also the abdominal muscles, especially the rectus abdominis and pyramidalis muscles. Long-lasting tendinitis of these muscles may evolve into a general and vague picture of diffuse pain in the public bones and the symphysis region.

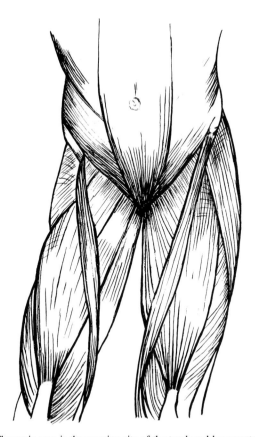

FIGURE 1. The groin area is the crossing site of the trunk and lower extremity muscles.

1. Etiopathogenesis

Bones, muscles, and tendons as a whole are actually the basis of a painful syndrome since these are the structures within which changes characteristic of overuse syndrome commonly develop.[18,22,23,29,33,34] According to Martens, the load-bearing capacity of a tendon and tendinous attachment differs from individual to individual. The limits of this capacity may be influenced by external and internal factors. The internal factors include insufficiency of the paravertebral and abdominal muscles, hip joint disorders, inequality of leg length, disorders in the sacroiliac joint, and foot deformities. The external factors include injuries in the adductor region, injuries in the hip joint, and inadequate athletic training.[22]

Several authors have reported[1,10,14,15,24,44] that the cause of groin pain lies in the disproportion between the strength of the abdominal wall muscles and the strength of the lower extremity muscles, as well as in a uneven load of all attachment in the symphysis and groin region. (Figure 3) Durey and Boeda[5] report that the painful groin syndrome is an injury, or more precisely, a lesion characteristically occurring in soccer players, since the symphysis region is the point of attachment and the point

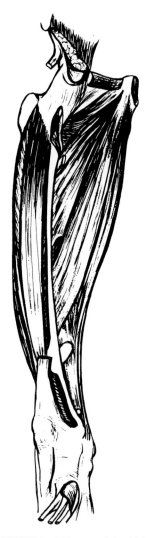

FIGURE 2. Adductors of the thigh.

of origin for groups of muscles with different functions; they are especially active during soccer playing. Adductors are under strain when side blows are performed and also when striking a ball with the interior side of the foot. Besides, they are especially under strain when "sliding starts" are performed (Figure 4). In the course of attempting a start, lower extremities become wide apart. The parting point is the symphysis region where the abdominal muscles contract simultaneously to prevent falling backward. Janković[16] also states that during the "sliding starts", the adductor muscles are involved to their maximum, resulting in their straining, microtraumas, and eventually inflammation of the region surrounding the tendinous attachment.[18] In 78.2% of patients, clinical examination reveals weakness of oblique abdominal muscles, so that during the "sliding starts" the upper leg muscles, especially the adductors, become extremely strained.[16] Sudden acceleration or change in direction

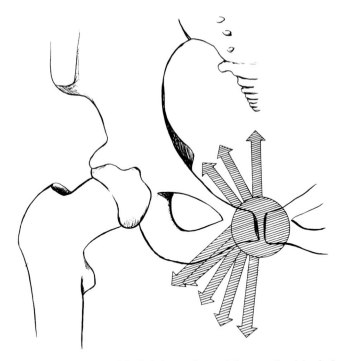

FIGURE 3. Graphic representation of the imbalance of strength between the abdominal muscles and muscles of the lower extremities.

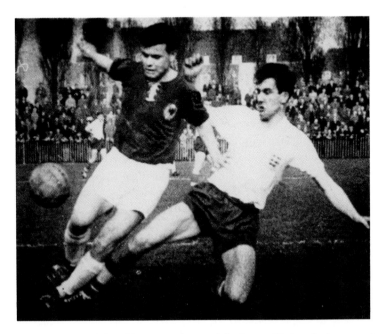

FIGURE 4. Maximal use of the adductor muscle, especially the gracillis muscle, is present in sliding tackles.

of movement and rough ground have been reported as other causes of adductor muscle overuse.[5,16] Pilardeau et al.[32] classify painful groin syndrome as the so-called *Lucy syndrome,* named after the fossil hominid remains of Australopithecus. The authors explain that due to the relatively more erect posture of modern man, when compared to Australopithecus, a change in the position of the pelvis, leading to the lowering of ischial bone tuberosity and to the lifting of the symphysis and anterior pelvic aspect, caused strain in the adductor muscles and the rectus femoris muscle.

2. Epidemiology

Painful groin syndrome is most commonly found in soccer players.[3,5,15,16,31,34,38] Cabot[5] reported that 0.5% of 42,000 examined soccer players complained of pain in the groin. Extrand and Gillquist[7] conducted a 1-year follow-up study of 12 soccer teams. Their results show that 13% of injuries are located in the groin region and 2.73% of cases are injuries of the adductor muscle. Nielsen and Yde[25] studied 123 soccer players; according to their report, 2.75% of cases are those of groin tendinitis. In a study sample of 1475 soccer players examined by Janković,[16] 6.24% of them had painful groin syndrome.

Besides soccer players, these injuries have also been reported in ice hockey, waterpolo, and handball players, fencers, high jumpers, bowlers, skaters, hurdlers, and triathletes.[4,8,27,28,29,34]

3. Clinical Picture and Diagnostics

Painful groin syndrome is characterized by pain in the inguinal and lower abdominal regions. Often the pain develops gradually, and the athlete is unaware of its connection with any injury. As time goes by, the pain becomes more severe and irradiates into the upper leg adductor zone, the pubic region, and the perineum, spreading toward the hips and the anterior abdominal wall. Overuse only increases the pain. The pain restricts certain motions during training and the game, especially reducing the speed of the player. In adductor overuse, the pain occurs during sprint, ball kicking, sliding starts, and pivoting.[5,16,22,44] Furthermore, the motion performed during entering or exiting a car may cause pain. In abdominal muscle overuse, the pain occurs in the lower abdominal region, especially during sprint and sudden motion, e.g., a rapid change of direction when running.[22] Pain may appear bilaterally as well. In persistent cases, pain occurs simultaneously in the lower abdominal area and the adductor region.

Similar to other overuse syndromes, painful groin syndrome is also characterized by specific developmental stages. Initially, the pain is unilateral and appears shortly after the strain. It disappears until the time of the next training session so that it does not prevent the athlete from actively participating in training and matches. With time, the pain lasts longer and is not relieved by the time of the next athletic event. During that period, even a minor strain may cause severe pain. Then the pain becomes bilateral, i.e., it occurs in the other groin. This causes greater difficulties for the athlete even in everyday life, especially when climbing up and down stairs or hills, getting up from a sitting position, or attempting to get up from bed. Coughing, sneezing, defecation, urination, and sexual activity also cause pain in the groin. The pain is not strictly limited to the origin or insertion of a given muscle but diffusely extends over a wider area, thus justifying the term *pubalgia*. This may be understood as a developmental stage of the adductor or rectus abdominis muscles tendinitis, but also of the gracillis and pyramidalis muscles tendinitis. These events only confirm the complexity of a pathological condition, i.e., best described by the term *painful groin syndrome*. Mental difficulties of these patients should by all means be added to the clinical picture for they are too often blamed for malingering.

Clinical examination reveals pain during palpation of the pubic bone occurring above the gracillis and adductor longus muscle attachments.[10,16,22] The patient feels pain during passive elevation of the foot at external rotation and in maximum abduction of the upper leg. When testing adductors, the patient is lying on his back with slightly abducted lower extremities so that a fist may be inserted between the knees (Figure 5). The patient is then asked to hold the fist tightly by contracting the adductor muscles of the upper leg. This motion causes pain in the typical site of the upper leg adductor muscle attachment on the pubic bone.[16,31,34]

In tendinitis of the rectus abdominis muscles, pain following palpation appears in the region of the attachment to the ramus superior pubis (superior pubic branch). In a great number of patients, the inspection of the abdominal wall shows weakness of the oblique abdominal muscles. The so-called "sausage and spindle-like prominences" above the iliac crest and the inguinal ligament (in literature commonly referred to as Malgaigne's sign) appearing during contraction of the abdominal muscles are also signs of abdominal wall weakness.[16]

For the testing of rectus abdominal muscles, the patient is lying on his back and lifting his lower extremities up to the height of 45° from the surface (Figure 6).

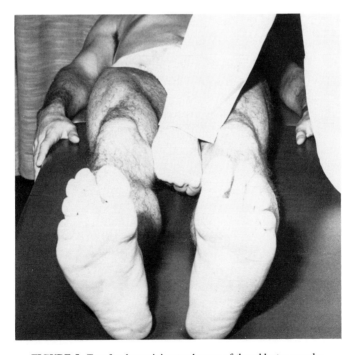

FIGURE 5. Test for determining tenderness of the adductor muscles.

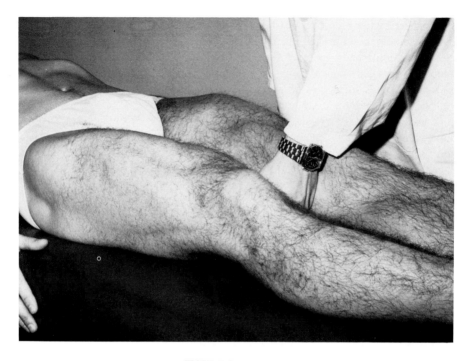

FIGURE 5 (continued).

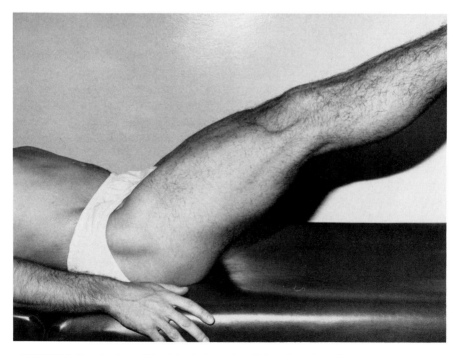

FIGURE 6. Test for the straight abdominal muscles: lift legs from the surface to form a 45° angle.

During these motions, pain occurs in the lower abdominal region and at the point of the muscle attachment to the pubic bone. The pain also appears when the patient is asked to sit up. (Figure 7)

When painful groin syndrome is identified, X-rays of the pelvis, showing pubic bones, symphysis, and both hips are necessary. It enables the physician to rule out arthrotic changes in the hip as causes of pain; it also enables rough analysis of sacroiliac joints and the caudal segment of the lumbosacral spine. A centered scanning of the symphysis is recommended for that purpose in the standing position on one leg (the affected side) and then on the other leg. The scans may show pathological mobility of the symphysis. It is an established fact that during an athletic activity (e.g., running, jumping, kicking), the symphysis moves cranially, caudally, anteriorly, posteriorly, and to a lesser degree, rotatively. These motions of the symphysis are especially observable in soccer players and long-distance walkers.[21] According to Janković,[16] radiologically identified changes in the symphysis and pubic bones may be classified into four stages that correspond to the developmental stages of the painful groin syndrome clinical picture.

During the first stage, the os pubis is characterized by larger, semioval or semicircular transparencies directed toward the symphyses (Figure 8). The transparencies are not limited strictly to the gracillis muscle attachment; they also appear at the attachments of the adductor longus and brevis muscles. In the gracillis muscle attachment to the counter pubic bone, rare osteolithic changes may be seen. Any greater asymmetry of the symphyseal regions is absent at this stage. In the second

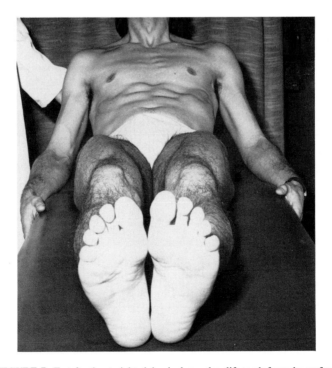

FIGURE 7. Test for the straight abdominal muscles: lift trunk from the surface.

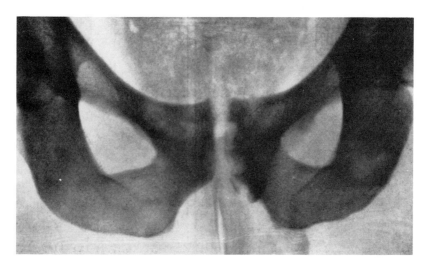

FIGURE 8. The first stage of radiologically visible changes in the pubic symphisis. Translucency is visible on the affected (painful) side of the groin.

stage, the symphyseal region is clearly asymmetrical (Figure 9). The pathological changes in the pubic bone show unclear borders. Scan of the distal symphyseal half shows oblique borderline of the bones with the disappearing symphyseal angle (bone) so that now it is an oblique line extending medially and proximally toward the distal and lateral directions. The third stage is characterized by irregularly undulated symphyseal region of both pubic bones, partially protruded edge borderline, and a clear condensation of osseous structure (Figure 10). At the site of Cooper's pubic ligaments, a borderline swelling or borderline indentation of the osseous apposition may be seen bilaterally. The symphyseal fissure may be vertical or extremely

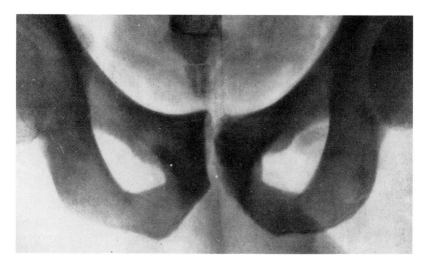

FIGURE 9. The second radiologically visible stage is characterized by asymmetry of the pubic symphisis and saw-like bone on the pathologically changed side.

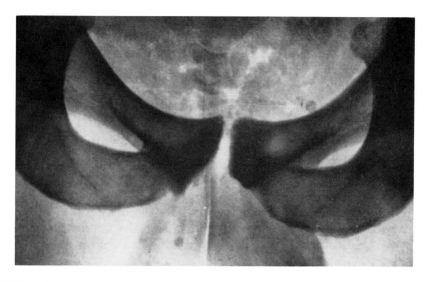

FIGURE 10. Shape of the pubic bones is irregular and undulating with clearly visible bone condensation (characteristic for the third radiological stage).

oblique. The scan resembles that of a secondary osteoarthritis. Besides changes occurring in the symphyseal region during the third stage, the fourth stage is additionally characterized by osseous areas assuming the form of lines or drops in the foramen obturatum area or symphyseal part of the pubic bone branch. According to the X-ray morphological criteria, these correspond to the finding of myositis ossificans.[44] The sclerosing bone regions are primarily found on the side showing an old posttraumatic pubic osteonecrosis (Figure 11).

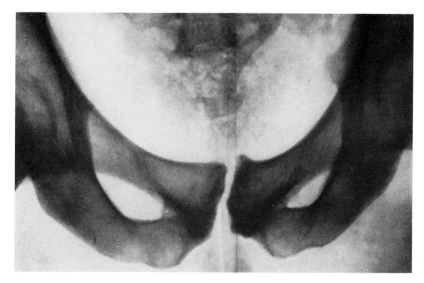

FIGURE 11. The fourth radiologically visible stage, besides the changes described in the third stage, is characterized by clearly visible radiological signs characteristic for posttraumatic pubic osteonecrosis.

Scintigraphy has proved highly valuable in the diagnosis. It helps to identify stress fracture and avulsions in the pubic branch region.[6,19] Le Jeune et al.[19] state that in the case of radiologically invisible changes in the symphysis and a negative scintigraphic finding, it is the condition of long adductor muscle tendinitis.

Ultrasound diagnostics are very useful in differential diagnosis of acute trauma to overuse injuries (Figure 12).

If inguinal hernia is suspected as a cause of pain, herniography should be performed.[37,38]

4. Treatment

Treatment of painful groin syndrome is as complex as the causes of its development. Similar to many other situations in medicine, the best possible treatment is based upon the elimination of causes and prevention of development of the syndrome. Since painful groin syndrome is not of unique etiology, it is very hard to establish unique principles of treatment. However, in our opinion, it should always be started with nonoperative procedures; only when these fail, strictly selective surgery should be contemplated, i.e., depending upon the cause of the syndrome. The following are some common principles of nonoperative treatment of painful groin syndrome regardless of its cause: (1) alleviate pain and control inflammation in the myotendinous apparatus; (2) hasten healing of the myotendinous apparatus; and (3) control further activities.

We would like to emphasize that it is of utmost importance to commence treatment as early as possible, i.e., when the first symptoms occur.[28,33] Not paying due attention to initial symptoms and continuation with athletic activity at the same intensity are the most common mistakes. When the athlete contacts his physician during the initial stage of overuse syndrome development, the training intensity

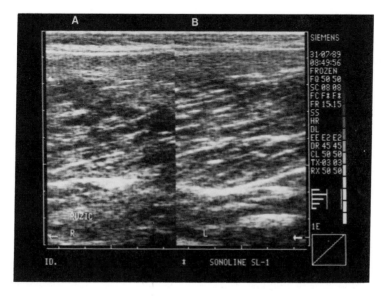

FIGURE 12. Sonogram shows partial rupture of adductor muscles. (A) Rupture; (B) normal muscles.

should be decreased and all motions causing pain avoided (i.e., sudden acceleration or change of direction; an easy-going straight-line run is allowed). When the syndrome is at a later stage of development, the athlete should discontinue his training altogether.

Local cryotherapy of the painful site is aimed at alleviating inflammation. Ice should be applied 4 to 5 times a day for 15 to 20 min (never directly on the skin). Before the activity, heparin or similar ointments together with those causing local hyperemia, i.e., heating, are locally applied.[22,29,33,34] Anti-inflammatory nonsteroid medications are given orally, also with the aim of relieving inflammation. Some authors[13,22,34] recommend local corticosteroid infiltrations. Stretching exercises should be commenced at the same time, starting with static stretching exercises for the adductor muscles. These exercises are performed in a way that the muscle is stretched to the point of pain and kept in the position for 15 to 20 s. The athlete should do the stretching exercises several times a day, but at minimum 3 times. It is especially important that the stretching exercises do not cause additional pain; along with the exercises, cryotherapy is recommended (local application of ice).

The athletes with weak abdominal muscles should work on their strengthening. An equal strengthening is required for both the rectus and oblique abdominal wall muscles.[29,31] The exercises should be performed several times a day. At the beginning, the exercises are repeated only a few times and without any load. Gradually, the number of repetitions and the load are increased.

Athletes who have discontinued their specific training may engage in supplemental activities, purposely maintaining general physical fitness [bicycle riding, swimming (on the back or freestyle)].

The purpose of rehabilitation is to preserve strength, elasticity, and contractual abilities of the tissues along with the improvement of mechanical and structural characteristics of the tissues.

At the beginning of rehabilitation, isometric or static strengthening exercises for the adductor muscles are introduced.[13] When performing isometric exercises, the contraction force should not cause any pain. The training begins with only a few contractions daily; further on, training gradually increases the number of contractions and the total load.

At the stage when isometric training may be performed without pain, a dynamic strength training may be introduced. At the beginning of the adductor muscle dynamic training, the weight of the leg itself is used as a load. Gradually, the load may be increased by adding weight, although this should not be done too fast. Isokinetic training is actually the best one, although it requires special equipment (Cybex). Isokinetic training includes working at a constant speed and maximum resistance along the whole range of movement. At the end of rehabilitation, the athlete may commence with his specific training. The common error is that many tend to resume full athletic engagement too soon, which may lead to repeating treatment. In such a case, instead of approximately 3 months, the treatment may be prolonged to 12 or more months.

Operative treatment of painful groin syndrome, to a certain extent, depends upon the attitude in approaching this complex problem.[1,10,14,16,36,44] The authors who consider tendinitis as the most important feature of the painful groin syndrome recommend operative treatment in terms of disinsertion, i.e., cutting (tenotomy) of the adductor, gracilis, rectus abdominis, piramidalis, and other muscles. The authors who believe that painful groin syndrome is primarily caused by disproportion in strength between the abdominal wall muscles and the upper leg muscles, especially emphasizing weak abdominal muscles (oblique and transverse abdominal muscles in particular), recommend surgical strengthening of the anterior abdominal wall by the method applied for inguinal hernia, i.e., by the Bassini's method.[24]

We agree with the opinion of Quilles,[44] who by praising this operative method, said, "It is more fair to enrich the poor than to impoverish the rich", meaning that it is better to strengthen or support the abdominal muscles than to weaken the adductor muscles by tenotomy. Nevertheless, on the basis of our experience, we have realized that sometimes the disequilibrium and difference are so great that the muscular balance may be achieved only by a combination of "enriching the poor and impoverishing the rich". The fact is that in certain cases, beside strengthening the anterior abdominal wall, the tenotomy of the adductor needs to be done, especially when tendinitis is clinically obvious, e.g., the upper leg long adductor tendinitis. Similar to all other surgeries, postoperative rehabilitation procedure is essential here as well. On the second or third day following surgery, the patient gets up and starts with a moderate dose of static exercises for abdominal muscles accompanied by general physical therapy measures, such as breathing exercises, exercises for proper circulation in the lower extremities, etc. After the stitches are removed and the wound appears satisfactory, swimming, easy walking, and gradual increase in the intensity of exercises for the strengthening of the abdominal wall muscles are recommended. One month after the operation (sometimes even 3 weeks after), the patient is allowed to run easily and to perform regularly his exercises for abdominal wall muscles, gradually increasing the load, but only to the pain limit. After 6 weeks (sometimes 5), a soccer player is allowed to begin with ball training. After 8 weeks (sometimes 6), he is allowed to participate in a training match, while after 10 to 12 weeks (sometimes 8), full participation in athletic activity is allowed. Eventually, it should be pointed out that when discussing treatment of painful groin syndrome, whether operative or nonoperative, the approach should always be an individual one. In this regard, it should be emphasized that procedures may and should be combined and that there is no unique scheme of painful groin treatment. It is also essential to bear in mind that prevention is of utmost importance, especially in young patients, and should be aimed at strengthening the abdominal muscles, particularly the obliques. Exercises for strengthening abdominal muscles are often done so that only the rectus abdominal muscles get strengthened. If exercises are exaggerated, tendinitis may result, i.e., the development of painful groin syndrome. We would like to add here that stretching exercises should be intensified for the upper leg muscles and for the whole lower extremity muscle, especially before and after the athletic activity. The biggest mistake is made when the athlete, his coach, and his physician lose patience, and he returns to his full strain too soon, thus repeatedly causing the recurrence of painful groin syndrome. Such course of events may continue for several years only to end up in definite cessation of any engagement in athletic activities.

From the etiological, diagnostic, and therapeutic points of view, painful groin syndrome is further complicated by the many origins and insertions of muscles and tendons in the pelvic, hip joint, and proximal segment of the upper leg regions as well as the bursal sacs (synovial sacs), all of which may be the site of pathological changes in terms of overuse syndrome. The possibility of stress fracture of bones in these regions should be taken into account, while in younger persons, the possibility of epiphysiolysis and apophysitis should not be ruled out. The nerve entrapment syndromes are also of importance in differential diagnosis.[30]

B. Osteitis Pubis

Osteitis pubis was reported for the first time in 1923 by Rochet.[10] The term itself indicates that inflammatory changes are taking place, although in the majority of cases, no causative agent has been isolated (identified). A number of different terms and phrases have been used in the past with the purpose of avoiding the connotation of inflammation (e.g., osteitis necroticans pubis, syndroma rectus-adductor, traumatic inguino-leg syndrome, anterior pelvic joint syndrome, groin pain in athletes, osteoarthropathy of the pubic symphysis, traumatic pubic osteitis, Pierson's syndrome, pubic chondritis, and posttraumatic osteonecrosis of the pubic bone.[35,43] However, these expressions were also used to denote pelvis stress fractures, adductor tendinitis, avulsion injuries of the adductor tendons, postoperative changes occurring without infection, stress changes in the symphyseal region, and various arthrotic changes.

In a large number of cases, the link between osteitis pubis and urological problems was described as well as postpartal complications.[28]

The condition was reported for the first time as occurring in an athlete (fencer) in 1932 by Spinelli.[39] Only in the early 1960s, to a greater extent, did the study of the condition in athletes begin. Osteitis pubis has been reported in soccer players, U.S. football players, basketball players, long-distance runners (marathon), and long-distance walkers.[28,29,43] As Lloyd-Smith et al.[21] reported on the basis of their research, the condition is more common in men. Among the total number of osseous lesions in the pelvic bones, osteitis pubis ranks third in frequency (14% in males, 6.3% in females). These authors further reported that in 43% of patients, varus alignment has been observed while in 29% of cases, different leg length has been found. So far, etiology is unknown. Steinbach et al.[40] reported that venous obstructions caused by trauma might be the cause, while Goldstein and Rubin[11] reported that osteitis pubis is caused by chronic infection. Wheeler[41] reported on aseptic necrosis as the cause of pubic osteitis.

The patient complains of pain in the lower abdomen and in the groin, but cannot link it to any known injury. At a later stage, the pain spreads in a fan-like manner into the adductor region. The principal characteristics of the pain are that its onset is linked to the athletic activity, then diminishes, and gradually disappears upon resting. The pain may also occur or become more intense when coughing, sneezing, or laughing.[38]

Palpation during clinical examination causes pain along the pubic bone and the symphysis itself.

X-ray of the pelvis shows no changes in the initial phase of the disorder, while later on, the alterations are visible in the symphyseal region (fraying and sclerosis).[28]

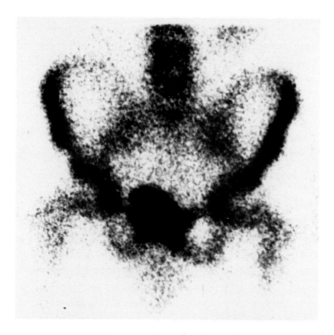

FIGURE 13. Bone scan demonstrating osteitis pubis.

Scintigraphic scan shows increased bilateral accumulation of radionuclides around the pubic bone already in the initial stage of the disease (Figure 13). Scintigraphy helps in differential diagnosis, since in the case of avulsion or stress fracture in the pubic branch region, the accumulation of radionuclides is a unilateral one.[35] Le Jeune[19] reported that in the case of a negative scintigraphic scan and positive clinical signs, the adductor longus and rectus muscles tendinitis is usually in question.

The treatment recommended is reduced athletic activity or complete rest if the pain is too severe. As supplementary activity, swimming may be recommended (free and backstyle only). Pearson[28] recommends administration of nonsteroid anti-inflammatory medication in combination with corticosteroids (10 mg of prednisone daily for 10 d). Prospects for recovery are very good. When athletic activities are avoided, the disease subsides spontaneously. Only the duration of the recovery process may be variable.

II. ILIOPSOAS TENDINITIS AND BURSITIS (PSOAS SYNDROME)

Iliopsoas muscle tendinitis is caused by frequent repetitive flexions in the hip joint (Figure 14). It is common in weight lifters, ski runners, oarsmen, football players, long and high jumpers, and hurdlers.[24,27] Bursitis of the iliopsoas is more common in gymnasts, wrestlers, and uphill runners. The principal clinical sign is pain in the groin region on the anterior aspect of the hip joint, in the small pelvis, and sometimes in the back as well; this is accounted for by the fact that tendinitis and bursitis of the iliopsoas develop as a result of hypertonic muscle and prolonged strain. Overuse or excessive strain may be the consequence of disturbed biomechanical

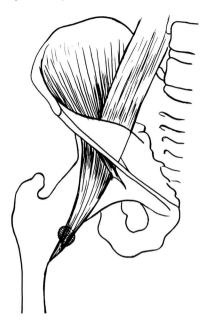

FIGURE 14. Insertion of the iliopsoas tendon to the lesser trochanter. Broken lines indicate the bursa between the tendon and joint capsule.

relations in the lumbar spine and in the hip joint. Initially, the pain is mild in intensity, but the repetitive strain makes it increasingly intense to the degree that the athletic activity becomes impossible. Often the patient cannot find the link between the pain and injury. Palpation of the tendinous attachment to the small trochanter causes pain. If in a patient's sitting position the affected leg is put over the healthy one, i.e., with its heel touching the knee of the unaffected leg, a painful and tense iliopsoas muscle may be palpated. During flexion of the upper leg in the hip joint against resistance, pain occurs at the point of the muscle attachment. The motion should be attempted in a sitting position (Figure 15) because then the iliopsoas muscle is the chief and only flexor of the upper leg in the hip joint. Between the iliopsoas tendon and the anterior aspect of the hip joint articular capsule, there is a nut-size synovial sac; when irritated, it produces a clinical picture of a typical bursitis, reaching its peak on the fourth or fifth day from the onset of pain during and after the athletic activity. Eventually, the activity has to be discontinued entirely.

In differential diagnosis, the following should also be considered: tendinitis of the adductor longus muscle and rectus femoris muscle; rupture and avulsion of the iliopsoas muscle, rectus femoris muscle, and adductor longus muscle.[2] Rupture of the iliopsoas muscle is extremely rare. In most cases, the attachment of the muscle to the small trochanter is the rupture site. The injury most commonly occurs when the upper leg in flexion is forcibly extended. At the moment of injury, the athlete complains of severe pain in the groin region. After the injury, the upper leg is usually kept in flexion, adduction, and external rotation since it is the position of least pain.[31] Each attempt of extension and internal rotation causes severe pain and so does the active contraction of the muscles. At the site of the injury, pain occurs on palpation. Besides ultrasound, X-ray should be made and attention paid to the probability of the avulsion of the small trochanter.[9,42] It is especially important for the younger age groups since in these patients, the epiphysis of the small trochanter is not yet united with the bone shaft. In

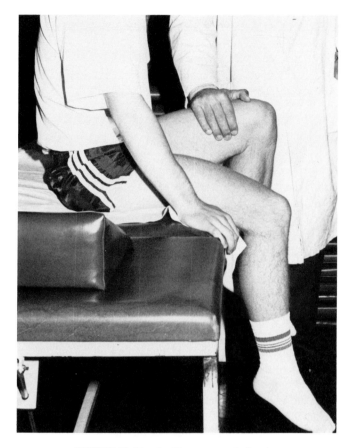

FIGURE 15. Test for iliopsoas muscle function.

the case of complete avulsion, surgery is the only recourse available.[12,26,29] Tendinitis of the iliopsoas muscle is treated nonoperatively. When the patient contacts his physician during the initial stage of the disorder, training should not be completely discontinued but only reduced in intensity. However, if the athlete contacts his physician at a later stage, a restful period from 3 to 4 weeks is necessary. During this time, the athlete may engage in substitute activities, such as swimming or riding on a bicycle. The site of injury is treated with ice for at least 15 min, 3 to 4 times a day (the ice should not come into direct contact with the skin), and anti-inflammatory nonsteroid drugs are administered orally. Renstrom et al.[34] recommend an additional local infiltration of corticosteroids followed by a 2-week rest. At the very beginning of treatment, stretching and static strengthening exercises without load or weight bearing should be commenced.[13] At a later stage, dynamic exercises for strengthening may be introduced, although care should be taken that the patient feels no pain. When the pain is absent, even during maximum load, the athlete is ready to continue his training at full intensity as required for participation in competitions.

III. TENDINITIS OF THE RECTUS FEMORIS MUSCLE

Tendinitis of the rectus femoris muscle usually occurs as a result of prolonged, repetitive, and sudden increase in strengthening exercises training or intensive goal-shooting training, e.g., in soccer. The athlete feels pain in the region above the hip joint at the point where the rectus femoris muscle attaches anteriorly and inferiorly to the iliac spine. The patient is unable to make any connection between the onset of pain and an injury.

Pain appears on palpation of rectus femoris muscle tendon attachment. The pain may also be provoked by resisting the upper leg flexion and lower leg extension.

In differential diagnosis, the following should be taken into consideration: rupture or avulsion of the rectus femoris or iliopsoas muscles, tendinitis of the iliopsoas or adductor longus muscles, stress fracture of the femoral neck, changes in the hip joint (e.g., arthrosis, rheumatoid arthritis, osteochondritis dissecans, loose body in a joint, synovitis), and bursitis.[31,34] Pain in the groin region may develop as a consequence of the rupture at the attachment point or in the proximal third of the rectus femoris muscle. At the moment of injury, the pain is so severe that the athlete is compelled to discontinue his activity. If complete rupture takes place, the muscle cannot be contracted. During palpation of the injured site, pain appears, and often a defect may be palpated on the belly of the muscle. In the attempt of the upper leg flexion against resistance, pain occurs at the site of the injury. Pain in the muscle during extension of the lower leg against resistance is an additional sign of the trauma.

Ultrasound will confirm the diagnosis and enable the evaluation of the severity of injury (Figure 16). X-ray should also be made in order for bone avulsion to be ruled out.

Complete rupture, especially if in combination with avulsion fracture, is treated operatively.[26] Partial rupture is usually treated nonoperatively; during the initial stage, rest, cryotherapy, compression, elevation, and nonsteroid anti-inflammatory medication are prescribed.

Rehabilitation in terms of strengthening the muscles may begin when pain and swelling disappear.[17]

Treatment of rectus femoris muscle tendinitis is very similar to the treatment of overuse syndromes, e.g., tendinitis of the iliopsoas muscle.

IV. HIP EXTERNAL ROTATOR SYNDROME

Although not very often, external hip rotator syndrome presents a complicated problem, with regards to both diagnosis and treatment.[45] It is most frequently found in hurdlers and ballet dancers where the symptoms consist of a vague pain in the buttocks and the greater trochanter area. The inflexibility of the hip external rotators (Figure 17), primarily the piriformis, gemellus superior, and gemellus inferior muscles, together with the internal rotation contracture of the hip, is thought to lead to chronic overuse of these muscles.

To locate the exact area of pain, the upper leg is maximally and externally rotated during physical examination; pressure is applied to the greater trochanter

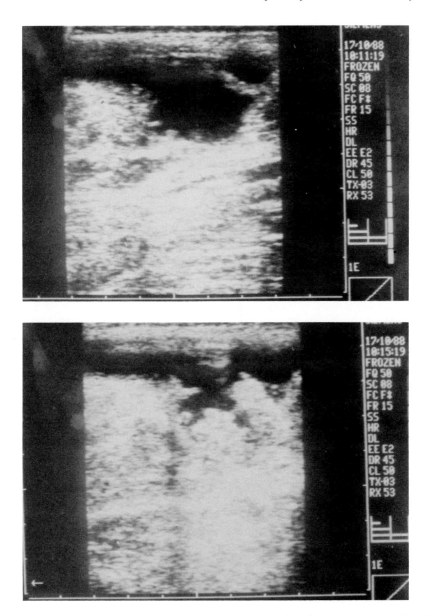

FIGURE 16. Sonogram showing rupture with hematoma of rectus femoris muscle. (A) Relaxation; (B) contraction.

area, producing intense pain. Differential diagnosis must take into account the possibility of piriformis muscle syndrome[46] and trochanteric bursitis, which can be confirmed by ultrasound.

Nonoperative treatment of short external hip rotator syndrome is based on stretching exercises for the afflicted muscle groups and neighboring muscles, with the aim of increasing their flexibility and concurrently the flexibility of the whole hip.

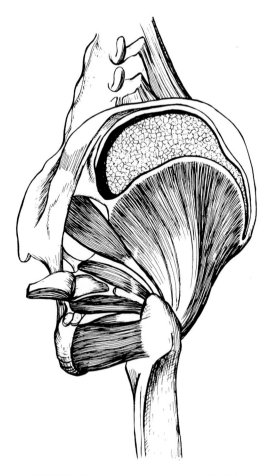

FIGURE 17. External rotator muscles of the hip.

Other nonoperative measures include rest, ice, and nonsteroidal anti-inflammatory drugs. Steroid injections can also be administered.

V. SNAPPING HIP SYNDROME

Snapping hip syndrome is a symptom complex characterized by an audible snapping sensation and usually, but not necessarily, associated with hip pain during certain movements of the hip joint. A number of different etiologies, both intra-articular and extra-articular, have been described.[54,59,61,62] Intra-articular causes for the snapping hip include loose bodies, osteocartilaginous exostosis, osteochondro-matosis, and subluxation of the hip.[57,62] The most frequent extra-articular cause of the snapping hip is the snapping of the iliotibial band over the greater trochanter. For a long time, this was considered to be the only extra-articular cause of snapping hip syndrome, but further researches have indicated other extra-articular etiologies. These include the snapping of the iliopsoas tendon over the iliopectioneal eminence of the pelvis, the iliofemoral ligaments over the femoral head, and the tendinous origin of the long head of the biceps femoris muscle over the ischial tuberosity. Taking into account the localization of the causes for the snapping hip, we recognize three different snapping hip syndromes: medial (internal), lateral (external), and posterior snapping hip syndrome (Table 2).

Medial (internal) snapping hip syndrome is caused either by the snapping of the iliopsoas tendon over the iliopectioneal eminence of the pelvis, as described by Nunziata and Blumenfeld[56] in 1951, or by the snapping of the iliofemoral ligaments over the femoral head, as reported by Howse[52] in 1972. This type of snapping hip syndrome is frequently found in ballet dancers.[59] When leaving the pelvis, the iliopsoas tendon lies in a groove between the anterior-inferior iliac spine laterally and the iliopectineal eminence medially. From there, the tendon inserts on the lesser trochanter passing over an anteromedially placed bony ridge. The snapping of the iliopsoas tendon occurs when the hip is extended from a flexed, abducted, and externally rotated position. The snapping can take place over the anterior-inferior iliac spine, the iliopectioneal eminence, or at the point where the iliopsoas tendon passes over the bony ridge on the lesser trochanter. Besides an audible snapping sound, this movement is also, in some cases, accompanied by a painful sensation in the frontal hip area.

Differential diagnosis includes consideration of psoas bursitis. Frequent movements of the iliopsoas tendon can lead to irritation of the iliopsoas bursa situated between the iliopsoas tendon and the anterior hip capsule; communication exists between them in about 15% of adult hips.[61] This irritation is accompanied by pain in the frontal hip area, which increases typically with resisted hip flexion. Psoas muscle syndrome, which consists of psoas bursitis, enthesitis, and tenosynovitis of the iliopsoas muscle, is therefore a clinical entity that should be differentiated from snapping hip syndrome.

Treatment of medial snapping hip syndrome depends on whether the syndrome is asymptomatic, accompanied only by audible snapping sounds, or whether it is associated with hip pain. Nonoperative treatment consists of reduction of (or tempo-

TABLE 2
Extra-Articular Causes of Snapping Hip

Localization	Etiology
Medial (internal)	Iliofemoral ligament over femoral head
	Iliopsoas tendon over the anterior-inferior iliac spine
	Iliopsoas tendon over the iliopectineal eminence
	Iliopsoas tendon over the bony ridge on the lesser trochanter
Lateral (external)	Iliotibial band over the greater trochanter
	Gluteus maximus tendon over the greater trochanter
Posterior	Tendinous origin of the long head of the biceps femoris muscle over the ischial tuberosity

rary cessation of) painful activities and movements, nonsteroidal anti-inflammatory medication, and stretching exercises.[61] Good results are sometimes obtained by steroid injections. Surgical treatment is indicated in those patients whose painful symptoms persist after prolonged nonoperative therapy. The operative procedure consists of resection of the lesser trochanter bony prominence, transection of the tendinous slip at the level of the groove between the iliopectineal eminence, and anterior-inferior iliac spine, and/or partial or total release of the iliopsoas tendon.[55,57,61]

Lateral (external) snapping hip syndrome is the most frequent, and consequently the best known snapping hip syndrome. It is caused by the slipping of the iliotibial band over the posterior part of the greater trochanter (Figure 18), and is frequent in runners, dancers, and basketball players.[53,57,59–62] It can be asymptomatic or accompanied by pain; it is especially intense in those cases which develop trochanteric

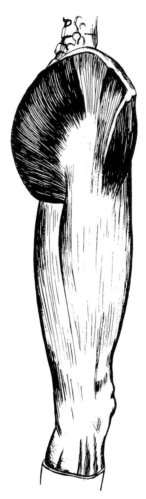

FIGURE 18. Iliotibial band.

TABLE 3
Operations for Painful Snapping Hip

Author (year)	Operation	Ref.
Dickinson (1928)	Simple release of the band	48
Orlandi et al. (1981)	Incision of the band and suturing of the cut ends to the greater trochanter	48
Bruckl et al. (1984)	Diagonal notching of the band and fixation of band to the greater trochanter	49
Fery and Sommelet (1988)	Cruciate incision of the band over the greater trochanter and the four flaps produced are sutured back on themselves or to adjacent structures	51
Asai and Tonnis (1979)	V-Y-plasty	47
Dederich (1983)	Z-plasty	50
Brignall and Stainsby (1991)	Z-plasty	48
Larsen and Johansen (1986)	Resection of the posterior half of the band	54
Zoltan et al. (1986)	Excision of an ellipsoid-shaped portion of the band overlying the greater trochanter	62

bursitis. Besides the audible snapping phenomenon, the symptomatic form is characterized by pain in the region of the greater trochanter, which sometimes radiates to the buttocks and/or lateral thigh. The snapping can best be observed by placing the palm of one's hand on the greater trochanter area of the patient during walking. Another maneuver which will consistently reproduce the patient's symptoms is to have the patient stand on the healthy leg and imitate running motions on the affected side. In some cases, the snapping can only be demonstrated by having the patient lay on the unaffected side with a large pad under the pelvis so that the affected hip is in adduction. Keeping the knee in extension, which tightens the fascia lata, the affected hip is then actively flexed and extended. The iliotibial band can then be felt to flip anteriorly over the greater trochanter as the hip is flexed. The most common cause of the slipping of the iliotibial band over the greater trochanter is its excessive tightness (shortening), which can result from leg length discrepancies, pelvic tilt, or certain activities such as habitual running on the sides of roads. In the latter case, it occurs on the so-called "downside leg", because the drainage pitch of the road causes increased tension in the iliotibial band in this extremity. Tightness of the iliotibial band is diagnosed using Ober's test. Excessive tightness of the iliotibial band causes greater friction between the band, the greater trochanter, and the bursa, which is normally located there; this in turn leads to chronic trochanteric bursitis. Characteristic symptoms of this bursitis include intense pain in the greater trochanter area and limping.

Nonoperative treatment of the lateral (external) snapping hip syndrome consists of rest, avoidance of painful movements, iliotibial band stretching exercises, nonsteroidal anti-inflammatory medication, and correction of the disturbed biomechanical

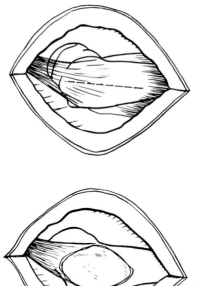

FIGURE 19. Schematic representation of the operative procedure described by Zoltan et al.[62]

relationships of the lower extremities (arch supports, adequate shoes, etc.). Injections of local anesthetics and soluble steroids are also sometimes effective. In refractory cases that do not respond to nonoperative therapy, surgical treatment is indicated. Numerous operative procedures have been described. Operative procedures include resection of a large portion of the greater trochanter or various surgical alterations of the iliotibial band. The latter include the simple release of the iliotibial band, the release and fixation of the cut ends of the band to the greater trochanter, lengthening of the band, and excision of a portion of the band in the greater trochanter area (Table 3).[47–51,61–63] We have successfully used the operative procedure described by Zoltan et al.[62] on our patients (Figure 19). The procedure consists of excising an ellipsoid-shaped portion of the band overlying the greater trochanter; we have termed this procedure as *fenestration* of the iliotibial band.

Posterior snapping hip syndrome is caused by the snapping of the tendinous origin of the long head of the biceps femoris muscle over the proximal part of the ischial tuberosity. Rask[58] has described cases in which the subluxation of this tendon was accompanied by an audible snapping sound, a condition which he termed *snapping bottom*. Differential diagnosis must include considerations of the developed bursitis in this area and enthesitis of the tendon, which we classify as belonging to the hamstring syndrome. Treatment is usually nonoperative.

VI. HAMSTRING SYNDROME

Hamstring syndrome is a condition that affects muscles of the posterior thigh, primarily the semitendinosus, semimembranosus, and biceps femoris muscles (Figure 20). It is frequent in sprinters, hurdlers, and both long and high jumpers, but can also be found in other athletes, especially those who engage in rapid acceleration and short intense sprinting, such as baseball players, football players, tennis players, and others.[67,79] Hamstring syndrome is caused either by the overuse of the muscles at their insertion on the ischial tuberosity, or by the partial or total rupture of an individual muscle. It is a very common sports injury and numerous studies have been devoted to determining the causative factors and possible preventive measures of this typical self-induced injury. One of the reasons for this attention is the well-documented propensity of this syndrome to reoccur (as epitomized by the old saying "once a strain, always a strain").

A. Etiopathogenesis

Numerous authors have tried to determine the predisposing factors that might cause the hamstring muscle group to become strained.[82] O'Neil summarizes some of

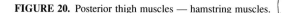

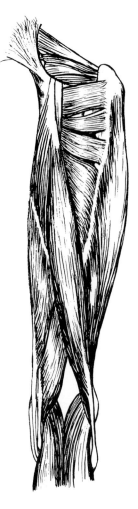

FIGURE 20. Posterior thigh muscles — hamstring muscles.

these factors, such as fatigue, poor posture, improper warm-up, overuse, abnormal muscle contraction, improper conditioning, magnesium imbalance, sepsis, and anatomical variations, as primary causes leading to hamstring strain. Most authors today agree that the basic causative reason for the development of hamstring syndrome is the muscle strength imbalance between the hamstring muscle group and the quadriceps femoris muscle. The normal biomechanics of the lower extremity depend on the smoothly coordinated reciprocal action between the quadriceps and the hamstring muscle group. Unusual stress is placed on the quadriceps and hamstrings mechanism at certain points within the range of motion; this suddenly precipitates injury. Hamstring syndrome will develop, in various forms, when there is a relative weakness of the hamstring muscle group in relationship to the quadriceps femoris muscle. The relationship between the hamstring muscle group and the quadriceps femoris muscle has changed during evolution. Pilardeau et al.[77,78] speculate that the hamstring syndrome is caused by the still inadequate adaptation of modern man to an upright position. For this reason, they classify hamstring syndrome as belonging to *Lucy syndrome,* named after the fossilized remains of an Australopithecus who lived approximately 3 million years ago. The osseous remains of Lucy indicate that she walked in a semi-crouch with habitually flexed knees. Modern man's upright position caused a permanent elongation of the posterior thigh muscles and at the same time shortened the quadriceps muscle in relation to the Australopithecus.

Studies have indicated that the hamstring muscles should have at least 60% of the strength of the quadriceps[18] in athletes; this is often not the case with the hamstrings, which have 40%, and sometimes even less, of the strength of the quadriceps. Unlike the quadriceps, however, hipotrophy of the hamstring muscles is not readily visible, and unlike the unstable knee syndrome, weakened hamstring muscles do not cause severe clinical symptoms. This is one of the basic reasons why strengthening of the hamstring muscle group does not receive enough attention. Hamstring-to-quadriceps muscle strength ratios change during movements in the hip and knee joint. This is further complicated by the fact that the hamstring muscles are primarily biarticular structures that act on both of these joints. During a 60° flexion of the knee, the quadriceps-to-hamstring strength ratio corresponds to 2:1. A ratio of 3:1 is considered a predisposition to hamstring strain. At a 30° knee flexion, the quadriceps-to-hamstring strength ratio becomes 1:1. During the last 20° of this flexion, the mechanical efficiency of the quadriceps muscle in extending the knee begins to decline. However, extension of the knee is enhanced at this point by the synergistic action of the gastrocnemius and hamstring muscles, creating a paradoxical extension moment at the knee in a closed kinetic chain. This example best illustrates the complex relationship existing between the quadriceps and the hamstring muscle group. Hamstring syndrome can also develop as a result of strength deficit between the right and left hamstring muscle groups. A 10% or greater muscle strength deficit between the two sides is also thought to be a predisposition for hamstring strain. Besides the relative or absolute weakness of the hamstring muscles, another, and fairly frequent cause of hamstring syndrome is the decreased flexibility of these muscles. The flexibility of the hamstring muscles is determined by a number of individual characteristics, including sex, age, type and duration of athletic activity, and the specific types of training programs (during the on and off season). Flexibility of the hamstring muscles is commonly measured by the Well's "sit-and-reach" test (Figure 21). The sit-and-reach test calls for the athlete to bend forward while sitting, in an effort to reach to or beyond his toes with his ankles supported in a neutral position. Performance is measured on a ruler placed in front of the athlete's toes. The basic fault of this test is that while it does present a general picture of trunk flexion capability, the results are dependent on the mobility of multiple joints and the extensibility of various soft-tissue structures. The test also does not allow for the relative length of body segments (i.e., in the case of basketball players), or for unilateral conditions. A more appropriate test for the flexibility of the hamstring muscle group has been described by Wallace (Figure 22). The athlete is positioned

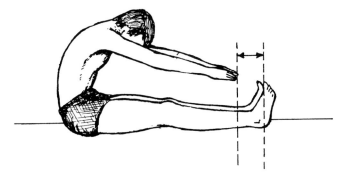

FIGURE 21. Well's test ("sit-and-reach test").

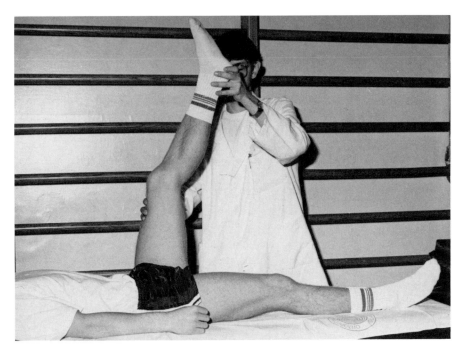

FIGURE 22. Wallace's test.

supine with both hips and knees extended. The athlete flexes the tested hip and knee to 90°, stabilizing the thigh in that position with his hands. From this position, the athlete attempts to straighten the knee into full extension. Decreased flexibility is demonstrated by the number of degrees the athlete lacks from completing full extension of the knee.

The speed at which various muscle fibers contract is also a factor that can contribute to the development of hamstring syndrome. Histochemical studies[65] indicate that the hamstring muscles have a relatively high proportion of type 2 fibers, which are involved with exercises of higher intensity and force production. Strength at high velocities of movement or power can be measured by the high-speed stress test. Aided by various testing equipment, of which the Cybex II is most commonly used, the strength of the hamstring muscles and the hamstring-to-quadriceps muscle strength ratio are isokinetically determined. This test also allows the evaluation of the muscle strength torque curve which typically decreases in size. Isokinetic studies have shown that the quicker loss of strength in the hamstring muscles, when compared to the quadriceps, is a factor that can predispose an athlete to hamstring strain.

In summary, the causes of hamstring strains have been attributed to various factors, the most important of which are muscle strength. This includes both the quadriceps-to-hamstring muscle strength ratio and the strength deficit between the right and left hamstring muscle groups. It also includes the flexibility of both the hamstring muscles and the lower extremities. Generally, when observing levels of flexibility and strength within an athletic population, attention should be directed toward individual variation with respect to such factors as age, level of maturity, sex, specific event or position, and demands that a particular activity place on the individual. An athlete who is below the standards of a specific group of players in flexibility and muscle strength should not be allowed to compete with that group of players as this predisposes him to hamstring injury. Studies have shown[67] that a combination of testing on the Cybex II and moderate training and/or rehabilitation (also with the aid of Cybex II) can help to prevent the development of hamstring syndrome in athletes or its recurrence in already injured athletes.

B. Clinical Picture and Diagnostics

Clinical features of hamstring syndrome that have resulted from overuse of the hamstring muscles at the point of their insertion at the ischial tuberosity include constant pain in the lower gluteal area, which radiates down the posterior thigh to the popliteal area. The pain typically increases during the performance of forcible or sudden movements, which stretch the hamstring muscles (i.e., in sprinting or hurdling). Another characteristic complaint is pain felt while sitting, e.g., while driving a car or sitting during lectures. The pain is often relentless, causing the patient to change position or stand up for relief.

During physical examination, the pain can be reproduced by applying pressure to the ischial tuberosity area. In some cases, it is possible to palpate the tautness of the hamstring muscles. Various clinical tests that cause the stretching of the hamstring muscles also induce pain in the ischial tuberosity area.[69] One of the most common tests has the patient stand by a table and lift the outstretched affected leg on the table. Bending the body forward produces intense pain at the site of the ischial tuberosity. Well's and Wallace's tests also produce pain in the same area. Pećina[76] uses the more exact "shoe wiping" test (Figure 23) The test consists of having the patient imitate movements typically used when wiping shoes on a doormat. The hip and knee are in a position of maximal extension while the hamstring muscles are in retroflexion in the hip. While performing these movements, the hamstring muscles are stretched and, at the same time, in motion, which gives an additional value to this test; this enables the patient to score positive even when scoring negative on other tests. A positive score is indicated by pain in the ischial tuberosity area or along one

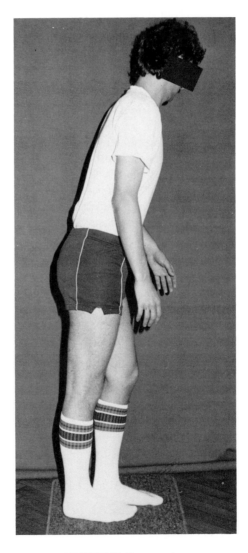

FIGURE 23. Doormat sign.

of the hamstring muscles. Another frequently used test has the patient lie in a prone position with legs extended in the knees and attempt to flex the knee of the afflicted leg. The examiner holds the leg by the ankle and applies a gradually increasing amount of resisting pressure to the flexion which, at a given degree of flexion and resisting pressure to that flexion, produces pain in the ischial tuberosity area. Research done at our department indicates that this is a less reliable test than tests incorporating passive stretching of the hamstring muscles. The best test, in our opinion, is the "shoe wiping" test according to Pećina; this test combines testing the hamstring muscles in a stretched position and in motion. Any diagnosis of hamstring syndrome should include a neurological examination since differential diagnosis includes ruling out the possibility of spinal sciatica. Radiological, electrodiagnostical (EMG), CT, and MRI examinations can be used to achieve this. Piriformis syndrome presents a special problem in differential diagnosis.[74,75] Gluteal pain is the most frequent symptom of this syndrome, although in this case, the tenderness is located more proximally at the buttock, over the belly of the piriformis muscle. Pain caused by resisted abduction in conjunction with external rotation of the thigh (Pace's sign) and the test for piriformis syndrome, according to Pećina, are commonly used tests for this syndrome. The latter test is performed by having the patient stand in an upright position with the afflicted leg maximally rotated internally and then bending forward. This typically causes pain as the ischiadicus is stretched over the passively extended piriformis. The test can also be performed in a lying position with the patient lying supine with his leg maximally and internally rotated and extended in the knee. Pain is produced by trying to lift the afflicted leg from the surface. Ischiogluteal bursitis also causes buttock pain similar to that of hamstring syndrome. It differs from it in that the pain is also felt at rest, and patients have difficulties in finding a comfortable position at night. Chronic compartment syndrome also causes pain in the posterior thigh, especially during exercise, but there is no gluteal pain while sitting.

Hamstring syndrome, as we have already mentioned, can also be caused by a partial rupture of one of the hamstring muscles. Most authors agree that the most commonly ruptured muscle is the biceps femoris. The patient usually remembers the exact moment he heard the sound, or felt the "tearing", or simply felt a sharp pain in the posterior thigh. Depending on the degree of rupture, which some authors divide into slight, moderate, and severe, the patient can, in some cases, resume athletic activities. However, the pain will intensify during the following 3 to 6 h in moderate and slight ruptures and during the following 30 min in severe ruptures. Careful physical examination of the patient can reveal the exact location of the injury, which corresponds to the area of greatest pain. All movements causing greater stretching of the injured muscle typically produce pain along the whole muscle. In severe cases, visible bleeding on the skin will appear with characteristic changes in color from blue to brown descending all the way down to the knee. Ultrasound examination has greatly fascilated diagnosis.[64,68,71,73] Detailed ultrasound examination of the injured muscle, in both the longitudinal and transverse projections, and in a relaxed and contracted state, can reveal a hematoma in the muscle visible in the shape of a diffusely limited area of irregular shape (Figure 24). Ultrasound examination can also reveal fibrous scar tissue caused by previous hamstring muscle tear or tears. In

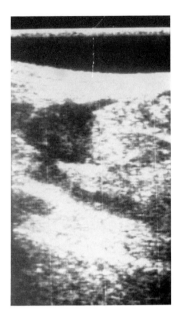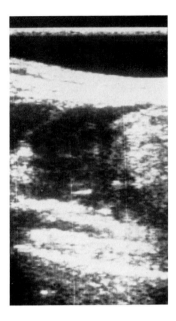

FIGURE 24. Sonogram of the posterior thigh demonstrating hematoma in the biceps femoris muscle. (A) Relaxation; (B) Contraction.

younger patients, roentgenographic diagnosis is also indicated because avulsions of the ischial tuberosity are possible, which manifests with similar symptoms.

C. Treatment

Treatment of injured hamstring muscles can best be summarized with the old saying "the best treatment is prevention". This applies both to injuries resulting from overuse at the insertion of the muscles on the ischial tuberosity and from rupture of the muscle. However, once an injury does take place, the starting therapy is based on the principles of RICE (*r*est, *i*ce, *c*ompression, and *e*levation). After 24 to 36 h, ice is removed and heat is applied to the injured area. This quickens the circulation to help the healing process. After a couple of days during which the pain gradually recedes, the patient begins stretching exercises. The proper execution of these exercises is of the greatest importance. The patient must remain in the position of greater nonpainful extension for 15 s. At this stage of treatment, nonsteroidal anti-inflammatory drugs can also be used. Strengthening of the hamstring muscles is also a part of the rehabilitation process. Garrick and Webb[66] note that the biggest mistake is to concentrate only on stretching exercises. The hamstring muscles, just like all the other muscles, regain their normal functional flexibility only and at the same time, when they regain their normal muscle strength. There is no better example for the saying "a weak muscle is a tightened muscle" than an injured hamstring muscle that has been inadequately rehabilitated. Another important factor in the rehabilitation process is advising both the athlete and his trainer that an unnecessarily quick return to full training accompanied by inadequate warm-ups while ignoring stretching exercises before and after training can, and often does, lead to the recurrence of a hamstring injury.[84] The return to normal training depends on the severity of the injury, and the final decision can be made only after a careful assessment of the whole rehabilitation program based on day-to-day examinations. Treatment of hamstring syndrome that has developed as a result of overuse at its origin on the ischial tuberosity is usually nonoperative. It consists of a rehabilitation program of stretching exercises and strengthening of the hamstring muscles.[72,83] Physical procedures commonly applied to all chronic overuse syndromes are also applicable as are nonsteroidal anti-inflammatory drugs. On rare occasions, corticosteroids are locally applied. Surgical treatment as recommended by Puranen and Orava[79] consists of cutting and dividing the tendinous tissue near the site of origin of the hamstring muscles without loosening the muscles from the ischial tuberosity. After division, the tendon ends should be completely separated from each other. The sciatic nerve must also be freed from any tendinous parts of the hamstring muscle. Puranen and Orava[80] reported that 52 of the 59 operated patients were completely relieved following this operation.

REFERENCES

Groin Pain

1. **Benezis, C.** Syndrome de surmenage inguino-pubiens. In: *Microtraumatologie du Sport.* Rodineau, J. and Simon, L. Paris: Masson, 1990.
2. **Booher, J. M. and Thibdeau, G. A.** *Athletic Injury Assessment.* St Louis: Mosby College Publishing, 1986.
3. **Brunet, B., Imbert, J. C., and Brunet-Guedj, E.** Les pubalgies: etiopathogenie, diagnostic et traitement medical. In: *Muscles, Tendons et Sport.* Benezis, C., Simeray, J., and Simon, L. Paris: Masson, 1990.
4. **Collins, K., Wagner, M., Peterson, K., and Storey, M.** Overuse injuries in triathletes. A study of the 1986 Seafair Triathlon. *Am. J. Sports Med.,* 1989; 17:675–680.
5. **Durey, A., Boeda, A., Merville, L., Cabot, J. R., et al.** *Medicine du Football.* Paris: Masson, 1978.
6. **Ekberg, O., Persson, N. H., Abrahamsson, P., Westlin, N. E., and Lilja, B.** Long standing groin pain in athletes. A multidisciplinary approach. *Sports Med.,* 1988; 6:56–61.
7. **Ekstrand, J. and Gillquist, J.** Soccer injuries and their mechanisms: a prospective study. *Med. Sci. Sports Exerc.,* 1983; 15:267–270.
8. **Estwanik, J. J., Sloane, B., and Rosenberg, M. A.** Groin strain and other possible causes of groin pain. *Phys. Sportsmed.,* 1990; 18:54–65.
9. **Fernbach, S. K. and Wilkinson, R. H.** Avulsion injuries of the pelvis and proximal femur. *AJR,* 1981; 581–584.
10. **Fricker, A. P., Taunton, J. E., and Ammann, W.** Osteitis Pubis in athletes. Infection, inflammation or injury? *Sports Med.,* 1991; 12:266–279.
11. **Goldstein, A. E. and Rubin, S. W.** Osteitis pubis following suprapubic prostatectomy: results with deep roentgen therapy. *Am. J. Surg.,* 1947; 74:480–487.

12. **Grisogono, V.** *Sports Injuries.* London: John Murray, 1984.

13. **Hess, G. P., Capiello, W. L., Poole, R. M., and Hunter, S. C.** Prevention and treatment of overuse tendon injuries. *Sports Med.,* 1989; 8:371–384.

14. **Jaeger, J. H.** La pubalgie. Hypothese pathogenique, techniques operatoires, casuistique, resultats et indications. *Sport Med.,* 1982; 21:28–32.

15. **Jaeger, J. H.** La pubalgie. In: *Lesions Traumatiques des Tendons chez le Sportif.* Catonne, Y. and Saillant, G. Paris: Masson, 1992.

16. **Janković G.** Mehanika i etiopatogeneza nastanka oštećenja u područ ju simfize kod nogometa a. *Magisterij.* Zagreb: Medicinski fakultet Sveu ili´cta u Zagrebu, 1976.

17. **Kulund, D. N.** *The Injured Athlete,* 2nd ed. Philadelphia: J. B. Lippincott, 1988, 423–425.

18. **La Cava, G.** L'enthesite ou maladie des insertions. *Press Med.,* 1959; 67:9.

19. **Le Jeune, J. J., Rocheongar, P., Vazalle, F., Bernard, A. M., Herry, J. Y., and Ramee, A.** Pubic pain syndrom in sportsmen: comparison of radiographic and scintigraphic findings. *Eur. J. Nucl. Med.,* 1984; 9:250–253.

20. **Liebert, P. L., Lombardo, J. A., and Belhobek, G. H.** Acute posttraumatic pubic symphisis instability in an athlete. *Phys. Sportsmed.,* 1988; 16:87–90.

21. **Lloyd-Smith, R., Clement, D. B., McKenzie, D. C., and Taunton, J. E.** A survey of overuse and traumatic hip and pelvic injuries in athletes. *Phys. Sportsmed.,* 1985; 13:131–141.

22. **Martens, M. A., Hansen, L., and Mulier, J. C.** Adductor tendinitis and muscles rectus abdominis tendopathy. *Am. J. Sports Med.,* 1987; 15:353–356.

23. **Muckle, D. S.** Associated factors in recurrent groin and hamstring injuries. *Br. J. Sports Med.,* 1982; 16:37–39.

24. **Nešović, B.** Bolni sindrom simfize kod sportista i mogućnosti njegovog liječenja. U: Povrede u sportu i njihovo liječenja, SFKJ, Beograd, 1988; 104–113.

25. **Nielsen, A. B. and Yde, J.** Epidemiology and traumatology of injuries in soccer. *Am. J. Sports Med.,* 1989; 17:803–807.

26. **O'Donoghue, D. H.** *Treatment of Injuries to Athletes.* 4th ed. Philadelphia: W. B. Saunders, 1984.

27. **O'Toole, M. L., Hiller, D. B., Smith, R. A., and Sisk, T. D.** Overuse injuries in ultraendurance triathletes. *Am. J. Sports Med.,* 1989; 17:514–518.

28. **Pearson, R. L.** Osteitis pubis in a basketball player. *Phys. Sportsmed.,* 1988; 16:69–72.

29. **Pećina, M. and Bojanić, I.** Overuse injuries in track and field athletes. *Croat. Sports Med. J.,* 1991; 6:24–37.

30. **Pećina, M., Krmpotić-Nemanić, J., and Markiewitz, A. D.** *Tunnel Syndromes.* Boca Raton: CRC Press, 1991.

31. **Peterson, L. and Renstrom, P.** *Sports Injuries: Their Prevention and Treatment.* London: Martin Dunitz, 1988.

32. **Pilardeau, P., Richard, R., Pignel, R., Mussi, R., and Teillet, T.** Le syndrome de Lucy. *J. Traumatol. Sport.,* 1990; 7:171–175.

33. **Renstrom, P. and Johanson, R.** Overuse injuries in sports: a review. *Sports Med.,* 1985; 2:316–333.

34. **Renstrom, P. and Peterson, L.** Groin injuries in athletes. *Br. J. Sports Med.,* 1980; 14:30–36.

35. **Rold, J. F. and Rold, B. A.** Pubic stress symphysitis in a female distance runner. *Phys. Sportsmed.,* 1986; 14:61–65.

36. **Schneider, P. G.** Leistenschmerz: Operative Therapiemoglichkeiten, *Orthopade,* 1980; 9:190–192.

37. **Smedberg, S. G., Broome, A. E., Elmer, O., and Gullmo, A.** Herniography in the diagnosis of obscure groin pain. *Acta Chir. Scand.,* 1985; 151:663–667.

38. **Smedberg, S. G., Broome, A. E., Gullmo, A., and Ross, H.** Herniography in athletes with groin pain. *Am. J. Surg.,* 1985; 149:378–382.
39. **Spinelli, A.** Una nuova malattia sportiva: la pubalgia degli schermitori. *Ortop. Traumatol. Appar. Mot.,* 1932; 4:111–127.
40. **Steinbach, H. L., Petrakis, N. L., Gilfillan, R. S., and Smith, D. R.** Pathogenesis of osteitis pubis. *J. Urol.,* 1955; 74:840–846.
41. **Wheeler, W. K.** Periostitis pubis following suprapubic cystotomy. *J. Urol.,* 1941; 45:467–475.
42. **Wiese, H., Niers, B. A. M., Huisman, P. M., and Taconis, W. K.** An unusual swelling in the groin. *Eur. J. Radiol.,* 1990; 10:156–158.
43. **Wiley, J. J.** Traumatic osteitis pubis: the gracillis syndrome. *Am. J. Sports Med.,* 1983; 11:360–363.
44. **Witvoet, J.** *Lesions Osteotendineuses des Sportifs. Conf. d'Enseignement, No. 19.* Paris: Expansion Scientifique Francaise, 1979.

Hip External Rotator Syndrome

45. **Hunter, S. C. and Poole, R. M.** The chronically inflamed tendon. *Clin. Sports Med.,* 1987; 6:371–387.
46. **Pećina, M.** Piriformis syndrome in differential diagnosis of low back pain. *Acta Orthop. Iugosl.,* 1975; 6:196–200.

Snapping Hip Syndrome

47. **Asai, H. and Tonnis, D.** Die Verlangerung des Tractus iliotibialis zur Behandlung der Schnappenden Hufte. *Orthop. Praxis.,* 1979; 15:128–130.
48. **Brignall, C. G. and Stansby, G. D.** The snapping hip. Treatment by Z-plasty. *J. Bone Joint Surg.,* 1991; 73B:253–254.
49. **Bruckl, R., Rosemeyer, B., Schmidt, J. M., and Froschl, M.** Zur operativen Behandlung der Schnappenden Hufte. *Z. Orthop.,* 1984; 122:308–313.
50. **Dederich, R.** Die Schnappende Hufte erweiterung des Tractus Iliotibialis durch Z-plastik. *Z. Orthop.,* 1983; 121:168–170.
51. **Fery, A. and Sommelet, J.** La hanche a ressaut: resultats tardifs de vingt-trois cas operes. *Int. Orthop. (SICOT),* 1988; 12:277–282.
52. **Howse, A. J. G.** Orthopaedists aid ballet. *Clin. Orthop.,* 1972; 89:52–63.
53. **Jacobs, M. and Young, R.** Snapping hip phenomenon among dancers. *Am. Correct. Ther. J.,* 1978; 32:92–98.
54. **Larsen, E. and Johansen, J.** Snapping hip. *Acta Orthop. Scand.,* 1986; 57:168–170.
55. **Lyons, J. C. and Peterson, L. F. A.** The snapping iliopsoas tendon. *Mayo Clin. Proc.,* 1984; 59:327–329.
56. **Nunziata, A. and Blumenfeld, I.** Cadeva a restorte. A proposito de una variedad. *Prensa Med. Argent.,* 1951; 38:1997–2001.
57. **O'Neill, D. B. and Micheli, L. J.** Overuse injuries in the young athlete. *Clin. Sports Med.,* 1988; 7:591–610.
58. **Rask, M. R.** Snapping bottom: subluxation of the tendon of the long head of the biceps femoris muscle. *Muscle Nerve,* 1980; 3:250–251.
59. **Reid, D. C.** Prevention of hip and knee injuries in ballet dancers. *Sports Med.,* 1988; 6:295–307.
60. **Sammarco, J. G.** Diagnosis and treatment in dancers. *Clin. Orthop.,* 1984; 187:176–187.

61. **Schaberg, J. E., Harper, M. C., and Allen, W. C.** The snapping hip syndrome. *Am. J. Sports Med.,* 1984; 12:361–365.
62. **Zoltan, D. J., Clancy, W. G., Jr., and Keene, J. S.** A new operative approach to snapping hip and refractory trochanteric bursitis in athletes. *Am. J. Sports Med.,* 1986; 14:201–204.
63. **Weyer, R. and Tonnis, D.** Eine Untersuchungsmethode zum Machweis der Schnappenden Hufte. *Z. Orthop.,* 1980; 118:895–896.

Hamstring Syndrome

64. **Fornage, B. D. and Rifkin, M. D.** Ultrasound examination of tendons. *Radiol. Clin. N. Am.,* 1988; 26:87–107.
65. **Garret, W. E., Califf, J. C., and Bassett, F. H. III.** Histochemical correlates of hamstring injuries. *Am. J. Sports Med.,* 1984; 12:98–103.
66. **Garrick, J. G. and Webb, D. R.** *Sports Injuries: Diagnosis and Management.* Philadelphia: W. B. Saunders, 1990.
67. **Heiser, T. M., Weber, J., Sullivan, G., et al.** Prophylaxis and management of hamstring muscle injuries in intercollegiate football players. *Am. J. Sports Med.,* 1984; 12:368–370.
68. **Hannesschlager, G. and Rudelberger, W.** Real-Time-Sonographie bei sportspezifischen Sehnenverletzungen. *Sportverletzung Sportschaden,* 1988; 2:133–146.
69. **Kibler, W. B., Chandler, T. J., Uhl, T., et al.** A musculoskeletal approach to the preparticipation physical examination. *Am. J. Sports Med.,* 1989; 17:525–531.
70. **Kulund, D. N.** *The Injured Athletes.* 2nd ed. Philadelphia: J. B. Lippincott, 1988.
71. **Matasović T., et al.** Diagnostic *Ultrasound of the Locomotor System.* Zagreb: Skolska Knjiga, 1990.
72. **Mattalino, A. J., Deese, J. M., Jr., and Campbell, E. D., Jr.** Office evaluation and treatment of lower extremity injuries in the runner. *Clin. Sports Med.,* 1989; 3:461–475.
73. **Mellerowicz, H., Stelling E., and Kefenbaum, A.** Diagnostic ultrasound in the athlete's locomotor system. *Br. J. Sport Med.,* 1990; 24:31–39.
74. **Pećina, M.** Contribution to the ethiological explanation of the piriformis syndrome. *Acta Anat. (Basel),* 1979; 105:181–187.
75. **Pećina, M., Krmpotić-Nemanić, J., and Markiewitz, A. D.** *Tunnel Syndromes.* Boca Raton: CRC Press, 1991.
76. **Pećina, M. and Bojanić, I.** Overuse injuries in track and field athletes. *Croat. Sports Med. J.,* 1991; 6:24–37.
77. **Pilardeau, P., Richard, R., Pignel, R., Mussi, R., and Teillet, T.** Le syndrome de Lucy. *J. Traumatol. Sport.,* 1990; 7:171–175.
78. **Pilardeau, P., Pignel, R., Sezneec, J. C., Sardi, O., Cereuil, V., and Teillet, T.** L'appareil extenseur de la jambe dans le syndrome de Lucy. *Actual. Sport Med.,* 1991; 12:45–47.
79. **Puranen, J. and Orava, S.** The hamstring syndrome. *Am. J. Sports Med.,* 1988; 16:517–521.
80. **Turanen, J. and Orava, S.** The hamstring syndrome — a new gluteal sciatica. *Ann. Chir. Gynaecol.,* 1991; 80:212–214.
81. **Soldmonow, M., Baratta, R., and D'Ambrosia, R.** The role of the hamstrings in the rehabilitation of the ACL deficient knee in athletes. *Sports Med.,* 1989; 7:42–48.
82. **Sutton, G.** Hamstring by hamstring strains. A review of the literature. *J. Orthop. Sport. Phys. Ther.,* 1984; 5:184–195.

83. **Torg, J. S., Vegso, J. J., and Torg, E.** *Rehabilitation of Athletic Injuries: An Atlas of Therapeutic Exercise.* Chicago: Year Book Medical Publishers, 1987, 107–110.
84. **Williford, H. N., East, J. B., Smith, F. H., et al.** Evaluation of warm-up for improvement in flexibility. *Am. J. Sports Med.,* 1986; 14:316–319.

Chapter 7

The Knee

I. OVERUSE INJURIES AROUND THE KNEE JOINT

The knee is a frequently injured joint in athletic and recreational activities. According to some statistics, one half, or possibly even more, of all sports-related injuries incurred in the knee joint. The precise statistics differ between various athletic activities and depend upon the specific movements habitually performed in these activities. Overuse injuries are also frequent in the knee joint; the reasons for this are that the knee joint participates in all sports activities (running, jumping, kicking, etc.) plus its joint area is characterized by numerous attachment sites for muscles and their tendons as well as by numerous bursae. It is also because the specific joint between the patella and the femur (articulatio femoropatellaris) constitutes a part of the knee joint. The previous reasons amply explain why as much as 40% of all overuse injuries occurring in runners develop in the knee joint area. Overuse injuries in runners develop significantly less frequently in the Achilles tendon (15%), in the medial area of the lower leg (15%), in the hip and groin (15%), in the foot (10%), and in the lower back (5%). The impressive frequency of overuse injuries in the knee explains the existence of a special term to describe them, *runner's knee*. The term, runner's knee, however, is used to describe two different localizations of the overuse injuries in the knee. In recent times, this term has been used to describe the friction of the iliotibial band over the lateral femoral epicondyle, while today it is applied to the painful patellofemoral syndrome. This syndrome is also frequently described by the pathological changes in the cartilage of the joint surfaces of the patella as chondromalacia, or likewise, is also known as malalignment of the extensor system of the knee (malalignment of the patella). Speaking in general terms, all overuse injuries in the knee can be differentiated, depending on their anatomical localization, into four groups (Table 1).

As Table 1 shows, there are numerous possible reasons for anterior knee pain. We would, however, like to stress at this point that Table 1 primarily consists of chronic causes that lead to the development of anterior knee pain. The reason for this is that anterior knee pain caused by acute reasons (i.e., meniscus injury) completely disappears after a certain period of time if correct therapy is applied.

Irregularities in the course of the patella and malalignment of the extensor system of the knee are all described when talking about pain in patellofemoral syndrome (chondromalacia patella). For this reason, we feel it is imperative to clearly

TABLE 1
Overuse Injuries Around the Knee Joint

Anterior aspect
Patellofemoral pain syndrome
Jumper's knee
Osgood-Schlatter's disease
Sinding-Larson-Johansson's disease
Stress fracture of the patella
Fat pad syndrome

Medial aspect
Plica syndrome
Semimembranosus tendinitis
Pes anserinus tendinitis/bursitis
Breastroker's knee
Medial retinaculitis

Lateral aspect
Iliotibial band friction syndrome
Popliteal tendinitis
Bicipital tendinitis

Posterior
Fabelitis
Gastrocnemius strain

define the terms *patellar malalignment, chondromalacia of the patella*, and *anterior knee pain.*

II. PATELLOFEMORAL JOINT

A. Patellar Malalignment

Malalignment of the extensor system of the knee is difficult to define, a fact which perhaps will be easier to understand when one takes into consideration that it is equally difficult to define a well-aligned extensor system of the knee. Perhaps the easiest way to define it is to say that malalignment of the extensor system of the knee entails changes in the architecture of the patellofemoral joint, which in turn changes the relationship between the patellar stabilizers leading to excessive tightness in some and insufficiency in others. Malalignment of the extensor system of the knee also leads to an incorrect distribution of strain in the patellofemoral joint, resulting in increased pressure in certain areas of patellofemoral contact.

Until the 1980s, malalignment of the knee extensor system was nondynamically investigated while the relationship between the patella and the femoral trochlea was studied solely by means of axial radiographic pictures of the patella.

The first significant contribution to solving the problem of malalignment of the knee extensor system was made in 1979 by Larson.[9] His research indicated that in evaluating the orientation of the extensor system of the knee, special emphasis must be placed on the patellar stabilizers and their function, as well as to the orientation of the lower extremity, i.e., anatomical deviations of the lower extremity. Larson[9] differentiated between three groups of causative factors that resulted in malalignment of the knee extensor system: (1) changed (disturbed) relationships in the patellofemoral joint, (2) irregularities in the patellar stabilizers, and (3) malalignment of the lower extremity which affects the function of the patellofemoral joint. In the first group of causative factors resulting in malalignment of the knee extensor system, Larson cites abnormal tilting and/or displacement of the patella in the mediolateral direction, displasia and hypoplasia of the femoral trochlea, and displacement of the patella in the proximodistal direction — patella alta and patella infera. The second group consists of atrophy and/or high insertion site of the vastus medialis muscle ("dimple sign"[31]), excessive looseness of the medial stabilizers of the patella, which can result from trauma or a generalized lacity of the joints, and excessive tightness of the lateral stabilizers of the patella (vastus lateralis muscle, lateral patellar retinacul, and patellofemoral ligament). Anatomical deviations of the lower extremity which, ac-

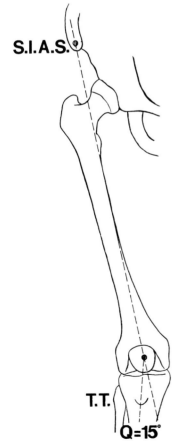

S.I.A.S.

T.T.

Q=15°

FIGURE 1. Schematic representation of the Q-angle.

cording to Larson[9], have an adverse effect on the function of the patellofemoral joint include excessive anteversion of the femoral head and neck, internal rotation of the femoral body, external rotation of the tibia, genu valgum, and lateral insertion of the patellar ligament. These causative factors can clinically be determined by an increased Q-angle (Figure 1). Larson[9] points out that in the vast majority of cases, a combination of the previously mentioned causes is present and that malalignment of the knee extensor system is not always accompanied by pain or other disturbances in the patellofemoral joint. It is also stressed that during clinical examination of a patient who exhibits the symptomatology characteristic of patellofemoral joint, the physician should direct his attention towards defining the underlying causative factors that led to the development of malalignment of the extensor system. The basic principle of therapy consists of correcting these underlying causative factors.

Based on the preceding differentiation of causative factors, Gecha and Torg[26] reported on deviations of the knee extensor system most frequently encountered in patients with patellofemoral pain:

A. Changed relationships in the patellofemoral joint:
  1. shallow femoral trochlea
  2. hypoplastic lateral femoral condyle
  3. deficient medial patellar facet
  4. chondromalacia of the patella and/or of the femoral trochlea
  5. osteochondral defect of the patella and/or the femoral trochlea

B. Parapatellar soft-tissue support abnormalities:
  1. tight lateral parapatellar soft tissue
    a) tight lateral retinaculum
    b) tight lateral patellofemoral or patellotibial bands
    c) presence of a band between patella and iliotibial or the vastus lateralis muscle
  2. vastus medialis obliquus muscle deficiency
  3. attenuated medial parapatellar soft tissue structures
  4. hypermobility of the patella
    a) isolated patellar hypermobility
    b) associated with generalized ligamentous lacity
    c) associated with patella alta
    d) associated with genu recurvatum

C. Lower extremity malalignment:
  1. increased Q-angle (greater than 15°)
  2. increased femoral anteversion
  3. increased external rotation of the tibia
  4. increased genu valgum
  5. foot hyperpronation

In 1988, Teitge pointed out[72] all of the mistakes made during the evaluation of the orientation of the knee extensor system. His investigation showed that the orientation should be evaluated in all three planes — both in rest and during active movement. According to Teitge,[72] this is necessary because the characteristics of some factors that determine the orientation of the knee extensor system change when placed under stress, when the knee is in a bent position, when changes occur in the rotation of the femur and/or tibia, and when under some other circumstances. Teitge reported[72] that in the frontal plane, the physician should take into consideration the value of the Q-angle, the rotation of the patella (clockwise or counterclockwise), and the orientation of the tibiofemoral joint — genu valgum or genu varum. An evaluation of the orientation in the sagittal plane should consider the position of the patella: its height (patella alta or infera), inclination (proximal or distal), and displacement (anterior or posterior). Besides the preceding, a detailed investigation should define the possible presence of flexion or extension contracture of the knee, which can develop either as a consequence of bony changes, or more frequently, as a consequence of soft-tissue changes. Excessive tightness, i.e., shortening of some tissues such as the hamstrings, iliotibial band, and/or rotators of the hip, causes excessive strain to the patellofemoral joint. In the horizontal plane, special emphasis must be placed on identifying the possible presence of anatomical deviations of the femur, tibia, and the upper and lower foot joints, such as excessive anteversion of the femoral head and neck, internal torsion of the femur, excessive external rotation of the lower leg, and hyperpronation of the foot. Consideration should also be placed on the position of the patella, its possible displacement (either medially or laterally), and tilt of the patella (medial or lateral) (Figure 2).

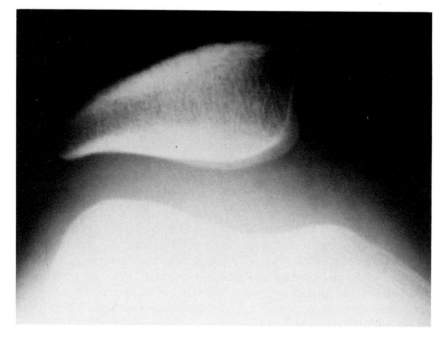

FIGURE 2. Axial roentgenogram of 30° knee flexion demonstrating tilt of the patella.

B. Chondromalacia of the Patella

The term *chondromalacia patellae* (chondromalacia of the patella), was introduced into medical literature by Konig in 1924.[28] Dugdale and Barnett[18] are, however, of the opinion that the term was first used by Aleman[18] and that the term chondromalacia of the patella became generally known and used only after the publication of Aleman's paper in 1927. Six years later, in 1933, Kulowski[18] introduced this term into English medical literature.

Budinger[22] was the first (in 1906) to notice changes in the patellar cartilage. Budinger, as well as Ludloff and Axhusen,[22] later attributed these changes to the effects of trauma. Numerous authors have investigated the causes leading to the development of chondromalacia of the patella. In our opinion, the most concise report is the one submitted by Morscher,[56] according to whom the etiology of chondromalacia of the patella can be classified into six groups:

1. trauma and mechanical overloading
2. anatomical variations (Wiberg types 3 and 4 and "Hunter's hat" form; Outerbridge ridge, bipartite patella, high riding patella, etc.)
3. disturbance in alignment of the patella
4. alteration of the gliding path of the patella
5. nutritional disturbance of cartilage
6. hormonal factors

Because changes in the patellofemoral joint cartilage are not always clinically visible, it is hard to get a reasonable idea of the incidence of these changes. Aleman,[18] based on 220 arthrotomies of the knee in a population of soldiers, reported a 33% incidence rate.

In 1926, Heine[18] reported an 80% frequency of patellar cartilage change in his sample of patients between the ages of 50 to 59 years. Owre noticed an even greater frequency of patellar cartilage change in his sample of patients belonging to the same age group, but also reported a slight incidence of patellar cartilage change in adolescents.[18]

Wiles et al.[18] pointed out that patellar cartilage change was, to some degree, present in all of the adult knees they examined. Contrary to the results obtained by Wiles et al., Outerbridge[58] has found patellar cartilage change in only 56 out of 133 patients who have undergone open medial meniscectomy. Analysis of the patellofemoral joint of the knee after meniscectomy showed a decrease of contact surfaces, and altered distribution and magnitude of stresses on the side of meniscectomy.[19] An investigation carried out by Marrara and Pillay, which also deserves to be mentioned, indicated only a 50% frequency of patellar cartilage change in their group of patients with a mean age of 68 years.[18] Similar results were obtained by Casscells in 1978,[10] who noticed significant patellar cartilage changes in 37% of his patients and slight patellar cartilage changes in 25% of his patients. The analyzed sample consisted of elderly patients with a mean age of 70 years.

Numerous and different categorization systems of chondromalacia of the patella are found in medical literature, depending on the state and characteristics of the change in the cartilage of the patellofemoral joint and with regards to the size and localization of these changes.[33] Table 2 shows the most frequent ones encountered today. Besides the men-

TABLE 2
Review of Classification Symptoms of Articular Cartilage Lesions

Author	Surface descriptions of articular cartilage		Diameter		Location
Outerbridge	I:	softening and swelling	I:	none	Starts most frequently on medial facet of patella; later extends to lateral facet 'minor' lesion on intercondylar area of femoral condyles; upper border medial femoral condyle.
	II:	fragmentation and fissuring	II:	<1/2 in.	
	III:	fragmentation and fissuring	III:	>1/2 in.	
	IV:	erosion of cartilage down to bone	IV:	none	
Bentley	I:	fibrillation or fissuring	I:	<5 cm	Most common at junction of medial and odd facets of patella.
	II:	fibrillation or fissuring	II:	5 -1.0 cm	
	III:	fibrillation or fissuring	III:	1.0–2.0 cm	
	IV:	fibrillation with or without exposure of subchondral bone.	IV:	>2.0 cm	
Casscells	I:	superficial area of erosion	I:	< or =1 cm	Patella and anterior femoral surfaces.
	II:	deeper layers of cartilage involved	II:	1–2 cm	
	III:	cartilage is completely eroded and bone is exposed	III:	2–4 cm	
	IV:	articular cartilage completely destroyed	IV:	"wide area"	
Insall	I:	swelling and softening of cartilage (closed chondromalacia)	None		I–IV: midpoint of patellar crest with extension equally onto medial and lateral patellar facets.
	II:	deep fissures extending to subchondral bone			
	III:	fibrillation			IV: also involves opposite or mirror surface of femur.
	IV:	erosive changes and exposures of subchondral bone (osteoarthrosis)			Upper and lower 1/3 nearly always spared (patella); femur never severe.

tioned classification systems, Outerbridges classification is most frequently used.[58] The categorizations of Fulkerson and Hungerford[22] and Noyes and Stabler[57] should also be mentioned. The arthroscopic categorization, from Johnson,[40] is shown in Figure 3.

Fulkerson and Hungerford[21] differentiate between closed chondromalacia, open chondromalacia, chondrosclerosis, surface changes in the cartilage, and development of tufts.

1. Closed Chondromalacia

This change is characterized by a slight softening of the joint cartilage, which begins its development in a localized area (usually consisting of a 1 cm area), and

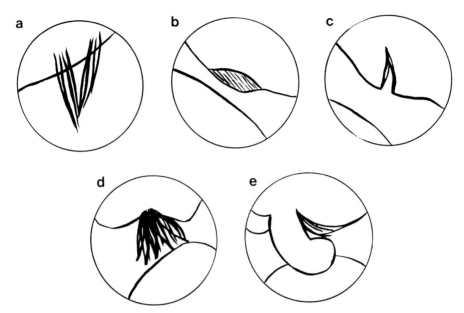

FIGURE 3. Schematic representation of arthroscopically visible developmental stages of chondromalacia of the patella. (a) Bacon strip changes; (b) "bubble" defect; (c) fissuring; (d) fragmentation; (e) chondronecrosis.

later radiates equally in all directions. The surface area remains intact. In some cases, small "blisters" appear and represent the first changes. Closed chondromalacia is, in most cases, localized on the lateral facet of the patella.

2. Open Chondromalacia

This change is characterized by having two basic types:

Fissure — one or more fissures are encountered, usually on the surface but in some cases penetrating deep into the cartilage, all the way to the subchondral bone. These fissures are usually accompanied by greater or smaller areas of softened cartilage.

Ulceration — by which term we describe a loss of cartilage that can be of a greater or lesser degree. In cases of greater cartilage loss, the subchondral bone is usually visible and has a polished appearance (eburnated).

Closed chondromalacia is usually localized on the medial facet of the patella.

3. Chondrosclerosis

Chondrosclerosis is characterized by the presence of hard cartilage. This hard cartilage develops in the whole touching area of the joint and is so hard that it cannot be indented with a surgical probe. In appearance, the cartilage is yellow, translucent, and shiny.

4. Superficial Surface Changes

Superficial surface changes are characterized by a furrowed appearance of the joint surface of the patella; the furrows are oriented in a longitudinal direction.

5. Tuft Formation

Tuft formation is characterized by the appearance of numerous "projections" of the patellar cartilage, which usually develop on the "odd" border and the medial facet of the patella; this takes the form of tufts. These tufts leave cracks of varying length and depth on the joint surface of the patella.

Lindberg et al.[46] have shown the need for a more precise and more reproducible classification system for joint cartilage injury. Presently, in our opinion, the best existing classification system that mets both these criteria and the practical considerations encountered in everyday clinical examinations, i.e., routine arthroscopy, was devised in 1989 by Noyes and Stabler[57] (Table 3).

C. Anterior Knee Pain

After the first reports of chondromalacia of the patella, which were all based on intraoperatively visible changes in the patellar cartilage, this principal criteria was gradually abandoned and more authors diagnosed chondromalacia of the patella clinically, on the basis of some very unreliable indicators, e.g., Freund's sign (percussion of the patella). During the mid-1970s interest renewed concerning the patellofemoral joint, while proof of cessation of pain solely after cutting through the lateral retinaculum, with the patellar cartilage injured, provoked further investigations concerning the precise localization of the pain. Numerous authors, among them Blazina et al.,[57] Goodfellow et al.,[27] Radin,[64] Fulkerson et al.,[24] and Dandy et al.,[12] noticed other localizations of the pain, resulting in a new clinical syndrome — anterior knee pain [dolor peri(para) patellaris]. One of the most influential papers concerning this problem was published in 1985 by Radin.[64]

Although some physicians compare the diagnosis of anterior knee pain to a "large wastepaper basket", these physicians still agree that it is better to begin treatment, even with this "provisory" diagnosis, and try to determine the precise localization of the injury and/or damaged area while monitoring the development of the syndrome. The leading symptom of this injury, pain in the anterior knee area, is included in the term used to describe this syndrome. The term does not, however, answer two important questions, namely (1) the precise localization of the pain and (2) the etiology of the injury. For this reason, different authors describe numerous and different injuries under the term used to describe this clinical syndrome.

To illustrate the large number of different injuries that "hide" under the name "anterior knee pain", we will show a number of classifications currently available in medical literature.

According to the classification proposed by Ireland[37], when defining anterior knee pain, one should take into consideration the etiology of the pain. Ireland[37] recognizes mechanical, inflammatory, and mixed causes of pain (Table 4). Contrary to the preceding classification, Dandy[12–14] recommends a classification based on the localization of the injured area, which leads to the development of pain and discomfort. According to Dandy,[13] the synovial membrane can be the cause of pain in cases of traumatic synovitis, while a much more frequent cause of pain is the synovial shelf syndrome, primarily the medial synovial shelf syndrome (medial plica syndrome).

TABLE 3
Noyes and Stabler's Classification of Articular Cartilage Lesions[57]

Surface description	Extent of involvement	Diameter (mm)	Location	Degree of knee flexion
Cartilage surface intact	Definite softening with some resilience remaining Extensive softening with loss of resilience (deformation)	<10 ≥15 ≥20 ≥25 >25	Patella Proximal 1/3 Middle 1/3 Distal 1/3 Odd facet Middle facet Lateral facet	Degree of knee flexion where the lesion is in weightbearing contact (e.g., 20-45°)
Cartilage surface damaged: cracks, fissures, condyle fibrillation, or fragmentation	<1/2 thickness ≥1/2 thickness		Trochlea Medial femoral condyle Anterior 1/3 Middle 1/3 Posterior 1/3 Lateral femoral condyle	
Bone exposed	Bone surface intact Bone surface cavitation		Anterior 1/3 Middle 1/3 Posterior 1/3 Medial tibial condyle Anterior 1/3 Middle 1/3 Posterior 1/3 Lateral tibial condyle Anterior 1/3 Middle 1/3 Posterior 1/3	

TABLE 4
Differential Diagnosis of Anterior Knee Pain[37]

Inflammatory

Bursitis
  Prepatellar
  Retropatellar
  Pes anserinus
Tendonitis
  Pes anserinus
  Semimembranosus
  Patellar
Synovitis

Mechanical

Hypermobility
Subluxation
Dislocation
Patellofemoral stress syndrome
Pathologic plica syndrome
Osteochondral fracture
Arthrosis

Miscellaneous

Reflex sympathetic dystrophy
Osteochondritis dissecans
Fat pad syndrome
Systematic arthritis
Muscle strain
Stress fracture
Meniscal tear
Iliotibial band syndrome

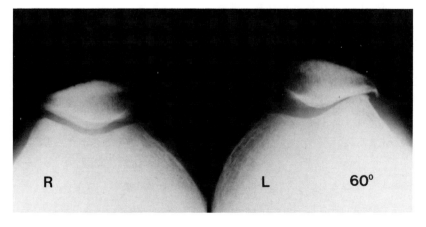

FIGURE 4. Axial view showing patellofemoral arthrosis.

Pain can also be caused by changes on the patella, principally on the patellar cartilage — chondromalacia, arthrotic changes (Figure 4), osteochondral fractures, chondral flaps, osteochondritis dissecans patellae (Figure 5), and divided patella (patella partita) (Figure 6). Dandy states[14] that in this group of causative factors, the most frequent cause of anterior knee pain is the excessive lateral pressure syndrome. Certain tendon injuries can also cause anterior knee pain, the most frequent, according to Dandy,[12–14] is injury to the patellar ligament (jumper's knee). Reflex sympathic distrophy is another common cause of anterior knee pain, and according to Dandy,[12–14] it repre-

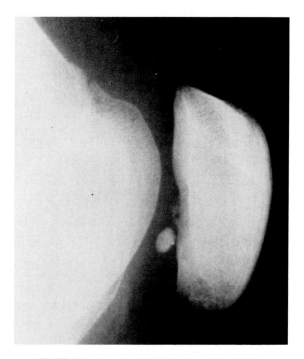

FIGURE 5. Osteochondritis dissecans of the patella.

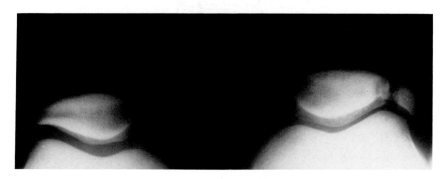

FIGURE 6. Bipartite patella.

sents an exceedingly complex diagnostic and therapeutic problem. In this group, in which pain results as a consequence of changes in or on the bone, Dandy[12-14] also includes Osgood-Schlatter's disease, Sinding-Larson-Johansson's disease, and stress fractures of the patella. Possible causative factors are also the so-called internal injuries of the knee, i.e., injuries of cruciate ligaments and meniscuses. A special group of causative factors consists of less frequently encountered causative factors of anterior knee pain such as inflammation or injury of the infrapatellar bursa and some tumors which develop in the knee area: ganglion, hemagiom, neurinom, etc.

Jacobson and Flandry[39] proposed a different classification and recommended that when evaluating patients with anterior knee pain, the physician should always have in mind all of the possible causative factors. According to these authors, they include instability of the patellofemoral joint, synovial shelf syndromes,[59] inflammatory changes of the peripatellar tissue, injury to the patellofemoral cartilage, arthrotic changes in the cartilage of the patellofemoral joint, and trauma.

Macnicol[47] reported the numerous causes of anterior knee pain with regards to the localization of the injury (Table 5). Fulkerson[24] has shown that patients with

TABLE 5
Different Pathological Conditions Producing Anterior Knee Pain[47]

Site	Pathology
Patellar	Trauma (osteochondral fracture)
	Abnormal pressure or stress
	Increased or decreased
	With or without patellofemoral instability
	With or without patellar tilting
	Osteodystrophy
	Abnormal ossification center
	Sinding-Larson-Johansson's disease
	Patellofemoral arthropaty
	"True" chondromalacia patellae
	Osteoarthritis
Prepatellar	Synovial finge lesion
	Medial fat pad syndrome
	Synovitis
	Loose body
	Plica syndrome
Quadriceps mechanism	Chronic quadriceps weakness
	Quadriceps tendon partial rupture
	Patellar tendinitis
	Ligament laxity
Superficial	Prepatellar, infrapatellar, or suprapatellar bursitis
	Neuroma (especially of the infrapatellar branch of the saphenous nerve)
	Scarring
	Skin conditions
Other	Referred pain (meniscal tear, ligament rupture, hip pathology, lumbar disk herniation)
	Psyhosomatic
	Idiopathic

anterior knee pain frequently localize the area of greatest tenderness in the lateral retinacul area and at the insertion site of the vascus lateralis muscle. This phenomenon, according to Fulkerson,[24] results because of injury to the nerve endings in the retinaculum caused by malalignment of the extensor system of the knee. Johnson[40] also considers "retinacular pain" to be a possible causative factor of anterior knee pain. Fulkerson and Hungerford[22] stressed that it is equally important, when dealing with patients suffering from anterior knee pain, to keep in mind other possible localizations of the injury and/or damaged area, which can manifest themselves as anterior knee pain. These consist of primarily injury or damage to the hips or spine such as Legg-Calve-Perthes' syndrome, epiphysiolysis of the femoral head, idiopathic aseptic necrosis of the femoral head, osteoarthritis of the hip, protrusion or prolapse of the intervertebral disk, and lumbosichialgies of various etiologies.

As we have already pointed out in the beginning of this chapter, a synergistic effect and definite correlation exists between malalignment of the knee extensor system, instability of the patella, chondromalacia of the patella, and anterior knee pain; this explains why the terms used to describe these syndromes are often incorrectly applied (Scheme 1).

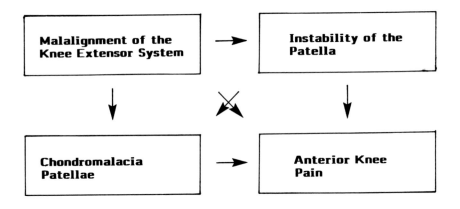

Malalignment of the knee extensor system does not, for instance, necessarily mean that instability of the patella, anterior knee pain, and chondromalacia of the patella are also present. Malalignment of the knee extensor system, can, however, contribute to the development of instability of the patella, principally because of the changed relationship between the patellar stabilizers characterized in most cases by insufficiency in the medial stabilizers of the patella. In cases of malalignment of the knee extensor system, the architecture of the patellofemoral joint is also changed, which results in an incorrect distribution of the strain, increased pressure in certain areas of patellofemoral contact, and the consequent development of chondromalacia in these areas. The synergistic effects of malalignment of the knee extensor system therefore lead to pain in the anterior knee area. The point that we are stressing here, however, is that neither instability of the patella, nor chondromalacia of the patella, nor anterior knee pain can be considered to be causes leading to the development of malalignment of the knee extensor system. Malalignment of the extensor system of the knee results exclusively as a result of anatomical deviations. Instability of the patella causes pain in the anterior area of the knee due to overuse and excessive strain to the surrounding tissue. Likewise it leads to chondromalacia of the patella due to injury to the cartilage of the patellofemoral joint. Chondromalacia of the patella leads to pain in the anterior knee area due to the development of secondary synovitis. We would also like to point out at this time that a definite diagnosis of chondromalacia of the patella can only be reached intraoperatively (nowadays usually arthroscopically). Direct trauma can also cause pain in the anterior knee area. Anterior knee pain is primarily a clinical symptom and cannot be a cause of either malalignment of the knee extensor system, instability of the patella, or chondromalacia of the patella. The reverse, however, is quite possible.

From all that we have put forth in the preceding parts of this chapter, it is obvious that after a provisory, symptomatic diagnosis of anterior knee pain, the physician should attempt to diagnose the cause leading to the development of this syndrome. In diagnosing the cause leading to the development of anterior knee pain, a detailed and targeted clinical examination is of the utmost importance.[8] Specific clinical signs must also be examined to establish the possible presence of instability of the patella, malalignment of the knee extensor system, chondromalacia of the patella, patellar tendinitis ("jumper's knee", Osgood-Schlatter's disease), and other syndromes. Radiological examinations are of great help[2,4,6,9,11,15,16,20,32,36,45,53,54,63] in discovering anatomical deviations and irregularities in the patellofemoral joint [excessively high or low placed patella, inclination of the patella, Wiberg's angle (Figure 7), angle of the femoral trochlea, etc.]. A CT examination of the lower extremity is of immeasurable help when evaluating and assessing rotation deformations in the hip and knee area and the related changed kinematic relations in the patellofemoral joint.[17,23,51,68] (Figure 8). The usefulness of kinematic analysis in the study of motion of the patellofemoral joint *in vivo* is proved by Matijašević et al.[50] The future of functional examinations of the patellofemoral joint is closely related to the use of MRI techniques. This method allows examination of the femoropatellar joint during movements from 0 to 140° (Figure 9) and also allows analysis of the state of the joint facet patellar cartilage.[38,43,69,70] Scintigraphic analysis can also be used in the diagnosis of anterior knee pain, i.e., in cases of reflex sympathic distrophy of the patella. Sympathic reflex distrophy of the patella can also be diagnosed with the computerized telethermograph method. This method can objectively determine the presence of anterior knee pain and can also enable the monitoring of the course of the disease and the results of the applied treatment. Arthroscopy of the knee is, of course, of the utmost importance and is basically an unavoidable examination method.[12,13,40,46,48,57,66,71] Arthroscopy is also, at present, the only sure way to confirm the existence of suspected chondromalacia of the patella and other intra-articular causes of anterior knee pain, such as plica synovialis medialis. A definite decision about the causes leading to the development of anterior knee pain, despite the auxillary input of numerous diagnostic examination methods, can only be reached on the basis of history and a detailed physical examination.[65] A diagnosis of, for instance, plicae synovialis medialis does not as yet mean that we have precisely defined the cause leading to the development of pain. Simi-

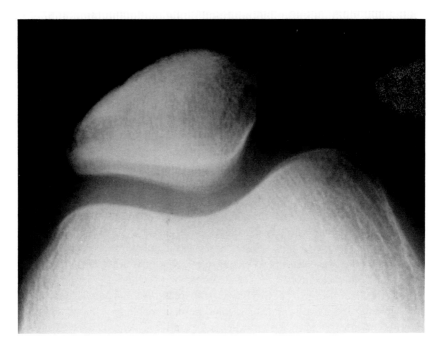

FIGURE 7. Wiberg type 4: Alpine hunter's cap deformity.

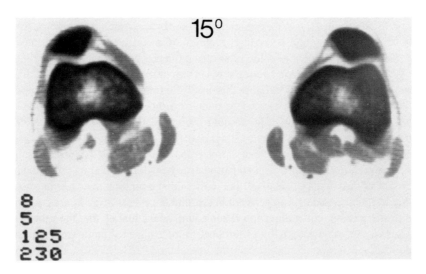

FIGURE 8. CT image of the patellofemoral joint.

larly, a diagnosis that confirms the presence of pathological changes on the patellar cartilage does not necessarily mean that these changes are the cause of pain. It is quite possible that these changes are a side-effect and that the real cause of pain is, for instance, Hoffa's disease or patellar tendinitis (jumper's knee). The preceding parts of this chapter illustrate the complexity related to the anterior knee pain syndrome

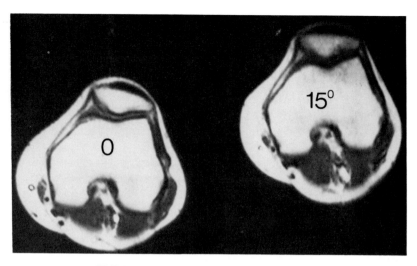

FIGURE 9. MRI image of the patellofemoral joint.

and likewise explain the complexity present when treating this syndrome.[3,14,28,29,30,31,32,49] After a precise diagnosis, the physician should, if possible, prescribe causative treatment that can be either nonoperative or operative. If, for instance, the primary cause of pain is excessive pressure on the lateral part of the patella (the lateral patellar joint facet) caused by malalignment of the knee extensor system, then the physician can attempt to correct this malalignment with nonoperative treatment such as electrostimulation of the vastus medialis muscle or by having the patient wear a brace designed for stabilizing the patella (Figure 10). If nonoperative treatment does not lead to any appreciable results, the physician can attempt to resolve the problem of malalignment of the knee extensor system and the syndrome of lateral hyperpressure of the patella operatively. Nowadays, this usually entails arthroscopic releasing of the lateral retinacul of the patella. When the pain is caused by plicae synovialis medialis, the latter can be arthroscopically resected while softened patellar cartilage can be arthroscopically shaved (shaving of the patella). In the beginning stages, when the precise etiology of anterior knee pain is not yet known, immediate treatment consists of ceasing all physical activities that cause pain. This, however, does not necessarily entail a complete cessation of all athletic activities. If, and when, the symptoms grow in intensity, which usually happens when the athlete persists in his athletic activities despite the pain, a complete unburdening and relaxation of the knee, including walking with crutches for a short period of time, can be recommended. Complete immobilization of the affected knee with a plaster of Paris cast is rarely necessary. Classical treatment, in the sense of recommending cryotherapy (ice), nonsteroidal anti-inflammatory drugs, and isometric exercises for the quadriceps muscle is a necessary part of any treatment for anterior knee pain. When performing exercises for the quadriceps muscle, the patient's knee should be in a position of flexion that is comfortable, i.e., in a position where contraction of the quadriceps muscle is painless. Electrotherapy, either for the purposes of stimulation or for its analgesic effect, is another nonoperative treatment method that can be prescribed. Special knee braces that stabilize the patella and prevent its lateral displacement, as well as special

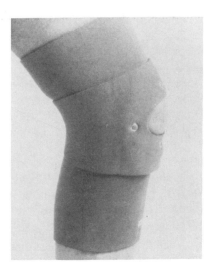

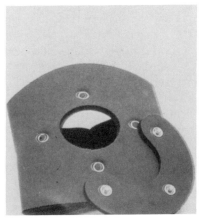

FIGURE 10. Knee brace for patellar instability.

bands used when treating patellar tendinitis, are other methods that fall into the domain of nonoperative treatment. Another important step in the treatment of anterior knee pain is the slow and gradual return to sports activities, beginning at first with fast walking and progressing gradually to jogging, sprinting, running with sudden changes of direction, and finally jumping. However, some exercises and procedures routinely carried out during training will have to be permanently banned. These include lifting weights from a crouched position, performing deep knee bends, and running up and down a hill. In the treatment of anterior knee pain syndrome, an important place is reserved for stretching exercises, especially for the quadriceps muscle and hamstrings. The latter enables complete extension of the knee which has the effect of decreasing the pressure in the patellofemoral joint. When all of the aforementioned methods fail to produce significant results, in the sense of lessening the intensity or alleviating the painful symptoms, surgical treatment is, perforce, the only remaining option. Surgical treatment can be complex, and during the course of one intervention, a number of surgical procedures can be performed. It is not uncommon to perform a releasing of the lateral patellar retinaculum, a shaving of the patellar cartilage, a transposition of the tibial tuberosity and its ventralization,[61] and an apicotomy of the patella, all during one surgical intervention. A valuable contribution to the field of surgical treatment for anterior knee pain syndrome has been made by Morscher[56] who introduced longitudinal (sagittal) osteotomy of the patella into clinical practice. We have been successfully applying longitudinal osteotomy of the patella since 1980.[60,62] Up until 1991, we performed 89 longitudinal osteotomies of the patella, of which 16 were performed on top-level athletes or ballet dancers.[62] The mean value of Wiberg's patellar angle was 112° preoperatively, and 142° postoperatively. The results, judged on the basis of criteria evaluation compiled by Bandi and Ficat, were excellent. Our successful application of longitudinal osteotomy of the patella is confirmed by the fact that all of the operated athletes, except one (karate), returned to competitive sports, and that three ballerinas returned to professional dancing. After every surgical intervention, an adequate postoperative rehabilitation program, including a slow and gradual return to sports activities, must be carried out. In some cases, however, a complete return to the normal state before the injury (restitutio ad integrum) will not be obtainable.

III. PATELLAR TENDINITIS (JUMPER'S KNEE)

Patellar tendinitis (jumper's knee) is an overuse injury characterized by pathological changes in the distal parts of the extensor system of the knee joint: the quadriceps tendon and the patellar tendon (patellar ligament). Other terms are also found in medical literature which apply to the same syndrome: patellar or quadriceps tendinitis, patellar apicitis, and enthesitis apicis patellae.[77,78,81] The first description of patellar tendinitis dates from 1921 when Sinding-Larson and Johansson first described pathological changes on the proximal insertion of the patellar tendon. However, only in 1962 did Smillie describe this clinical entity in adults.[77] In 1973, a detailed description of the clinical picture and a form of therapy were published by Blazina,[77] who, at the same time, also introduced in medical literature the term *jumper's knee.*

Jumper's knee is a clinical entity most commonly found in athletes who, during their athletic activities, habitually place excessive strain on the extensory system of their knees with numerous jumps or long periods of running.[84,89,94,140] The high frequency of patellar tendinitis in volleyball players was first noticed by Maurizio in 1963.[89] Ferretti,[86] who was himself a volleyball player, carried out an epidemiological study, the results of which showed that jumper's knee accounted for 28% of all sports-related injuries in volleyball and that fully 40% of top-level volleyball players suffer from this syndrome at least once during their athletic career. A high incidence of jumper's knee was also noticed in other athletic activities, primarily in the so-called "jumping sports" such as the high jump, the long jump, the triple jump, and basketball.[98,99,109,120] In other athletic activities, this syndrome is noted in lesser frequencies but is encountered occasionally in soccer players, weight lifters, and bicyclists.[13] Pećina et al.[119] reported that jumper's knee is also found in top-level skaters because of the numerous jumps now being performed in this athletic activity. Jumper's knee can also develop in athletes who habitually run for long periods of time and in hockey players.[111] Painful symptoms very similar to patellar tendinitis can be present during the postoperative treatment of patients who have had various surgical procedures performed on their knee joints. With these patients, however, the clinical symptoms disappear as soon as the quadriceps femoris muscle regains its initial strength. Kujala et al.[111] reported in their retrospective study that during a 5-year interval in a test sample of 2672 ambulatorly treated patients with various knee injuries, fully 26.4% (252 patients) suffered from complications related to jumper's knee. These findings led them to believe that jumper's knee is the most common athletic injury to the knee joint and that it is encountered in higher frequencies than either meniscal or anterior cruciate ligament injuries.

A. Etiopathogenesis

Jumper's knee is usually noticed in athletes who have taken part in strenuous athletic activities that place strong and repeated mechanical strain on the extensory system of their knees. Repeated mechanical excessive strain is, without doubt, the basic prerequisite for the development of this syndrome. However, it should be noted that of different athletes who participate in the same sport, play in the same position in the team, and are placed under the same repeated mechanical stresses, some develop jumper's knee while others remain free from any symptoms.[84,86,110] For this reason, it is necessary to discover the factors which predispose some athletes to develop this syndrome.

The main athletic activity that substantially increases the amount of mechanical strain placed upon the knee extensory system are various types of jumps. These consist of both sudden and strongly performed jumps from a stationary position (e.g., when performing a block in volleyball), and jumps taken while running (e.g., in the high or long jump). Both of these jumps are performed with one or with both feet stationary during take off. It is important to note that the maximal amount of mechanical strain is placed on the tendon during the deceleration phase of the landing — on the landing knee(s) — during the time the quadriceps femoris muscle is overcoming the force of gravity with its eccentric contraction.[135,141] Precisely, these contractions of the quadriceps femoris muscle are one of the basic causative factors in the development of jumper's knee.[88] In practice, these contractions are present when, e.g., performing exercises in which the athlete jumps on a barrier 1 to 2 m in height and then lands from that height on the floor to immediately take off from the floor in a new jump.

The development of jumper's knee is significantly correlated to the weekly amount of strain placed on the knee during training. The results of a study carried out by Ferretti et al.[86,88,89] confirm this: 40% of the top-level volleyball players they have treated who train at least 4 times a week, develop clinical symptoms due to overstrain of the patellar tendon. At the same time, it was noticed that athletes who train on hard surfaces (e.g., concrete) develop clinical symptoms in 37.5% of the cases, while those athletes who train on floor develop jumper's knee in only 4.7% of the cases.[88] This difference is attributed to the poor absorptive qualities of hard surfaces which place increased strain on the muscle-tendon unit of the knee extensory system. Another characteristic of jumper's knee is that it develops with equal frequency in adolescents (beginner athletes) and in mature athletes.[89] For this reason, it is believed that the length of time the athlete has been engaged in a particular athletic activity has little to do with the potential development of this syndrome. There are, however, some indications that the syndrome has a tendency to develop in the third year of intensive training.[89]

An analysis of training methods and procedures has indicated that the type of training method used has no significant bearing on the development of jumper's knee. A much more important causative factor was found in the amount of training (both the amount of time and the amount of mechanical strain placed upon the knee) that the athlete habitually carries out.[87] An interesting fact noticed with regards to the development of jumper's knee was that the syndrome has a tendency to develop after relatively longer breaks in the training process, e.g., when renewing intensive physical activities after the summer holidays. Jumper's knee has an equal propensity for developing in both sexes and to develop in ages older than 15 years — in other words, when growth and development are finished.[89] In the younger age groups (younger than 15 years), mechanical overstrain is more often followed by the appearance of juvenile osteochondrosis of the knee joint. This is due to the fact that in those age groups, the bony centers of growth are delicate and therefore prone to injury through excessive mechanical strain.[89]

The development of jumper's knee also, to a large degree, depends on the somatic characteristics of the athlete, of which the best known and most intensively studied are the anatomic features of the lower extremities.[110] Studies carried out with this in mind have shown that athletes suffering from patellar tendinitis sometimes also have concomitant genu valga, genu vara, and a varus position of the proximal tibia.[76,87] In a small number of patients, increased anteversion of the femoral neck and a prominent tibial tuberosity were also noted.[89] Martens et al.[114] have shown, by studying the physical height of athletes afflicted with jumper's knee, that there is no physical height of athletes afflicted with jumper's knee, that there is no physical constitution of the organism which predisposes an athlete to develop this syndrome. Kujala et al.[110] reported that an unequal length (inegality) of the lower extremities and patella alta can significantly increase the likelihood of developing patellar tendinitis. They believe that in these cases, the patella is unable to fully perform its function as a movable center of force between the quadriceps femoris tendon and the patellar tendon, which leads to increased mechanical strain on the extensor system of the knee joint. A frequently analyzed (especially in recent times) possible causative factor of patellar tendinitis is the orientation of the extensor system of the knee.[84,86,88,119–121] On X-rays of the knee joint in 30, 45, 60, and 90° flexion in the axial projection, it is possible to analyze the orientation of this system based on the position tilting or lateralization of the patella and the congruence of the patella and the femoral trochlea.[107] From a clinical standpoint, the orientation of this system is determined by the value of the angle of the quadriceps femoris muscle or the Q-angle. The normal value of this angle is up to 10° in males and no more than 15° in females. The Q-angle is slightly greater in females because of the width of the female pelvis. Pećina et al.[119] reported a significant correlation between a pathological Q-angle and the development of jumper's knee, while Ferretti et al.[88] reported a 50% presence of pathological values for the Q-angle in their total sample. Another clinical indication of a badly oriented extensor knee system is the so-called *bayonet symptom*. Pećina et al.[120] reported a 70% presence of this symptom in athletes suffering from patellar tendinitis. Although a pathological value of the Q-angle and the bayonet symptom are generally present in athletes afflicted with jumper's knee, Ferretti et al.[89] reported that a badly orientated knee extensor system need not be a risk factor because an athlete should be encouraged to take up other nonjumping sports. A badly oriented extensor system is, however, without doubt an important factor that should be taken into account when prescribing treatment for this syndrome.

The functional imbalance of the muscles that stabilize the pelvis and the lower extremity is another factor that needs to be analyzed in the context of predisposing an athlete to developing jumper's knee. It is a well-known fact that strong and shortened muscles of the posterior part of the thigh (hamstring muscles) cause significant mechanical overstrain to the extensor system of the knee joint. A biomechanical and kinematographical analysis of a typical jump performed by a basketball player,[132] showed that a weak iliopsoas, gluteus maximus, and rectus abdominis muscle contribute to increased strain of the extensor musculature of the knee. The reason for this is the inadequate distribution of force during the jump. For this reason, Sommer[132] recommended strengthening the abdominal muscles and stabilizing the muscles of the pelvis in patients suffering from this syndrome.

Based on what is reported in medical literature, we feel safe in concluding the following. Although most of the studies carried out to date have been less interested in the external factors causing jumper's knee, it is without any doubt quite certain that excessive strain caused by training and exercising on hard surfaces contributes significantly to the development of this syndrome. With regards to the group of anatomical changes of the lower extremity, the inegality of the lower extremities and patella alta are causative factors for the development of jumper's knee. In spite of this, it seems that the underlying causes of patellar tendinitis are based not on anatomical or biomechanical changes in the knee joint, but on the mechanical characteristics of the tendon and the area of insertion of the tendon into the bone (its elasticity and its ability to stretch). In conclusion, the basic etiopathogenetic course of events leading to the development of overuse syndrome of the quadriceps tendon and the patellar tendon, i.e., jumper's knee, can be defined as the state that arises when mechanical overstrain overcomes the adaptive ability of the excessively strained tissue.

B. Clinical Picture and Diagnostics

The clinical picture of jumper's knee is characterized by the presence of pain as the basic symptom, and a decreased functional ability of the afflicted lower extremity.[117,118,127] The pain can appear either in the area of the upper or lower pole of the patella, or in the area of the tibial tuberosity. Pećina et al.[120] reported the appearance of pain at the junction of the quadriceps tendon to the base of the patella present in 20% of their patients, at the insertion of the patellar tendon to the tibial tuberosity in 12% of their patients, and at the insertion site of the patellar tendon at the tip of the patella in 68% of athletes suffering from jumper's knee. The main features of this pain consist of sharpness of varying intensity that gradually evolves and appearance that is not connected with evident trauma.

In the beginning stages of the disease, the pain appears only after training/ competition or after running down an incline[77,99] and disappears after a short period of complete rest (a couple of hours or 1 d).[137,138] In later stages, pain felt at the insertion areas of the quadriceps tendon and the patellar tendon becomes continuous and is present before, during, and long after athletic activities. The appearance of pain is quite frequent after long periods of sitting with the knees in a flexed position, e.g., when driving a car for long periods of time or when watching a movie at the theater. The appearance of this pain is sometimes called the *movie sign*[77,89,120] and can usually be relieved by rubbing the painful area and stretching the leg in the knee with the sole of the foot in supination. Some patients complain of a feeling of weakness and feebleness in the knee when this joint is subjected to stronger mechanical strain.[111] The functional inability of the afflicted lower extremity is accompanied by intense pain and shows a range from slight to complete inability to participate in athletic activities.

In very rare cases, a continuation of intensive athletic activities, despite the presence of evident symptoms of the disease, leads to a complete break (rupture) of the patellar ligament.[126,128,130] Ferretti et al.[89] describe this state in 3 out of 110 patients (2.7%) suffering from jumper's knee. Although considerably less frequent, a complete rupture can sometimes be seen at the junction of the quadriceps tendon to the base of the patella. Kelly et al.[106] describe one-sided ruptures of the quadriceps tendon in 3 patients, and a complete break of the patellar tendon in 11 patients with jumper's knee. They also reported that, in their opinion, important causative factors leading to the development of this rupture are the degeneration of the tendon caused by mechanical overstrain, as well as structural changes in the tendon tissue caused by aging. Tarsney[136] reported the appearance of sudden bilateral ruptures of the quadriceps tendon and the patellar tendon in athletes while they were playing basketball. These bilateral ruptures should be diagnostically differentiated from complete tendon breaks which develop during the course of rheumatic diseases.[113] It has also been noted that a complete tendon break is very frequently preceded by the local application of corticosteroid medication.[106,136]

Based on histological analysis of tendon tissue of the knee extensor system performed during the course of overuse syndrome, Ferretti et al.[85] note that the basic pathological changes develop on the insertion sites of the quadriceps tendon and patellar tendon to the patella and tibial tuberosity. The changes consist of a thickening of the transition cartilages between the tendon and the bone, the appearance of cystic cavities, and the loss of the border between the two transition cartilages (the blue line). Further research has shown that histopathological changes are also evident in the tendon structure.[123] For this reason, it is nowadays believed that there exists, during the course of jumper's knee, an enthesitis (insertion tendinopathy) as well as a change in the tendon structure (tendinosis) of varying intensity.

The main clinical symptom of jumper's knee, in patients suffering from that disease, is the presence of a very intense, palpatory, pain in the lower or upper pole of the patella or on the tibial tuberosity. In some cases, a cystic fluctuation is present in one of three predilected areas.[77,109,125,139] Intense pain can be produced by extending the lower leg against pressure.[77] Jumper's knee is also characterized by the presence of concomitant ligament or meniscus lesions, while chondromalacia of the patella is very rarely seen.[89] Blazina,[77] Krahl,[109] and Roels[125] have suggested the categorization of jumper's knee into different stages, based on the prevalence of the main clinical symptoms — pain and loss of function in the extremity (Table 6). This categorization is, however, based on subjective evaluation and as such does not represent a sure base on which a definite decision, regarding the type and method of therapy to be employed, can be made.

Radiographic analysis of patients suffering from jumper's knee can reveal bony changes on the poles of the patella and the tibial tuberosity, as well as ossification in the tendon structure[96] (Figure 11). The range of possible pathological changes seen in radiographic analysis is described by Blazina et al.[77] and Kelly et al.[106] (Table 7). The most characteristic radiological indications of jumper's knee are elongation of the poles of the patella, irregular centers of ossification seen in the patellas of adolescents, stress fractures of the lower patellar pole, and a marked spiking of the anterior surface of the patella. Elongation of the lower pole of the patella is referred to as the "beak" of the patella, while the spiky anterior surface of the patella, which can be seen in axial radiographical pictures, is called[95] the *tooth sign.* Scintigraphic

TABLE 6
Classification of the Patellar Tendinitis According to
Incidence and Progression of Symptoms

Stage	Symptoms	Ref.
Stage 1:	Pain after activity only	77
	No undue functional impairment	
Stage 2:	Pain during and after activity	
	Still able to perform at a	
	satisfactory level	
Stage 3:	Pain during and after activity	
	and more prolonged	
	Patient has progressively	
	increasing difficulty in performing	
	at satisfactory level	
Stage 1:	Pain only after sports activity	125
Stage 2:	Pain at the onset of sports	
	activity, disappearing after warm-up	
	and reappearing at fatigue	
Stage 3:	Constant pain at rest and during activity	
	Inability to participate in sports at	
	previous level.	
Stage 4:	Complete rupture of patellar tendon	
Stage 1:	Pain only after sports activity	109
Stage 2:	Pain at the beginning of sports activity,	
	disappearing after warm-up and reappearing	
	after activity	
Stage 3:	Pain at the beginning, during, and after	
	sports activity	
Stage 4:	Constant pain at rest and during activity	
	Inability to participate in sports	
Stage 5:	Complete rupture of patellar tendon	

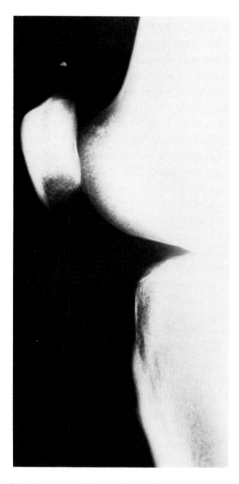

FIGURE 11. Changes of the lower pole of the patella in chronic patellar tendinitis (jumper's knee).

TABLE 7
Radiological Signs of the Patellar Tendinitis

	Ref.
1. Radiolucency at the involved pole	77
2. Irregular centers of ossification	
3. Periosteal reaction at the anterior surface	
4. Elongation of the involved pole with an occasional fracture at the junction of the elongation with the main portion of the patella	
5. Stress fracture of the inferior pole of the patella	
6. Calcification of the involved tendon	
1. Calcification in the quadriceps tendon	106
2. Elongation of the proximal pole of the patella	
3. Tooth sign (anterior surface of the patella)	
4. Elongation of the distal pole of the patella	
5. Calcification in the patellar tendon	
6. Osteophytes in the area of the tibial tubercule	

analysis of patients suffering from jumper's knee can reveal pathological changes at the insertion sites of the tendon into the bone, in which there exists increased vascularization and an accumulation of radionuclides.[104] This accumulation of radionuclides is not, however, unique in jumper's knee, a fact which should be kept in mind when interpreting the results of the scintigraphic analysis.

In recent times, there have been reports in the medical literature about the use of CT with the aim of achieving an objective diagnosis of jumper's knee.[113,114,115] King et al.[108] reported that by using this method, they were able to see pathological changes of the real tendon structure such as the localized thickening of the tendon and the presence of cystic cavities within the tendon.

The diagnosis of jumper's knee is facilitated by the use of ultrasound examination of the quadriceps tendon and the patellar ligament.[83,90–92,97,101–103,112,116,124,134] Fritchy et al.[93] have used ultrasound examination to analyze the patellar ligament of patients in whom jumper's knee was clinically diagnosed. They note that in the beginning stages of this syndrome, there is swelling of the tendon, usually found in the area of the proximal insertion site of the patellar tendon. The later stages in the tendon take the form of a heterogeneous tendon structure accompanied by an unclear definition of the tendon sheath. Concomitant ultrasound examination of the knee patellar bursae, which are clearly defined when using this technique, is also performed. Ultrasound examination also enables examination of the tendon structure during contraction of the muscle; this allows a dynamic examination of the knee extensor system.[93] The thickening of the tendon in the area of its insertion, which remains present during muscle contraction, is called a *vacuola* and is a characteristic sign of the acute stage of jumper's knee (Figure 12). According to Kalebo et al.,[103] a cone-shaped poorly echogenic area exceeding 0.5 cm in length in the center of the patellar tendon in combination with its localized thickening proved to be a reliable indicator of jumper's knee. In the tendon itself, hematoma, degenerative changes, and the beginnings of ossification (Figure 13) can be seen. At this stage of the disease, these changes are not visible by radiographic examination. For a detailed analysis of the extensor system of the knee, a comprehensive knowledge of the clinical picture and the anatomy of the afflicted area is mandatory. Fritchy et al.[93] and Jeroch et al.[102] have recommended an ultrasound classification of jumper's knee with the aim of facilitating diagnosis and making it more objective and reproducible (Table 8). Ultrasound diagnostics is becoming an important and invaluable tool in diagnosing jumper's knee due to the following qualities:[112] noninvasive, inexpensive, wide range of application, and safety.

Diagnosis of overuse injury of the knee extensor system can also be achieved by thermography and MRI.[79] Thermographic analysis distinguishes the temperature difference between the affected and healthy part of the knee. This enables the physician to evaluate the severity of the symptoms and also affords him the opportunity to monitor the course and success of the prescribed treatment.

Up until now, there have been few reports concerning the success of MRI diagnostics of jumper's knee. Bodne et al.[79] claim that they are able to differentiate pathological changes, both in the bony and tendinous part of the knee extensor system by using this diagnostic method. They feel that based on these results, they are better able to objectively prescribe the most suitable therapy.

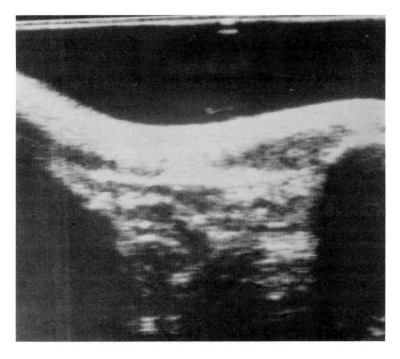

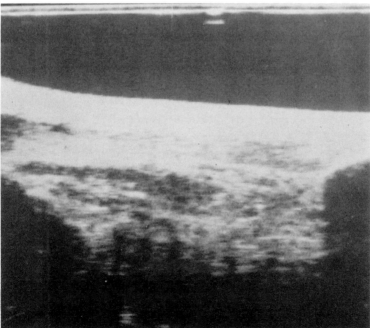

FIGURE 12. Sonogram of the patellar tendon showing acute form of patellar tendinitis (jumper's knee). (A) Relaxation; (B) Contraction.

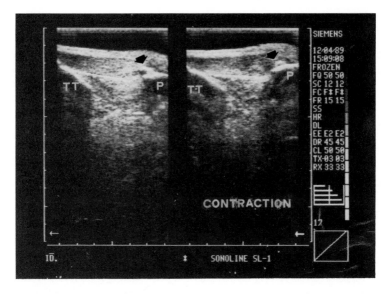

FIGURE 13. Sonogram of the patellar tendon showing chronic form of patellar tendinitis (jumper's knee). (P) Patella; (TT) tibial tubercle.

TABLE 8
Ultrasound Classification of the Patellar Tendinitis

		Ref.
1. Pure inflammatory stage	Initial stage characterized by edema of the tendon fibers. Tendon is swollen and thickened but still presents a homogenous appearance	93
2. Stage with irreversible anatomical lesions	Tendon has a heterogenous appearance. There are hypoechoic and hyperechoic images with or without edema. Tendinous envelope is more or less well defined but may have a variable appearance.	
3. Final stage of lesion	Tendinous envelope is irregular and thickened and the tendon fibers appear heterogeneous, but the swelling has disappeared	

		Ref.
Stage 1:	Normal tendon	102
Stage 2:	Edema of the tendon at the distal patellar pole	
Stage 3:	Edema of the whole tendon; normal echogenicity; tendon sheath smooth	
Stage 4:	a. Edema of the whole tendon; hyperechogenicity; tendon sheath smooth	
	b. Edema of the whole tendon; hyperechogenicity; irregular tendon sheath	
Stage 5:	Rupture of the tendon	

C. Treatment

The basic principles of treating jumper's knee consist of reducing the local inflammatory process, encouraging and facilitating tissue healing, and completely rehabilitating the afflicted extremity with the aim of returning the athlete as soon as possible to his normal athletic activities.[76,80] In acute stages of the disease, the physician generally recommends the cessation of sporting activities which place strain on the afflicted extremity. In the first 72 h after injury, cryotherapy is applied, along with a compressive bandage, and the afflicted extremity is placed in an elevated position. The inflammatory process facilitates healing during the first 3 d. This time interval is therefore the optimal time span during which the inflammatory process should be cured.

Inflammatory edemas, which last for longer periods of time, cause hypoxic changes, diminish tissue vascularity, lower the local pH, and lead to damage of the surrounding healthy tissue. It is believed that the application of cryotherapy reduces the inflammation by diminishing the edema and hematoma and eliminating pain. There are many different methods of applying cryotherapy. The safest and most effective method is crushed ice in a damp towel. However, ice-cold bandages, ice massage of the involved area, immersion in ice water, and application of ethyl chloride are also very effective. Ice should be applied for a limited time (less than 20 min) and repeated every 1 to 2 h in acute cases because continuous treatment may damage the surface tissue and result in unwanted consequences.

We have mentioned both the importance of the inflammatory reaction in initiating healing and the desirability of limiting this reaction if it is prolonged more than necessary. Oral nonsteroidal anti-inflammatory drugs are prescribed in order to decrease inflammation. Although local application of corticosteroids combined with prolonged-effect anesthetics is also recommended in the treatment of overuse syndrome of the soft tissues of the locomotor system, it is counterproductive when treating jumper's knee syndrome. Corticosteroids are not recommended because of the increased risk of total rupture of the patellar tendon. After the initial treatment of quickly soothing the inflammation, on the fourth day, heat therapy or contrast heat-cold therapy, in ratio 3:1 or 1:1, is applied to the knee. Heating facilitates vascularization and increases the speed of the healing process. The heating effect is produced by different methods, including the application of ointments, ultrasound, laser, electric stimulation, and many others. When inflammation and pain have been reduced, a rehabilitation program is introduced. The program consists of stretching exercises and strengthening of the extensor muscle system of the knee. Smith et al.[131] stress the importance of stretching exercises and the increased flexibility of the posterior area of the upper leg in successful nonoperative treatment. Apple[75] gives a detailed description of a stretching exercise program for the gradual strengthening of the afflicted limb. Exercises are conducted in such a fashion that the patient repeatedly performs one exercise (150 to 300 times), but with very light weights (1 to 5 kg). This promotes vascularization and the healing process and does not damage the tissue any further. The exercise program is called Progressive Resistance Exercise (PRE) and is characterized by fully extending the lower extremity in an elevated position, while burdened with a light weight (straight leg raising technique). There is also another approach to the strengthening of the extensor system of the knee joint — concentric and eccentric exercises.[100,101] When performing concentric contraction of the quadriceps femoris muscle, the force performed is antiparallel to the ground force, and the muscle fibers contract. This causes the muscle tissue to strengthen. An example of these exercises is when the body, appropriately loaded, is lifted from a semisquatting position to a standing position. Eccentric contraction, on the other hand, causes the extension of the muscle fibers since the force is parallel to the ground force. An example of this is when the body slowly descends from a standing to a semisquatting position. Apple[75] and Jensen and Fabrio[100] reported that eccentric exercises cause the greatest stress to the tendon tissue, thus preparing it to withstand further heavy mechanical loads. Proprioreceptive exercises (balance board) are included, depending on the progress of the rehabilitation program. These exercises stimulate the interaction of the nervous system, sensory receptors, muscles, tendons, and ligaments.[76] Wearing a patellar brace knee strap (Figure 14) is also highly recommended.[133] To conclude the description of nonoperative treatment for jumper's knee, we must point out the importance of alternative training constantly performed during the treatment.

Alternative training consists of workouts for uninjured body parts and is inevitable in order to maintain the cardiovascular abilities, stamina, and fitness of the body. The exercises include swimming, and strengthening and increasing the flexibility of the upper body. Nonoperative treatment of jumper's knee syndrome calls for persistence and commitment and is performed for several months.

Surgical treatment is indicated only if a prolonged and well-supervised conservative treatment program fails.[82,105] Surgical treatment is needed in cases of irreversible pathological changes of the knee extensor system appearing in the later stages of patellar tendinitis, but also in cases of total rupture of the quadriceps tendon and the patellar tendon. The general principle of surgical treatment consists of removing the devitalized tissue, initiating the healing process, and correcting the wrongly oriented knee extensor system. Patients encouraged to undergo surgery are usually highly motivated professional top athletes who will not give up their athletic careers.

There are numerous different operative approaches. One of them is reported by Smillie and consists of drilling the affected patellar apex to improve vascularization and healing of the damaged area.[121] Basset describes the excision of the degenerate part of the patella tendon, followed by restoration of the defect.[121] Blazina[77] outlines an operative technique concerning the resection of the affected patellar apex (apicotomy), patellar inspection, relegation of the patellar tendon, and retinacular strengthening. Ferretti et al.[87] suggest the following operative procedure based on their own experience: releasing the deep tendon fibers, drilling and "cleansing" the tendon insertion, and scarifying and excising the degenerate tendon tissue.

It is necessary to reorient the knee extensor system (if it is incorrectly oriented) by proximal realignment, lateral retinacular release, and advancement of the vastus medialis obliques muscle. According to Whitaker,[121] total disjunction of the quadriceps tendon and patellar tendon is treated surgically by nonresorptive tendon stitches, taking care to adequately correct the proximodistal position of the patella. Schelbourne[129] uses the resection of the middle third of the patellar ligament with a

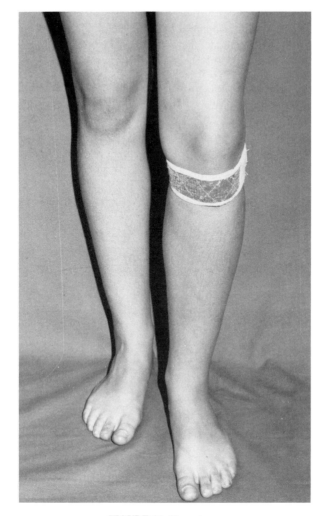

FIGURE 14. Knee strap.

small piece of bone on the apex of the patella; this is similar to the method of ACL reconstruction (bone-tendon-bone graft).

The method of our surgical intervention is decided upon individually, taking into consideration the localization of the pain, knee extensor mechanism alignment, ultrasound, and arthroscopic and intraoperative findings. When the pain is localized at the inferior pole of the patella, the resection of the nonarticular part of the apex (apicotomy) is made without further reinforcement of the ligament fibers (Figure 15). Upon resection (always by saw), we proceed with the drilling of the subcortical pole of the patella, depending on the changes of the patellar cartilage. In cases in which the pain is localized at the superior pole of the patella, multiple drilling of the affected pole combined with the excision of the degenerated tendon tissue and sometimes a lateral retinacular release is performed. When extensor mechanism malalignment is

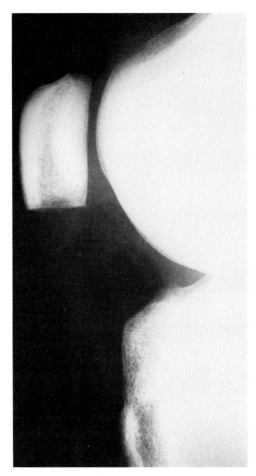

FIGURE 15. Lateral roentgenogram of the knee after patellar tendinitis surgery (apicotomy).

evident, the proximal (lateral retinacular release and VMO advancement) or distal realignment (anterior and medial displacement of the tibial tuberosity) of the patella is attempted. If degenerative changes of the tendon are diagnosed by ultrasonography or during surgery, the altered part is excised completely.

In cases where a totally enlarged and edematose patellar ligament is discovered, we use the method of longitudinal incision, i.e., decompression of the patellar ligament. If cartilage of the patella is changed, shaving of the damaged area of cartilage is effected; when necessary, additional surgical procedure is attempted. Thus, in the case of a patient with obvious dysplasia of the patella, we effect longitudinal osteotomy of the patella.

Postoperatively, when apical osteotomy is performed, we do not permit any active extension of the knee during the first 6 weeks following surgery. Three months after surgery, the patient starts with gradual sports training. However, full sports activity is allowed six to nine months after surgery. The ability of the athlete to return to sports varies considerably.

The results of surgical treatment of jumper's knee are more than satisfactory,[122] especially when the pathological changes are situated on the patellar apex or on the tuberositas tibiae. Nevertheless, let us not forget that the fundamental strategy is concentrating on intensive nonoperative treatment. Stretching exercise are important as an overuse preventive measure. Surgical intervention is always the last choice of treatment.

IV. BREASTSTROKER'S KNEE

In 1974, conducting a survey on the incidence of injuries to various parts of the musculoskeletal system of swimmers, Kennedy and Hawkins[145] noticed that a high percentage of breaststroke swimmers complained of pain in the medial knee. This condition has been termed breaststroker's knee, although further studies by Vizsoly et al.[150] on a population of 391 competitive swimmers showed that breaststroker's knee was diagnosed in 56 out of 77 breaststroke swimmers (73%), but also in 153 out of 314 (48%) swimmers who used either the freestyle, backstroke, or butterfly stroke.

Kennedy and Hawkins[145] believed that a tibial collateral ligament strain on the proximal femoral origin of the ligament, resulting from repeated stretching of the origin during breaststroke swimming, was the primary disorder leading to breaststroker's knee (Figure 16). In their opinion, the stretching of the ligament origin was caused by the extension of the knee during the "whip kick" phase of breaststroke swimming, accompanied by an excessive valgus stress on the knee joint and the outward rotation of the leg in the final phase of the stroke. Stulberg and co-

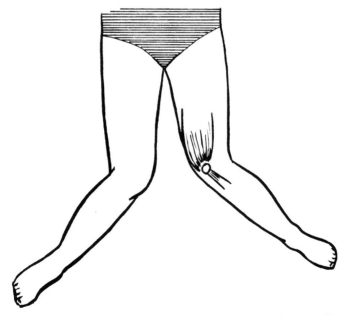

FIGURE 16. Biomechanical explanation of the causes leading to the development of breaststroker's knee.

workers[148] reported that, in most cases, the pain was localized in the lower area of the medial facet of the patella. The areas of the medial facet of the patella and the medial collateral ligament were indicated as the areas of greatest tenderness in 25% of the cases.[143] Rovere and Nichols[147] cite inflammation, thickening, and fibrosis of the medial parapatellar plica as potential causes of breaststroke knee pain.

Arthroscopic findings range from localized medial synovitis of the knee[146,151] to generalized synovitis and chondromalacic changes on the medial facet of the patella.[148]

Slow-motion analysis of the mechanics of the breaststroke showed that the primary cause of breaststroker's knee was the incorrect technique used in performing the "whip kick".[144,149] One group of authors believes that breaststroker's knee develops as a consequence of the amount of abduction in the hip joint in the beginning phase of the kick; both insufficient and excessive abduction lead to a strong valgus stress and excessive rotation of the lower leg in the final phase of the kick. Another group of authors are of the opinion that the final phase of the kick, characterized by extension of the lower leg with abducted legs, after which a sudden and strong abduction with excessive outward rotation follows, is the primary cause of breaststroker's knee.

Breaststroker's knee symptoms usually appear after 3 years of competitive breaststroke swimming. In most cases, both knees are affected. In the beginning stages, pain occurs only when performing the breaststroke. The area of greatest tenderness is localized in the proximal origin of the medial collateral ligament. The later phase is characterized by pain in the lower medial patellar facet area; this occurs regardless of swimming and inhibits other athletic and everyday activities, such as walking up steps and rising from a chair.

As with other overuse injuries, the ideal treatment of breaststroker's knee is prevention. Abnormal kick mechanics should be corrected as soon as possible. Proper warm-up exercises, local applications of ice, and ultrasound can be helpful. The symptomatic breaststroke swimmer should train infrequently with the "whip kick" and should use other kicks during workouts. In the early stages, stretching exercises of the hamstring muscles and strengthening exercises for the medial vastus muscle should also be performed. In more advanced stages of breaststroker's knee, breaststroke swimming should be stopped. Cryotherapy and nonsteroidal anti-inflammatory drugs can be prescribed. Surgical treatment is rarely indicated.

V. ILIOTIBIAL BAND FRICTION SYNDROME

Iliotibial band friction syndrome (IBFS) results from an activity comprised of many repetitive flexion and extension movements of the knee, during which rubbing of the band against the lateral femoral epicondyle occurs; this produces irritation and inflammatory reactions within the iliotibial band or the underlying bursa. IBFS is one of the most common overuse injuries in runners, not only professional athletes, but also in joggers and other athletes whose activities entail a lot of running.

Staff and Nilsson were among the first to describe the symptoms of IBFS in their paper published in 1971.[158] The term IBFS was introduced by Renne in 1975.[178] Orava[174] diagnosed IBFS in 6.4% of 1311 athletes with overuse injuries. Sutker et al.[181] found a 4.7% frequency of IBFS in 4173 injured runners. They also found a higher incidence of IBFS in long-distance runners than in middle-distance runners and sprinters. In a series of 200 knee injuries in long-distance runners, Noble et al.[172,173] found that 52% of the injuries were secondary to IBFS. IBFS was not unique to distance runners; it has been reported in cyclists, football players, skiers, hammer throwers, racquet sports participants, and ballet dancers.[160,166,169,174-177,179,184]

A. Etiopathogenesis

Iliotibial band or tract is a thickened band of fascia extending from the iliac crest down the lateral side of the thigh to its attachment on the lateral tibial condyle (Gerdy's tubercle).[159,183] At the level of the greater trochanter, the iliotibial band receives the insertions of the tensor fasciae latae muscle anteriorly and superficial tendinous layer of the gluteus maximus muscle posteriorly. It then attaches to the linea aspera of the femur through the lateral intermuscular septum, while its distal segment moves freely over the lateral femoral condyle. With the knee in the extended position, the iliotibial band lies anteriorly to the lateral femoral epicondyle; in knee flexion of 30° it lies behind the lateral femoral epicondyle (Figure 17A).

It is due to its movability that during the activities comprising many repetitive flexion and extension movements of the knee, rubbing of the band against the lateral femoral epicondyle takes place. This produces irritation and subsequent inflammatory reactions within the iliotibial band or formation of underlying bursae and secondary inflammation.

The etiology of IBFS, similar to other overuse injuries, is a multifactorial process, i.e., there are many interacting agents that contribute to the development of IBFS (Table 9.) Most commonly, the IBFS is a result of training errors and anatomical malalignment of the lower extremity.[153,154,170] According to Taunton et al.,[182] training errors and abrupt changes in intensity, duration, and/or frequency of training cause IBFS in 42%, and according to Grana and Coniglione,[157] in 35%. Malalignment conditions of forefoot varus and/or subtalar varus, tibia vara, and genu varum lead to excessive and/or prolonged forefoot pronation during the support phase of a running cycle; this, as research results show, seems to cause IBFS in more than 50% of cases.[155,158,161,168,181,182] During forefoot pronation, the tibia rotates inwardly. In the case of excessive and/or prolonged forefoot pronation, an excessive and prolonged internal rotation of the tibia occurs, producing excessive irritation to the iliotibial band. Other predisposing factors to IBFS, poor iliotibial band flexibility, leg length discrepancies, increased prominence of the lateral femoral epicondyle, hard and/or uneven running surface, and workout running shoes, are mentioned too.[153,169,172,173,180,181]

B. Clinical Picture and Diagnostics

The patient with IBFS experiences pain at the lateral side of the knee. Pain is stinging in nature, and is located at the lateral femoral condyle 2 cm above the joint line. In some cases, however, the pain may radiate downwards along the iliotibial band, or upwards along the lateral side of the thigh. As with other overuse injuries, there is characteristic onset and progression of symptoms. Initially, the pain appears immediately after engagement in activity necessitating repetitive flexion and exten-

TABLE 9
Predisposing Factors Leading to Overuse Injuries of the Musculoskeletal System in Runners

Training errors
Abrupt changes in intensity, duration, and/or frequency of training
Poorly trained and unskilled athlete

Muscle-tendon imbalance of
Flexibility
Strength

Anatomical malalignment
Leg-length discrepancy
Excessive femoral anteversion
Knee alignment abnormalities (genu valgum, varum, or recurvatum)
Position of the patella (patella alta or infera)
Excessive Q-angle
Excessive external tibial rotation
Flat foot

Footwear
Inappropriate running shoes
Worn-out running shoes

Surface
Hard
Uneven

Other
Growth
Disturbances of the menstrual cycle

sion movements of the knee (i.e., after running, bicycle riding, skiing) and usually disappears following a few hours of rest. The next phase is characterized by pain at the very beginning of the activity, its disappearance after warming up, and appearance again upon completion of the activity. It is common that the athletes do not seek medical attention in that time, but rather continue their activity at an unchanged intensity. This results in progressive development of the syndrome so that the pain appearing at the beginning of activity persists throughout the activity and intensifies upon its completion. In the final stage, the pain impairs even normal walking.

Lindenberg et al.[162] have proposed the following classification of injury grade according to symptoms in IBFS:

Grade 1: Pain comes on after the run but does not restrict distance or speed.
Grade 2: Pain comes on during the run but does not restrict distance or speed.

Grade 3: Pain comes on during the run and restricts distance or speed.
Grade 4: Pain is so severe that it prevents running.

The clinical history data are of great importance in the diagnosis of IBFS, especially those about the initiation of pain either during and/or after athletic activity consisting of many flexion and extension movements of the knee without previous knee injury, and disappearance of the pain during walking with a stiff knee in extension.

The most frequent sign is tenderness over the lateral femoral epicondyle of the injured leg (Figure 17B). Various provocative tests for IBFS have been described. In the Renne test, pain is provoked by having the patient support all of his weight on the affected leg with the knee in 30 or 40^0 flexion.[178] Compression test was described by Noble in 1979.[172] In this test, the patient is lying in a supine position and the knee is flexed to 90^0. The examiner holds the ankle of the affected leg by one hand and presses on the lateral epicondyle with the thumb of the other hand. While maintaining constant pressure, he slowly extends the leg (Figure 18). Pain appears when the knee is flexed to 30^0, and the patient usually reports that it is the kind of pain he experiences when running. The test modification according to Pe´cina consists of putting the lower leg in varus position when performing extension.[175]

In clinical examination, the Ober's test is used to diagnose flexibility of the iliotibial band (Figure 19). During the test, the patient lies on his ininjured side with that hip flexed to obliterate any lumbar lordosis. The affected knee is then flexed to 90^0, and the leg is held with one hand, while the pelvis is stabilized with the other. The hip is then passively abducted and extended so that the thigh is in line with the body and will catch the iliotibial band on the greater trochanter, maximizing its excursion. The leg is brought toward the table in adduction, and if iliotibial band shortening is present, the knee cannot reach the table. According to many reports and on the basis of our own experience, in practically all patients with IBFS, tightness of the iliotibial band takes place, although in varying degrees.[153,162,167,169,173,174,180,181]

All patients exhibit normal range of motion of the affected knee, while in some during extension and flexion movements of the knee and simultaneous pressure upon the lateral condyle, excursion of the band over the lateral femoral epicondyle may be felt and sometimes even heard.

As part of the differential diagnosis, other injuries of the knee joint and its structures should be taken into consideration, especially those primarily manifested by pain at the lateral side of the knee. These are popliteal tendinitis, rupture of the lateral knee joint capsule and/or lateral meniscus, meniscal degeneration, cyst of the lateral meniscus, lesion of the lateral collateral ligament, patellar chondromalacia, lateral patellar compression syndrome, patellar subluxation and/or dislocation, and arthritic changes of the knee joint. However, most often the differential diagnosis should be made between the IBFS and popliteal tendinitis.[153,158,160]

C. Treatment

The treatment of IBFS is usually nonoperative, although in some cases surgery may be required.

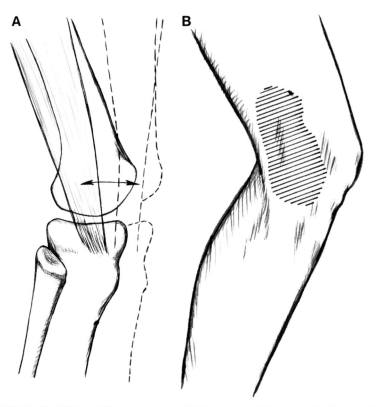

FIGURE 17. Iliotibial band friction syndrome. (A) Mechanism of development; (B) area of pain.

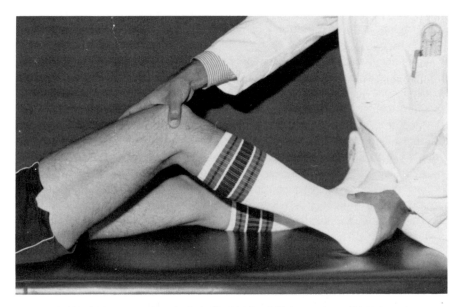

FIGURE 18. Provocation of pain in iliotibial band friction syndrome (Noble's test).

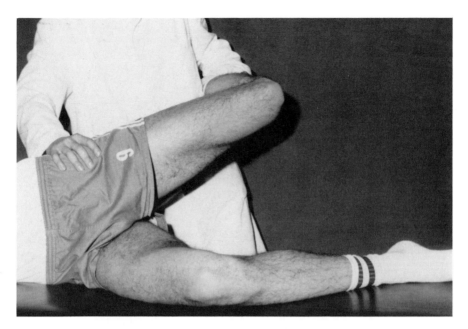

FIGURE 19. Ober's test — used for assessing the flexibility of the iliotibial band.

1. Nonoperative Treatment

Based on the most recent knowledge regarding the etiology of overuse injuries syndrome and evaluation of the applied treatment, a program of nonoperative treatment of IBFS has been conceived as follows:

- short-term cessation or modification of athletic activities
- iliotibial band stretching exercises
- ice massage of the painful area
- nonsteroidal anti-inflammatory drugs
- correction of predisposing factors — training errors, anatomical malalignment of the lower extremity, running shoes, etc.

Some authors[152,171,178,180] suggest complete rest from athletic activities for 3 weeks, while others[153,157,158,162,169,172,174,175,181] consider the period of rest to be from 1 week to 2 months, depending upon the severity of the condition. Our experience has shown that in the initial stages (stages 1 and 2[82]), it is not necessary to completely refrain from athletic activities but that besides other nonoperative treatment methods, it is sufficient to decrease training intensity, especially painful activities, e.g. running. In more advanced cases (stages 3 and 4), complete rest from athletic activities is needed from 3 to 4 weeks. Only alternative training activities are allowed to maintain functional abilities of the athlete — pool running and treading water in the deep end of the pool with or without a flotation device.

Stretching exercises, especially passive or static ones, are the basis in IBFS treatment (Figure 20). Passive stretching exercises necessitate a strictly defined

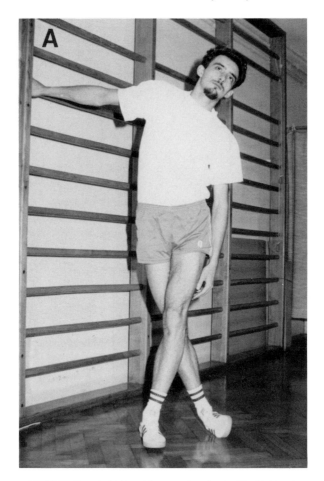

FIGURE 20. (A-D) Stretching exercises for the iliotibial band.

position for each exercise to be performed, slow movement until the sensation of stretching appears, and maintenance of the position for a given period of time. In doing these exercises, the idea of "no pain, no gain" should be disregarded. Keeping the stretching in a painful position decreases the possibility of longer maintenance of stretching, increases the possibility of reflex muscle contraction, and may sometimes cause damage of these muscles. On the other hand, remaining at the point of "initial" stretching enables complete relaxation of these muscles and keeping of the position for a longer period of time. The athlete who is beginning to do the stretching exercises is recommended to keep stretching at the point of initial stretching for 15 s, gradually increasing the time to a maximum of 25 s.

In both treatment and prevention of IBFS, predisposing factors and their correction have a significant role. It should be pointed out again that the most common predisposing factors to IBFS are the following: excessive and/or prolonged pronation of the foot during running, training errors, genu varum, excessive tightness of iliotibial band, and uneven and hard running surface. Although the infiltration of

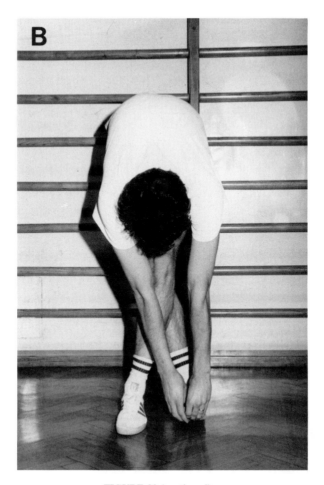

FIGURE 20 (continued).

steroids combined with local anesthetic into the site of most intense pain is recommended as a method of choice by some authors,[165,172,173] it is our opinion that this method should be utilized only in advanced stages. However, it should not be considered as the last resort but rather as part of a nonoperative treatment program. When the formation of bursa has been confirmed, the application of steroid injections is also indicated.

2. Surgical Treatment

Surgery is recommended in resistant cases, i.e., when following a long-term adequate nonoperative treatment, the IBFS symptoms do not disappear. Only a few authors have reported on surgical treatment for IBFS: Noble, [172,173] Pećina et al.,[153,175] Firer,[156] and Martens et al.[165].

As a method of choice, Noble[172,173] suggests surgery during which a transverse cut is made in the 2-cm long posterior portion of the iliotibial band at the level of lateral femoral epicondyle. In this way, a V-shaped defect is obtained, which de-

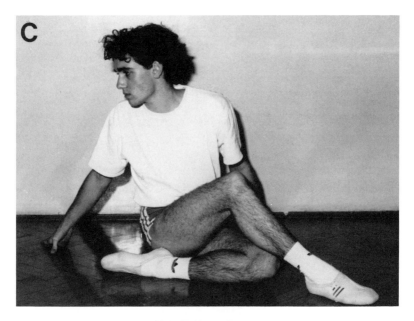

FIGURE 20 (continued).

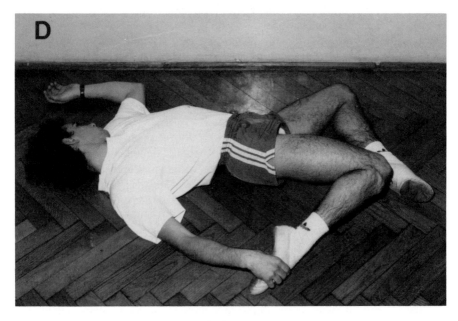

FIGURE 20 (continued).

creases tension in that part of the iliotibial band, preventing friction between the iliotibial band and lateral femoral epicondyle at knee flexion of 30°. Noble has used this surgical method in five athletes and has reported excellent results. All of the operated patients resumed training activities (running) 2 to 5 weeks following surgery; one patient completed a 32-km race without pain, 3 weeks after surgery.

Firer[156] used the same method in 64 athletes. He has also reported excellent results — disappearance of pain during running and the possibility of running an equally long or even longer race than before IBFS signs appeared; these results have been observed in 57 (89.5%) operated patients. Three patients (4.70%) reported temporary difficulties when running, while four patients (6.25%) could not continue with athletic activities. Our patients treated by this method have also shown excellent results.[153,175]

Martens et al.[165] have used a similar (modified) method of surgical treatment in 23 athletes and have reported excellent results in 19 regularly followed-up patients. Surgery was done with the knee held in 60^0 of flexion and consisted of a limited resection of a small triangular piece at the posterior part of the iliotibial band covering the lateral femoral epicondyle. The resected part concerns the iliotibial band fibers, measuring about 2 cm at the base and 1.5 cm in length toward the top of the triangle.

VI. OSGOOD-SCHLATTER'S DISEASE

The most often encountered overuse injuries in children and adolescents are the so-called traction apophysitis, among which the most common and best known is Osgood-Schlatter's disease.[191,207]

Osgood-Schlatter's disease is a traction apophysitis that develops during the adolescent growth spurt, most often at around 11 years of age in girls (because of their earlier bone growth development) and at about 13 years of age in boys.[185,186,199–201,203,207,210] It occurs slightly more often in boys; in large series, the ratio is 3:2.

The clinical picture consists of pain localized to the area of the tibial tubercle. In some cases, the tubercle may be swollen and hypertrophied. Most authors agree that rapid adolescent skeletal growth leads to relative "tightness" of the soft tissues, as skeletal growth is faster than the elongation of the muscle-tendon units. This in turn creates increased tensile forces on the muscles, tendons, and their attachment sites (the apophyses), which cause avulsion fractures of the bony part of the traction apophysis on the tibial tubercle.[190,199,200,207,210,214,216]

Physical examination reveals pain during palpation of the tibial tubercle. Resisted extension of the knee from the 90° flexed position will usually reproduce pain, but resisted straight-leg raising is usually painless. The Ely test, which proves excessive tightness of the quadriceps femoris muscle, is positive in all cases. Radiographic examinations of both knees should always be performed, in both the anterior-posterior (AP) and lateral (LL) projections, to rule out the possibility of tumors, fractures, or infections. The lateral radiograph generally shows the characteristic picture of prominent tibial tubercle with irregularly fragmented ossific nucleus, or a free bony fragment proximal to the tubercle (Figure 21). Nonoperative treatment of Osgood-Schlatter's disease, as with other traction apophysitises, is based on the same principles that apply to all overuse injuries.[185,186,190,191,199,200,207,217] Nowadays, there is

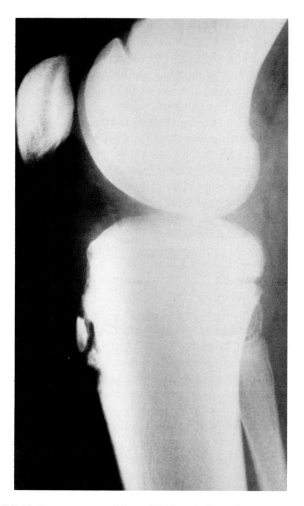

FIGURE 21. Roentgenogram of Osgood-Schlatter's disease in a young gymnast.

no need, in fact there is no excuse, for total immobilization, or for total refraining from athletic activities. Corticosteroid injections are not indicated because the condition is not primarily inflammatory and because of their numerous unwanted side-effects. Of vital importance is that the physician informs the parents, the coach, and the child athlete of the natural course of Osgood-Schlatter's disease. The child, who is an active athlete, should be allowed to continue with his normal athletic activities, to the limit that the pain allows it, but he should also be advised to take up, as secondary athletic activities, other sports that do not cause any discomfort, i.e., swimming. Besides other nonoperative methods of treatment, wearing knee braces is recommended.[199,207] The symptoms of Osgood-Schlatter's disease will generally decline and disappear in most patients if nonoperative treatment is carried out long enough, especially after bone growth is terminated. Persistent symptoms are followed by the development of loose fragments above the tibial tubercle, or within the patellar ligaments. In these cases, the symptoms will disappear only after these fragments are excised.[186,218,220]

VII. SINDING-LARSON-JOHANSSON'S DISEASE

Sinding-Larson-Johansson's disease is a traction apophysitis of the inferior pole of the patella (in rare cases it affects the superior pole also), which is in most respects similar to Osgood-Schlatter's disease.[190,201,206,207,210] It is more common in boys, generally between the ages of 10 to 15 years and is characterized by tenderness of the knee and limping.[206] Although it is basically an overuse syndrome, in most cases, some sort of trauma, e.g., falling on the knees, provokes the onset of the disease or intensifies the symptoms in which the disease has already manifested itself. Clinical examination reveals localized tenderness and swelling over the distal pole of the patella. Lateral radiograph reveals delayed ossification of the inferior pole of the patella (Figure 22). The treatment is the same as with Osgood-Schlatter's disease.[185,206,207]

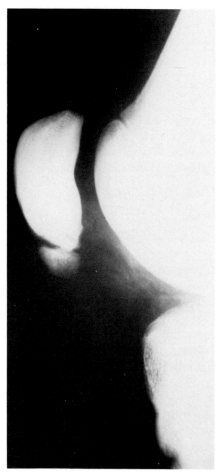

FIGURE 22. Roentgenogram of Sinding-Larson-Johansson's disease in a young athlete.

VIII. FAT PAD SYNDROME

Although the etiology of fat pad syndrome (Hoffa's disease) is not yet completely understood, most authors believe that the primary cause of fat pad syndrome
is the repeated traumatization of the infrapatellar fatty pad during activities that
require constant repetition of maximal extension in the knee.[188,193,197,201,202,209,215]
Diagnosis is usually made *per exclusionem* due to the fact that there are no specific
symptoms characterizing this disease. Unlike the asymptomatic projecting infrapatellar
fatty pad at the patella alta ("camel back sign"), fat pad syndrome is characterized by
contact tenderness of the fatty pad, as well as during palpation along the edge of the
patellar ligament. Fat pad syndrome is further characterized by the appearance of
pain during hyperextension of the knee — in other words, by a positive Smillie's sign
(appearance of pain during sudden passive hyperextension of the knee), by the
appearance of blockades that are hard to differentiate from meniscal blockades, and
by a normal X-ray.

In most cases, treatment is nonoperative; it involves rest, cryotherapy, nonsteroidal anti-inflammatory drugs, and elevation of the heels of the shoes which reduces,
and in some cases, completely disables hyperextension of the knee. In persistent
cases, surgical treatment is indicated — resection of the fatty pad.[212]

IX. PLICA SYNDROME

Fatty tissue pads located on the anterior wall of the joint capsule of the knee,
between the fibrous and synovial membrane, project the synovial membrane into the
cavity of the joint, forming plicae, the so-called plicae synovials (Figure 23). The
infrapatellar plica is the most constant of these plicae. It projects from the infrapatellar
fatty pad to the intertrochlear fossa and is also called the *mucosum ligament*. The

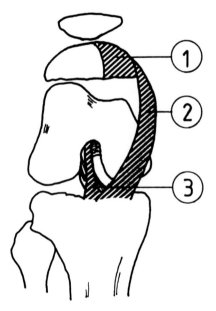

FIGURE 23. Schematic representation of plicae
synovials of the knee. (1) Suprapatellar; (2) medial; (3)
infrapatellar.

suprapatellar plica partially divides the suprapatellar recessus from the knee joint and is found in about 60 to 80% of the cases reported.[211] The medial plica, which can in some cases be joined to the suprapatellar plica, projects along the anteromedial part of the knee joint to the infrapatellar fatty pad and is found in 18 to 55% of the cases reported.[211]

The symptoms are, in most cases, caused by a chronically changed (fibrotic, enlarged, and sometimes calcified) medial plica, and only rarely by chronic changes of the suprapatellar plica.[192,194,211,215] While bending the knee, the affected plica strikes the medial facet of the patella; while extending the knee, it is in contact with the anteromedial part of the femoral condyle. Malacia, clinically manifested as chondromalacia, develops at the contact points. Anamnestic data of repeated audible effects described as explosive snaps and occasional blockades help in diagnosing the plica syndrome. Clinical examination sometimes reveals the plica during palpation, but in most cases, the only symptom is tenderness to palpation of the medial facet of the patella and medial femoral condyle. Nonoperative treatment consisting of rest, use of nonsteroidal anti-inflammatory drugs, stretching exercises for the hamstrings, strengthening exercises for the quadriceps, and wearing of special knee braces, generally supplies the results. In resistant cases, surgical treatment is indicated — arthroscopic excision of the plica.[192,194,201,211]

X. SEMIMEMBRANOSUS TENDINITIS

Semimembranosus tendinitis is not an uncommon entity and is often an overlooked cause of posteromedial knee pain. This entity is usually associated with other knee disorders caused by overuse, mostly chondromalacia of the patella, but may occur as an isolated syndrome. The main symptom is pain located at the very posteromedial corner of the knee just immediately below the joint line.[213] During physical examination, pain is produced by applying pressure to the anterior medial tendon of the semimembranous muscle, immediately below the knee joint, and at the insertion of the posterior medial tendon on the posterior part of the tibial medial condyle (Figure 24). Tenderness is amplified if the knee is in a 90° flexion and the lower leg in maximum outward rotation.

Semimembranosus tendinitis is often confused with injury of the medial meniscus. A proper diagnosis is reached by taking a detailed history and by the absence of pain during clinical tests for medial meniscus injuries.[187] Differential diagnosis includes ruling out the possibility of medial collateral ligament bursitis, which is characterized by pain and a slight swelling above the medial collateral ligament immediately below the knee joint.[198] The pes anserinus tendons should also be palpated to rule out the possibility of enthesitis of those tendons, and in some cases, the inflammation of the pes anserinus bursae. In most cases, treatment is nonoperative and surgical intervention is rarely indicated.

XI. PES ANSERINUS TENDINITIS AND BURSITIS

The tendons of the sartorius, semitendinosus, and gracillis muscles insert on the medial plane of the tibia, just below the condyle, forming the so-called pes anserinus (goose foot). Pes anserinus syndrome is frequently found in long-distance runners.

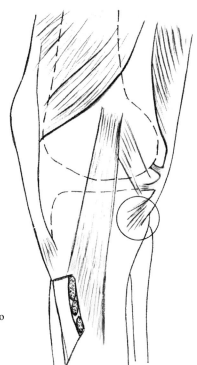

FIGURE 24. Insertion of the semimembranosus tendon to the posteromedial aspect of the tibia.

Predisposing factors for the development of this syndrome include incorrect training techniques, excessive tightness of the hamstring muscles, valgus alignment of the knee, and excessive rotation of the lower leg in the outward direction.[193,201,204,209]

Bursitis is more frequent and presents less problems, both in diagnosis and treatment. During physical examination, a slight swelling is usually found on the medial side of the knee joint at the level of the tibial tubercle. Ultrasound examination facilitates correct diagnosis of bursitis.

Diagnosing enthesitis presents more problems. In older athletes, medial meniscus injury must be ruled out as must arthrosis of the medial compartment of the knee. In some cases, scintigraphy is performed to rule out the possibility of stress fractures, which typically appear on the posteromedial part of the proximal tibia.[196] Treatment is usually nonoperative.[193,212]

XII. POPLITEAL TENDINITIS

Popliteal tendinitis is characterized by localized tenderness in the area above the origin of the popliteal muscle on the lateral part of the lateral femoral condyle.[189] Excessive and/or extended pronation of the foot during running is considered to be a predisposing factor in developing this syndrome.[201,216] Popliteal tendinitis is one of the many injuries to the knee joint that is characterized by tenderness in the lateral area of the knee. To localize the exact area of greatest tenderness, the afflicted leg is placed in the so-called "figure four" position (Figure 25), where the popliteus muscle tendon and the lateral collateral ligament are extended and thus accessible to

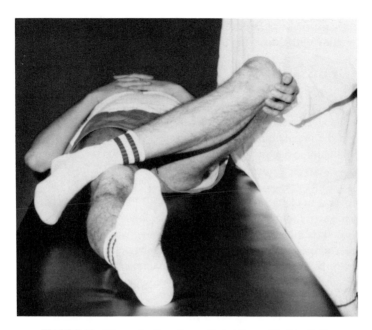

FIGURE 25. "Figure four" — diagnostic test for popliteal tendinitis.

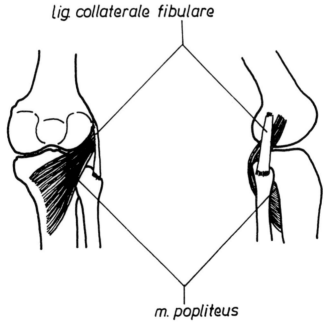

lig. collaterale fibulare

m. popliteus

FIGURE 26. Relationship of the lateral collateral ligament to the popliteal tendon.

palpation (Figure 26). Pain is produced by applying pressure with a finger to the area of the insertion of the popliteus muscle located slightly anteriorly and distally from the origin of the lateral collateral ligament.

Treatment is usually nonoperative and carried out according to the principles set down for treating enthesitis. Surgical treatment is rarely performed.[212]

XIII. FABELA SYNDROME (FABELITIS)

The fabela is a sesamoid bone located on the posterior side of the lateral femoral condyle in the lateral head of the gastrocnemius muscle (Figure 27). It is present in 10 to 18% of the population.[208] The fabela serves as an attachment site for strands from the popliteum arcuatum and popliteum obliquum ligaments. The anterior side of the fabela is covered in cartilage, which forms a joint with the lateral femoral condyle.

The presence of the fabela, and more specifically, injuries to the fabela can cause tenderness and sensations of radiating pain in the lower leg. The causes of this pain are multiple and include direct trauma to the fabela, overuse syndrome, changes on the fabelar cartilage, and arthritic changes in the fabela. In athletes, fabela syndrome is mostly the direct result of long-lasting microtraumas. Moyen et al.[208] reported that fabela syndrome makes up 1.7% of the pathological changes in athletes' knees. Excessive functioning of the lateral head of the gastrocnemius muscle, especially

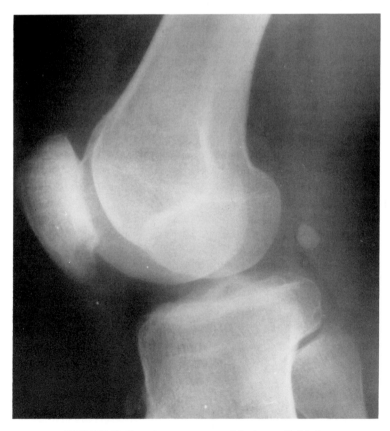

FIGURE 27. Lateral roentgenogram of the knee with fabela.

during the beginning stages of flexion in the knee and during outward rotation of the lower leg immediately before full extension, are thought to be related to the etiopathogenesis of fabela syndrome. Predisposing factors for developing fabela syndrome include existence of genu recurvatum accompanied by hypermobility of the lateral compartment of the knee.

Clinical manifestations are characterized by the gradual onset of pain which radiates into the lower leg, specifically the peroneus communis nerve dermatoma. The pain is usually moderate in intensity and associated with knee movements, either due to extension of the muscles during hyperextension of the knee or to direct pressure on the fabela, e.g., when sitting with legs crossed. Pain can be provoked by transverse movement of the fabela when the knee is extended or slightly flexed. Both the localized tenderness and the radiating pain can be amplified or provoked by applying pressure to the fabela, in the area posterior to the lateral femoral condyle, and above the joint line. Radiographic examination usually does not help, while arthroscopy, using the complicated posteroexternal approach, generally does.

Differential diagnosis must rule out the possibility of rupture of the posterior horn of the lateral meniscus and also tendinitis of the lateral head of the gastrocnemius muscle, the biceps femoris, and the popliteus muscle. Fracture of the fabela and hypertrophic and arthritic fabelas (which press the peroneus communis nerve) are rarely seen.

If the usual nonoperative treatment, including infiltration of anesthetics with corticosteroids, shows no improvement, surgical treatment, consisting of extirpation of the fabela, is indicated. Extirpation of the fabela must be accompanied by reconstruction of the posterior wall of the joint capsule.[219]

REFERENCES

Patellophemoral Joint

1. **Aglietti, P., Insall, J. N., and Cerulli, G.** Patellar pain and incongruence. I: Measurements of incongruence. *Clin. Orthop.,* 1983; 176:217–224.
2. **Bajraktarević-Ćiéin-Sain, T. and Pećina, M.** Radiološka istraživanja nestabilnosti patele. *Rad. Med. Fak. Zagrebu,* 1989; 30:41–50.
3. **Bandi, W.** Chondromalacia patellae und femoro-patellare Arthrose. *Helv. Chir. Acta (suppl.),* 1972; 1:3–70.
4. **Blackburne, J. S. and Peel, T. E.** A new method of measuring patellar height. *J. Bone Joint Surg.,* 1977; 59(B):241–242.
5. **Blazina, M. E., Kerlan, R. K., Jobe, F. W., Carter, V. S., and Carlson, J. G.** Jumper's knee. *Orthop. Clin. N. Am.,* 1973; 4:665–678.
6. **Bojanić, I. and Pećina, M.** Axial stress X-rays in diagnosing patellar instability. *Period. Biol.,* 1992; in press.
7. **Bourne, M. H., Hazel, W. A., Jr., Scott, S. G., and Sim, F. H.** Anterior knee pain. *Mayo Clin. Proc.,* 1988; 63:482–491.

8. **Burgess, R. C.** A new method of determining patellar position. *J. Sports Med.*, 1989; 29:398–399.

9. **Carson, W. G., Jr, James, S. L., Larson, R. L., Singer, K. M., and Winternitz, W. W.** Patellofemoral disorders: physical and radiographic evaluation. Part I and II. *Clin. Orthop.*, 1984; 185:165–186.

10. **Casscells, S. W.** Gross pathological changes in the knee joint of the aged individual: a study of 300 cases. *Clin. Orthop.*, 1978; 132:225–232.

11. **Caton, J., Deschamps, G., Chambat, P., Lerat, J. L., and Dejour, H.** Les rotules basses. A propos de 128 observations. *Rev. Chir. Orthop.*, 1982; 68:317–325.

12. **Dandy, D. J.** Arthroscopy in the treatment of young patients with anterior knee pain. *Orthop. Clin. N. Am.*, 1986; 17:221–229.

13. **Dandy, D. J.** *Arthroscopic Management of the Knee*, 2nd ed. Edinburgh: Churchill Livingstone, 1987.

14. **Dandy, D. J. and Griffiths, D.** Lateral release for recurrent dislocation of the patella. *J. Bone Joint Surg.*, 1989; 71(B):121–125.

15. **De Carvahlo, A., Andersen, A. H., Topp, S., and Jurik, A. G.** A method for assessing the height of the patella. *Int. Orthop. (SICOT)*, 1985; 9:195–197.

16. **Dejour, H., Walch, G., Neyret, P., and Adeleine, P.** La dysplasie de la trochlee femorale. *Rev. Chir. Orthop.*, 1990; 76:45–54.

17. **Delgado-Martins, H.** A study of the position of the patella using computerized tomography. *J. Bone Joint Surg.*, 1979; 61(B):443–444.

18. **Dugdale, T. W. and Barnett, P. R.** Historical background: patellofemoral pain in young people. *Orthop. Clin. N. Am.*, 1986; 17:211–219.

19. **Džolev, G., Simončev, V., Pećina, M., and Serafimov, L.** Finite elements method in the biomechanical analysis of the knee following meniscectomy. *Orthop. Trauma*, 1992; 23:27–33.

20. **Ficat, P. and Hungerford, D. S.** *Disorders of the Patellofemoral Joint.* Baltimore: Williams & Wilkins, 1977.

21. **Ficat, R. P., Philippe, J., and Hungerford, D. S.** Chondromalacia patellae: a system of classification. *Clin. Orthop.*, 1979; 144:55–62.

22. **Fulkerson, J. P. and Hungerford, D. S.** *Disorders of the Patellofemoral Joint.* Baltimore: Williams & Wilkins, 1990.

23. **Fulkerson, J. P., Schutzer, S. F., and Ramsby, G. R.** Computerized tomography of the ptellofemoral joint before and after lateral release or realignment. *J. Arthrosc. Rel. Surg.*, 1987; 3:19–24.

24. **Fulkerson, J. P. and Shea, K. P.** Disorders of patellofemoral alignment *J. Bone Joint Surg.*, 1990; 72(A):1424–1429.

25. **Garrick, J. G.** Anterior knee pain (chondromalacia patellae). *Phys. Sportsmed.*, 1989; 17:75–84.

26. **Gecha, S. R. and Torg, E.** Knee injuries in tennis. *Clin. Sports Med.*, 1988; 7:435–452.

27. **Goodfellow, J., Hungerford, D. S., and Zindel, M.** Patello-femoral joint mechanics and pathology. I. Functional anatomy of the patellofemoral joint. *J. Bone Joint Surg.*, 1976; 58(B):287–290.

28. **Graf, J., Neithard, F. U., and Cotta, H.** Zur Begriffsbestimmung von Chondropathia und Chondromalacia ptellae. *Z. Orthop.*, 1990; 128:289–294.

29. **Hehne, H. J.** Biomechanics of the patellofemoral joint and its clinical relevance. *Clin. Orthop.*, 1990; 258:73–85.

30. **Hughston, J. C.** Patellar subluxation. *Clin. Sports Med.*, 1989; 8:153–162.

31. **Hughston, J. C. and Deese, M.** Medial subluxation of the patella as a complication of lateral retinacular release. *Am. J. Sports Med.*, 1988; 16:383–388.

32. **Imai, N., Tomatsu, T., Takeuchi, H., and Noguchi, T.** Clinical and roentgenological studies on malalignment disorders of the patellofemoral joint. Part I. Classification of patellofemoral alignments using dynamic sky-line view arthrography with special consideration of the mechanism of the malalignment disorders. *J. Jpn. Orthop Assoc.,* 1987; 61:1–15.

33. **Imai, N. and Tomatsu, T.** Cartilage lesions in the knee of adolescents and young adults: arthroscopic analysis. *Arthroscopy,* 1991; 7:198–203.

34. **Inoue, M., Shino, K., Hirose, H., Horibe, S., and Ono, K.** Subluxation of the patella. *J. Bone Joint Surg.,* 1988; 70(A):1331–1337.

35. **Insall, J.** Patellar pain. *J. Bone Joint Surg.,* 1982; 64(A):147–151.

36. **Insall, J. N. and Salvati, E.** Patella position in the normal knee joint. *Radiology,* 1971; 101:101–104.

37. **Ireland, M. L.** Patellofemoral disorders in runners and bicyclists. *Ann. Sports Med.,* 1987; 3:77–84.

38. **Jackson, D. W., Jennings, L. D., Maywood, R. M., and Berger, P. E.** Magnetic resonance imaging of the knee. *Am. J. Sports Med.,* 1988; 16:29–38.

39. **Jacobson, K. E. and Flandry, F. C.** Diagnosis of anterior knee pain. *Clin. Sports Med.,* 1989; 8:179–195.

40. **Johnson, L. L.** *Arthroscopic Surgery: Principles and Practice.* St. Louis: C. V. Mosby, 1986.

41. **Karadimas, J. E., Piscopakis, N., and Syrmalis, L.** Patella alta and chondromalacia. *Int. Orthop. (SICOT),* 1981; 5:247–249.

42. **Kujala, U. M., Osterman, K., Kvist, M., Aalto, T., and Friberg, O.** Factors predisposing to patellar chondropathy and patellar apicitis in athletes. *Int. Orthop. (SICOT),* 1986; 10:195–200.

43. **Kujala, U. M., Osterman, K., Kormano, M., Kornu, M., and Schlenzka, D.** Patellar motion analyzed by magnetic resonance imaging. *Acta Orthop. Scand.,* 1989; 60:13–16.

44. **Kujala, U. M., Osterman, K., Kormano, M., Nelimarkka, O., Hurme, M., and Taimela, S.** Patellofemoral relationships in recurrent patellar dislocations. *J. Bone Joint Surg.,* 1989; 71(B):788–792.

45. **Laurin, C. A., Dussault, R., and Levesque, H. P.** The tangenital X-ray investigation of the patellofemoral joint: X-ray technique, diagnostic criteria and their interpretation. *Clin. Orthop.,* 1979; 144:16–26.

46. **Lindberg, U., Hamberg, P., Lysholm, J., and Gillquist, J.** Arthroscopic examination of the patellofemoral joint using a central, one-portal technique. *Orthop. Clin. N. Am.,* 1986; 17:263–268.

47. **Macnicol, M. F.** *The Problem Knee. Diagnosis and Management in the Younger Patient.* London: William Heinemann Medical Books, 1986.

48. **Main, W. K. and Hershman, E. B.** Chronic knee pain in active adolescents. *Phys. Sportsmed.,* 1992; 20:139–156.

49. **Maquet, P.** *Biomechanics of the Knee.* Berlin: Springer-Verlag, 1976.

50. **Matijasević, B., Pećina, M., Jelić, M., and Bajraktarević, T.** Kynematic analysis of the patellofemoral joint. *Orthop. Trauma,* 1992; 23:7–13.

51. **Martines, S., Korobkin, M., Fondren, F. B., Hedlund, L. W., and Goldner, J. L.** Computed tomography of the normal patellofemoral joint. *Invest. Radiol.,* 1983; 18:249–252.

52. **Merchant, A. C.** Classification of patellofemoral disorders. *Arthroscopy,* 1988; 4:235–240.

53. **Merchant, A. C., Mercer, R. L., Jacobsen, R. H., and Cool, C. R.** Roentgenographic analysis of patellofemoral congruence. *J. Bone Joint Surg.,* 1974; 56(A):1391–1396.

54. **Minkoff, J. and Fein, L.** The role of radiography in the evaluation and treatment of common anathrotic disorders of the patellofemoral joint. *Clin. Sports Med.,* 1989; 8:203–260.

55. **Moller, B. N., Krebs, B., and Jurik, A. G.** Patellofemoral incongruence in chondromalacia and instability of the patella. *Acta Orthop. Scand.,* 1986; 57:232–234.

56. **Morscher, E.** Osteotomy of the patella in chondromalacia. Preliminary report. *Arch. Orthop. Trauma Surg.,* 1978; 92:139–147.

57. **Noyes, F. R. and Stabler, C. L.** A system for grading articular cartilage lesions at arthroscopy. *Am. J. Sports Med.,* 1989; 17:505–513.

58. **Outerbridge, R. E.** The etiology of chondromalacia patellae. *J. Bone Joint Surg.,* 1961; 43(B):752–757.

59. **Patel, D.** Plica as a cause of anterior knee pain. *Orthop. Clin. N. Am.,* 1986; 17:273–277.

60. **Pećina, M.** Longitudinal osteotomy of the patella after Morscher. In: *Surgery and Arthroscopy of the Knee.* Muller, W., Hackenbruch, W. H., Eds. Berlin: Springer-Verlag, 1988; 471–476.

61. **Pećina, M., Bilić, R., and Koržinek, K.** Ventralisation der Patella unsere zehnjahrige Erfarung. In: *Das Kniegelenk.* Chapchal, G., Ed. Stuttgart: Georg Thieme Verlag, 1989; 118–120.

62. **Pećina, M.** Longitudinal osteotomy of the patella in the treatment of chondromalacia in the top-level athletes. 1st World Cong. Sports Trauma, Palma de Mallorca, 1992, Abstracts Book, 205–206.

63. **Perrild, C., Hejgaard, N., and Rosenklint, A.** Chondromalacia patellae. A radiographic study of the femoropatellar joint. *Acta Orthop. Scand.,* 1982; 53:131–134.

64. **Radin, E. L.** Anterior knee pain. The need for a specific diagnosis: stop calling it chondromalacia! *Orthop. Rev.,* 1985; 14:128–134.

65. **Reider, B., Marshall, J. L., and Ring, B.** Patellar tracking. *Clin. Orthop.,* 1981; 157:143–148.

66. **Roland, G. C., Beagley, M. J., and Cawley, P. W.** Conservative treatment of inflamed knee bursae. *Phys. Sportsmed.,* 1992; 20:67–77.

67. **Sandow, M. J., and Goodfellow, J. W.** The natural history of anterior knee pain in adolescents. *J. Bone Joint Surg.,* 1985; 67(B):36–38.

68. **Schutzer, S. F., Ramsby, G. R., and Fulkerson, J. P.** Computed tomographic classification of patellofemoral pain patients. *Orthop. Clin. N. Am.,* 1986; 17:235–248.

69. **Shellock, F. G., Mink, J. H., and Fox, J. M.** Patellofemoral joint: kinematic MR imaging to assess tracking abnormalities. *Radiology,* 1988; 168:551–553.

70. **Shellock, F. G., Mink, J. H., Deutsch, A. L., and Fox, J. M.** Patellar tracking abnormalities: clinical experience with kinematic MR imaging in 130 patients. *Radiology,* 1989; 172:799–804.

71. **Soejbjerg, J. O., Lauritzen, J., Hvid, I., and Boe, S.** Arthroscopic determination of patellofemoral malalignment. *Clin. Orthop.,* 1987; 215:243–247.

72. **Teitge, R. A.** Stress X-rays for patellofemoral instability. Monograph accompanying exhibit at the 3rd Eur. Congr. Knee Surgery (ESKA), Amsterdam, May 1988.

73. **Terry, G. C.** Office evaluation and management of the symptomatic knee. *Orthop. Clin. N. Am.,* 1988; 19:699–713.

74. **Wiberg, G.** Roentgenographic and anatomic studies of the patellofemoral joint. *Acta Orthop. Scand.,* 1941; 12:319–410.

Patellar Tendinitis (Jumper's Knee)

75. **Apple, D. F., Jr.** Progressive quadriceps strengthening — best cure for jumper's knee. *J. Muskuloskel. Med.,* 1987; 4:11.

76. **Beckman, M., Craig, R., and Lehman, R. C.** Rehabilitation of patellofemoral dysfunction in the athlete. *Clin. Sports Med.,* 1989; 8:841–861.
77. **Blazina, M. E., Kerlan, R. K., Jobe, F. W., Karter, V. S., and Carlson, G. J.** Jumper's knee. *Orthop. Clin. N. Am.,* 1973; 4:665–678.
78. **Black, J. E. and Alten, S. R.** How I manage infrapatellar tendinitis. *Phys. Sportsmed.,* 1983; 12:86–92.
79. **Bodne, D., Quinn, S. F., Murray, W. T.,** et al. Magnetic resonance images of chronic patellar tendinitis. *Skel. Radiol.,* 1988; 17:24.
80. **Brunet-Quedi, E. and Imbert, J. C.** Les tendinites du genou. In: *Lesions Traumatiques des Tendons chez le Sportif.* Catonne, Y. and Saillant, G., Eds. Paris: Masson, 1992; 100–106.
81. **Colosimo, A. J., Basset, F. H.** Jumper's knee. Diagnosis and treatment. *Orthop. Rev.,* 1990; 19:139–149.
82. **Combelles, F. and Saillant, G.** Place de la chirurgie dans le traitement des tendinites rotuliennes du sportif. *Lett. Chir.,* 1989; 77:28–30.
83. **Crass, J. R., Lucy van de Vegte, G., and Harkavy, L. A.** Tendon echogenicity: *ex vivo* study. *Radiology,* 1988; 167:499–501.
84. **Ferretti, A., Nevi, M., Mariani, P. P., and Puddu, G.** Ethiopathogenetic considerations on the jumper's knee. *Ital. J. Sports Trauma,* 1983; 5:101–105.
85. **Ferretti, A., Ippolito, E., Mariani, P. P., and Puddu, G.** Jumper's knee. *Am. J. Sports Med.,* 1983; 11:58–62.
86. **Ferretti, A., Puddu, G., Mariani, P. P., and Neri, M.** Jumper's knee. An epidemiological study of volleyball players. *Phys. Sportsmed.,* 1984; 12:97–106.
87. **Ferretti, A., Puddu, G., Mariani, P. P., and Neri, M.** The natural history of jumper's knee. *Int. Orthop (SICOT),* 1985; 8:239–242.
88. **Ferretti, A.** Epidemiology of jumper's knee. *Sports Med.,* 1986; 3:289–295.
89. **Ferretti, A., Papandrea, P., and Conteduca, F.** Knee injuries in volleyball. *Sports Med.,* 1990; 10:132–138.
90. **Fornage, B. D. and Rifkin, M. D.** Ultrasound examination of tendons. *Radiol. Clin. N. Am.,* 1988; 26:63–75.
91. **Fornage, B. D., Rifkin, M. D., Touche, D. H., and Segal, P. M.** Ultrasonography of the patellar tendon: preliminary observations. *AJR,* 1984; 143:179–182.
92. **Friedl, E. W. and Glaser, F.** Dynamic sonography in the diagnosis of ligament and meniscal injuries of the knee. *Arch. Orthop. Trauma Surg.,* 1991; 110:132–139.
93. **Fritchy, D. and Gautard, R.** Jumper's knee and ultrasonography. *Am. J. Sports Med.,* 1988; 16:637–640.
94. **Giacomelli, E., Grassi, W., and Zampa, A. M.** Le atlopatie nei pallavolisti. *Med. Sport.,* 1986; 39:425–434.
95. **Greenspan, A., Norman, A., and Kia-Ming, Tchang, F.** "Tooth" sign in patellar degenerative disease. *J. Bone Joint Surg.,* 1977; 59(B):483–485.
96. **Haller, W. and Lehner, K.** Bildgebende Verfahren zur Diagnostic von Kniegelenksverletzungen und — Erkraukungen. *Roentgenpraxis,* 1989; 42:198–204.
97. **Hannesschlager, G., Neumuller, H., Riedelberger, W., Reschauer, R.** Sonographische Diagnostic von Pathologischen Vernderungen des vorderen Kniegelenksbereiches. *Ultraschall,* 1990; 11:33–39.
98. **Henry, J. H.** Jumper's knee. *Sport Med. Actual.,* 1988; 3:10–13.
99. **Janssen, G.** Das Patellaspitzensyndrom. *Orthop. Praxis,* 1983; 19:12–15.
100. **Jensen, K., Di Fabrio, R. P.** Evaluation of eccentric exercises in treatment in patellar tendinitis. *Phys. Ther.,* 1989; 69:211–216.
101. **Jerosch, J., Castro, W. H. M., Sons, H. U., and Winkelman, W.** Der Aussagewert der Sonographic bei Verletzungen des Kneegelenkes. *Ultraschall,* 1989; 10:275–278.

102. **Jerosch, J., Castro, W. H. M., Sons, H. U., and Winkelman, W.** Moglichkeiten der Sonographic beim Patellaspitzen syndrom. *Ultraschall,* 1990; 11:44–47.

103. **Kalebo, P., Sward, L., Karlssen, J., and Peterson, L.** Ultrasonography in the detection of partial patellar ligament ruptures (jumper's knee). *Skel. Radiol.,* 1991; 20:285–289.

104. **Kahn, D. and Wilson, M. A.** Bone scintigraphic findings in patellar tendinitis. *J. Nucl. Med.,* 1987; 28:1769.

105. **Karlsson, J., Lundin, O., Lassing, I. W., and Peterson, L.** Partial rupture of the patellar ligament. Results after operative treatment. *Am. J. Sports Med.,* 1991; 19:403–408.

106. **Kelly, D. W., Carter, V. S., Jobe, F. W., and Kerlan, R. K.** Patellar and quadriceps tendon ruptures — jumper's knee. *Am. J. Sports Med.,* 1984; 12:375–380.

107. **Kettelkamp, D. B.** Management of patellar malalignment. *J. Bone Joint Surg.,* 1981; 63(B):1344–1347.

108. **King, J. B., Perry, D. J., Mowad, K., and Kumar, S. J.** Lesions of the patellar ligament. *J. Bone Joint Surg.,* 1990; 72(B):46–48.

109. **Krahl, H.** "Jumper's Knee". Atiologie, differential Diagnose und therapeutische Moglishkeiten. *Orthopade,* 1980; 9:193–197.

110. **Kujala, M. H., Osterman, K., Kvist, M., Aalto, T., and Friberg, O.** Factors predisposing to patellar chondropathy and patellar apicitis in athletes. *Int. Orthop. (SICOT),* 1986; 10:195–200.

111. **Kujala, M. H., Kvist, M., and Osterman, K.** Knee injuries in athletes, review of exertion injuries and retrospective study of outpatient sports clinic material. *Sports Med.,* 1986; 3:447–460.

112. **Laine, H. R., Harjube, A., and Peltokallio, P.** Ultrasound in the evaluation of the knee and patellar regions. *J. Ultrasound Med.,* 1987; 6:33–36.

113. **Maddox, P. A. and Garth, W. P.** Tendinitis of the patellar ligament and quadriceps (jumper's knee) as an initial presentation of hyperparathyroidism. A Case report. *J. Bone Joint Surg.,* 1986; 68(A):289–292.

114. **Martens, M., Wonkers, P., Bursens, A., and Mulier, J. C.** Patellar tendinitis. Pathology and result of treatment. *Acta Orthop. Scand.,* 1982; 53:445–450.

115. **Mourad, K., King, J., and Guggina, P.** Computed tomography and ultrasound imaging of jumper's knee — patellar tendinitis. *Clin. Radiol.,* 1988; 39:162–165.

116. **Mellerowicz, H., Stelling, E., Kafenbaum, A.** Diagnostic ultrasound in the athlete's locomotor system. *Br. J. Sports Med.,* 1990; 24:32–39.

117. **Noesberger, B., Fernandez, D., and Meyer, R. P.** Das jumper's knee. *Helv. Chir. Acta,* 1976; 43:447–450.

118. **Pećina, M. and Bilić, R.** Mogućnosti liječenja "koljena skakača". *ŠMO,* 1983; 20:143–148.

119. **Pećina, M., Dubravčić, S., Smerdelj, M., and Ribarić, G.** Doprinos etiologiji skakačkog koljena. *KMV,* 1988; 3:11–14.

120. **Pećina, M., Dubravčić, S., Smerdelj, M., and Ribarić, G.** Contribution to the etiological explanation of "Basketball knee". *Sport Med. Actual.,* 1988; 3:29–31.

121. **Pećina, M., Ribarić, G., Bojanić, I., and Dubravčić, S.** Jumper's knee. *KMV,* 1989; 4:15–21.

122. **Pećina, M. and Bojanić, I.** Surgical treatment of jumper's knee in top level athletes. In: *Sports, Medicine and Health.* Hermans, G. P. H., Ed. Amsterdam: Elsevier Science Publishers, 1990; 299–304.

123. **Perrugia, L., Pastacchini, F., and Ippolito, E.** *The Tendons: Biology — Pathology-Clinical Aspects.* Milano: Editrice Kurtis, 1986.

124. **Richardson, M. I., Selby, B., Montana, M. A., and Mack, L. A.** Ultrasonography of the knee. *Radiol. Clin. N. Am.,* 1988; 26:63–75.

125. **Roels, J., Martens, M., Mulier, J. C., and Burssens, A.** Patellar tendinitis (jumper's knee). *Am. J. Sports Med.,* 1978; 6:362–368.

126. **Rosenberg, J. M. and Whitaker, J. H.** Bilateral infrapatellar tendon rupture in a patient with jumper's knee. *Am. J. Sports Med.,* 1991; 19:94–95.

127. **Sala, H.** Jumper's knee: diagnosis and treatment. *Acta Orthop. Scand.,* 1985; 56:450.

128. **Schmidt, D. R. and Henry, J. H.** Stress injuries of the adolescent extensor mechanism. *Clin. Sports Med.,* 1989; 8:343–357.

129. **Shelbourne, K. D.** Personal communication,

130. **Siwek, C. W., and Rac, P. Y.** Ruptures of the extensor mechanism of the knee joint. *J. Bone Joint Surg.,* 1981; 63(A):932–937.

131. **Smith, A. D., Stround, L., and McQueen, C.** Flexibility and anterior knee pain in adolescent elite figure skaters. *J. Pediatr. Orthop.,* 1991; 11:77–82.

132. **Sommer, H.** Patellar chondropathy and apicitis and muscle imbalances of the lower extremities in competitive sports. *Sports Med.,* 1988; 5:386–394.

133. **Stanish, W. D., Rubinovich, R. M., and Curwin, S.** Eccentric exercise in chronic tendinitis. *Clin. Orthop.,* 1986; 208:65–68.

134. **Teitz, C. C.** Ultrasonography in the knee. Clinical aspects. *Radiol. Clin. N. Am.,* 1988; 26:55–62.

135. **Terry, G. C.** The anatomy of the extensor mechanism. *Clin. Sports Med.,* 1989; 8:163–179.

136. **Tarsney, F. F.** Catastrophic jumper's knee. A case report. *Am. J. Sports Med.,* 1981; 9:60–61.

137. **Urban, K. and Michalek, J.,** Mo˘znosti Diagnostiky a Le˘ceni Skokanskeno. Koleno. *Suppl. Sb. Ved. Pr. Lek. Fak. Karlovy Univ. Hradci Kralove,* 1989; 32:201–208.

138. **Van der Ent, A. and De Baere, A. J.** Jumper's knee: results of operative therapy. *Acta Orthop. Scand.,* 1985; 56:450.

139. **Voto, S. J. and Ewing, J. W.** Retrotendinous calcification of the infrapatellar tendon: unusual cause of anterior knee pain syndrome. *Arthroscopy,* 1988; 4:81–84.

140. **Walsh, W. M., Hunrman, W. W., and Shelton, G. L.** Overuse injuries of the knee and spine in girls gymnastics. *Orthop. Clin. N. Am.,* 1985; 16:329–334.

141. **Weinstabl, R., Scharf, W., and Firbas, W.** The extensor aparatus of the knee joint and its perpheral vasti: anatomic investigation and clinical relevance. *Surg. Radiol. Anat.,* 1989; 11:17–22.

142. **Wirth, M. A., De Lee, J. C.** The history and classification of knee braces. *Clin. Sports Med.,* 1990; 9:731–741.

Breaststroker's Knee

143. **Costill, D. L., Maglischo, W. E., and Richardson, B. A.** *Handbook of Sports Medicine and Science Swimming.* Oxford: Blackwell Scientific Publications, 1992.

144. **Johnson, J. E., Sim, F. H., and Scott, S. G.** Musculoskeletal injuries in competitive swimmers. *Mayo Clin. Proc.,* 1987; 62:289–304.

145. **Kennedy, J. C. and Hawkins, R. J.** Breaststroker's knee. *Phys. Sportsmed.,* 1974; 2:33–38.

146. **Keskinen, K., Eriksson, E., and Komi, P.** Breaststroke swimmer's knee. *Am. J. Sports Med.,* 1980; 8:228–231.

147. **Rovere, G. D. and Nichols, A. W.** Frequency, associated factors, and treatment of breaststroker's knee in competitive swimmers. *Am. J. Sports Med.,* 1985; 13:99–104.

148. **Stulberg, S. D., Shulman, K., Stuart, S., and Culp, P.** Breaststroker's knee: pathology, etiology, and treatment. *Am. J. Sports Med.,* 1980; 8:164–171.

149. **Taunton, J. E., McKenzie, D. C., and Clement, D. B.** The role of biomechanics in the epidemiology of injuries. *Sports Med.,* 1988; 6:107–120.

150. **Vizsoly, P., Taunton, J., Robertson, G.,** et al. Breaststroker's knee. An analysis of epidemiological and biomechanical factors. *Am. J. Sports Med.,* 1987; 15:63–71.

151. **Wethelund, J. O. and de Carvalho, A.** An unusual lesion in the knee of breaststroke swimmer. *Int. J. Sports Med.,* 1985; 6:174–175.

Iliotibial Band Friction Syndrome

152. **Andrews, J. R.** Overuse syndromes of the lower extremity. *Clin. Sports Med.,* 1983; 2:137–148.

153. **Bojanić, I., Pećina, M., and Ribarić, G.** Sindrom trenja iliotibijalnog traktusa. *Acta Orthop. lugosl.,* 1989; 20:68–75.

154. **Brody, D. M.** Running Injuries. *Clin. Symp.,* 1987; 39:1–36.

155. **Cook, S. D., Brinker, M. R., and Pocke, M.** Running shoes: their relationship to running injuries. *Sports Med.,* 1990; 10:1–8.

156. **Firer, P.** Aetiology and results of treatment of iliotibial band friction syndrome. 6th Congr. Int. Soc. Knee, Rome, Abstracts, Book 1989.

157. **Grana, W. A. and Coniglione, T. C.** Knee disorders in runners. *Phys. Sportsmed.,* 1985; 13:127–133.

158. **Jones, D. C. and James, S. L.** Overuse injuries of the lower extremity. *Clin. Sports. Med.,* 1987; 6:273–290.

159. **Kaplan, E. B.** The iliotibial tract. *J. Bone Joint Surg.,* 1958; 40 (A):817–832.

160. **Kujala, U. M., Kvist, M., Osterman, K.** Knee injuries in athletes. *Sports Med.,* 1986; 3:447–460.

161. **Lehman, W. L.** Overuse syndromes in runners. *AFP,* 1984; 29:157–161.

162. **Lindenberg, G., Pinshaw, R., and Noakes, T. D.** Iliotibial band friction syndrome in runners. *Phys. Sportsmed.,* 1984; 12:118–130.

163. **Lysholm, J. and Wikllander, J.** Injuries in runners. *Am. J. Sports Med.,* 1987; 15:168–171.

164. **Macintyre, J. G., Taunton, J. E., Clement, D. B., et al.** Running injuries: a clinical study of 4.173 cases. *Clin. J. Sport Med.,* 1991; 1:81–87.

165. **Martens, M., Libbrecht, P., and Burssens, A.** Surgical treatment of the iliotibial band friction syndrome. *Am. J. Sports Med.,* 1989; 17:651–654.

166. **Marti, B., Vader, J. P., Minder, C. E., and Abelin, T.** On the epidemiology of running injuries. *Am. J. Sports Med.,* 1988; 16:285–294.

167. **Mattalino, A. J., Deese, J. M., and Campbell, E. D.** Office evaluation and treatment of lower extremity injuries in the runner. *Clin. Sports Med.,* 1989; 8:461–475.

168. **McKenzie, D. C., Clement, D. B., and Taunton, J. E.** Running shoes, orthotics and injuries. *Sports Med.,* 1985; 2:334–347.

169. **McNicol, K., Taunton, J. E., and Clement, D. B.** Iliotibial tract friction syndrome in athletes. *Can. J. Appl. Sport Sci.,* 1981; 6:76–80.

170. **Micheli, L. J.** Lower extremity overuse injuries. *Acta Med. Scand. (suppl.),* 1986; 711:171–177.

171. **Newell, S. G. and Bramwell, S. T.** Overuse injuries to the knee in runners. *Phys. Sportsmed.,* 1984; 12:80–92.

172. **Noble, C. A.** The treatment of iliotibial band friction syndrome. *Br. J. Sports Med.,* 1979; 13:51–54.

173. **Noble, C. A.** Iliotibial band friction syndrome in runners. *Am. J. Sports Med.,* 1980; 8:232–234.

174. **Orava, S.** Iliotibial tract friction syndrome in athletes — an uncommon exertion syndrome on the lateral side of the knee. *Br. J. Sports Med.,* 1978; 12:69–73.
175. **Pećina, M., Bilić, R., and Buljan, M.** Tractus iliotibialis sindrom — koljeno trkača. *Acta Orthop. Iugosl.,* 1984; 15:91–93.
176. **Powell, K. E., Kohl, H. W., Caspersen, C. J., et al.** An epidemiological perspective on the causes of running injuries. *Phys. Sportsmed.,* 1986; 14:100–114.
177. **Reid, D. C.** Prevention of hip and knee injuries in ballet dancers. *Sports Med.,* 1988; 6:295–307.
178. **Renne, J. W.** The iliotibial band friction syndrome. *J. Bone Joint Surg.,* 1975; 57A:1110–1111.
179. **Rovere, G. D., Webb, L. X., Cristina, A. G., et al.** Muskuloskeletal injuries in theatrical dance students. *Am. J. Sports Med.,* 1983; 11:195–198.
180. **Staff, P. H. and Nilsson, S.** Tendoperiostitis in the lateral femoral condyle in long-distance runners. *Br. J. Sports Med.,* 1980; 14:38–40.
181. **Sutker, A. N., Barber, F. A., Jackson, D. W., et al.** Iliotibial band syndrome in distance runners. *Sports Med.,* 1985; 2:447–451.
182. **Taunton, J. E., McKenzie, D. C., and Clement, D. B.** The role of biomechanics in the epidemiology of injuries. *Sports Med.,* 1988; 6:107–120.
183. **Terry, G. C., Hughston, J. C., and Norwood, L. A.** The anatomy of the iliopatellar band and iliotibial tract. *Am. J. Sports Med.,* 1986; 14:39–45.
184. **Weiss, B. D.** Nontraumatic injuries in amateur long distance bicyclists. *Am. J. Sports Med.,* 1985; 13:187–192.

Subchapters VI.–XIII.

185. **Antičević, D.** Juvenilni osteohondritis. *Jugosl. Pedijatr.,* 1989; 32(suppl. 1):43–47.
186. **Bencur, O. and Oslanec, D.** Our experience with the Osgood-Schlatter disease. *Acta Chir. Orthop. Trauma,* 1990; 57:15–20.
187. **Bloom, M. H.** Differentiating between meniscal and patellar pain. *Phys. Sportsmed.,* 1989; 17:94–106.
188. **Bourne, M. H., Hazel, W. A., Jr., and Scott, S. G.** Anterior knee pain. *Mayo Clin. Proc.,* 1988; 63:482–491.
189. **Brody, D. M.** Running injuries. *Clin. Symp.,* 1987; 39:1–36.
190. **Clain, M. R. and Hershman, E. B.** Overuse injuries in children and adolescents. *Phys. Sportsmed.,* 1989; 17:111–123.
191. **Dalton, S. E.** Overuse injuries in adolescent athletes. *Sports Med.,* 1992; 13:58–70.
192. **Dandy, D. J.** *Arthroscopic Management of the Knee.* Edinburgh: Churchill Livingstone, 1987; 182–201.
193. **Grana, W. A. and Coniglione, T. C.** Knee disorders in runners. *Phys. Sportsmed.,* 1985; 15:127–133.
194. **Hardaker, W. T., Whipple, T. L., and Bassett, F. H., III.** Diagnosis and treatment of the plica syndrome of the knee. *J. Bone Joint Surg.,* 1980; 62(A):221–225.
195. **Hess, G. P., Cappiello, W. L., and Poole, R. M.** Prevention and treatment of overuse tendon injuries. *Sports Med.,* 1989; 8:371–384.
196. **Hulkko, A. and Orava, S.** Stress fractures in athletes. *Int. J. Sports Med.,* 1987; 8:221–226.
197. **Jacobson, K. E. and Flandry, F. C.** Diagnosis of anterior knee pain. *Clin. Sports Med.,* 1989; 8:179–195.
198. **Kerlan, R. K. and Glousman, R. E.** Tibial collateral ligament bursitis. *Am. J. Sports Med.,* 1988; 16:344–346.

199. **Krause, B. L., Williams, J. P. R., and Catterall, A.** Natural history of Osgood-Schlatter disease. *J. Pediatr. Orthop.,* 1990; 10:65–68.

200. **Kujala, U. M., Kvist, M., and Heinonen, O.** Osgood-Schlatter's disease in adolescent athletes. *Am. J. Sports Med.,* 1985; 13:236–241.

201. **Kujala, U. M., Kvist, M., and Osterman, K.** Knee injuries in athletes. *Sports Med.,* 1986; 3:447–460.

202. **Lehman, W. L.** Overuse syndrome in runners. *AFP,* 1984; 29:157–161.

203. **Main, W. K. and Hershman, E. B.** Chronic knee pain in active adolescents. *Phys. Sportsmed.,* 1992; 20:139–156.

204. **Mattalino, A. J., Deese, J. M., and Campbell, E. D.** Office evaluation and treatment of lower extremity injuries in the runner. *Clin. Sports Med.,* 1989; 8:461–475.

205. **McKeag, D. B. and Dolan, C.** Overuse syndrome of the lower extremity. *Phys. Sportsmed.,* 1989; 17:108–123.

206. **Medlar, R. C. and Lyne, D. E.** Sinding-Larson-Johansson disease. *J. Bone Joint Surg.,* 1978; 60(A):1113–1116.

207. **Micheli, L. J.** The traction apophysities. *Clin. Sports Med.,* 1987; 6:389–404.

208. **Moyen, B., Comtet, J. J., Genety, J., and De Mourgues, G.** Le syndrome de la fabela douloureuse. *Rev. Chir. Orthop.,* 1982; 68(suppl.):148–152.

209. **Newell, S. G. and Bramwell, S. T.** Overuse injuries to the knee in runners. *Phys. Sportsmed.,* 1984; 12:80–92.

210. **O'Neill, D. B. and Micheli, L. J.** Overuse injuries in the young athlete. *Clin. Sports Med.,* 1988; 7:591–610.

211. **Patel, D.** Plica as a cause of anterior knee pain. *Orthop. Clin. N. Am.,* 1986; 17:273–277.

212. **Pećina, M., Bojanić, I., Smerdelj, M., and Chudy, D.** Overuse injuries of the knee in basketball players. *Basketball Med. Per.,* 1990; 5:13–25.

213. **Ray, J. M., Clancy, W. G., Jr., and Lemon, R. A.** Semimebranosus tendinitis: an overlooked cause of medial knee pain. *Am. J. Sports Med.,* 1989; 16:347–351.

214. **Schmidt, D. R. and Henry, J. H.** Stress injuries of the adolescent extensor mechanism. *Clin. Sports Med.,* 1989; 8:343–355.

215. **Segal, P. and Jacob, M.** *The Knee.* London: Wolfe Medical Publications, 1989; 63–144.

216. **Taunton, J. E., McKenzie, D. C., and Clement, D. B.** The role of biomechanics in the epidemiology of injuries. *Sports Med.,* 1988; 6:107–120.

217. **Tehranzadeh, J.** Avulsion and avulsion-like injuries of the musculoskeletal system. In: *Avulsion and Stress Injuries of the Musculoskeletal System.* Tehranzadeh, J., Serafini, A. N., Pais, M. J., Eds. Basel: Karger, 1989; 1–64.

218. **Trail, I. A.** Tibial sequestrectomy in the management of Osgood-Schlatter disease. *J. Pediatr. Orthop.,* 1988; 8:554–557.

219. **Witvoet, J.** *Lesions Osteotendineuses des sportifs. Cahiers d'Enseignement de la SOFCOT.* Paris: Exp. Scien. Francaise, 1983; 70.

220. **Windhager, R. and Engel, A.** Zur operativen behandlung des Morbus Osgood-Schlatter. *Z. Orthop.,* 1988; 126:179–184.

Chapter
8

The Leg

I. SHIN SPLINTS (RUNNER'S LEG)

In sports medicine literature, the appearance of pain in the lower leg while running is referred to as *shin splints*. The term, shin spints, is commonly used by athletes, coaches, trainers, and physicians to describe all primarily chronic pains in the area between the knee and ankle not involving the triceps surae muscle and Achilles tendon. Obviously, the causes leading to the development of this syndrome are numerous and different in etiology,[28,29] but all of them share a common characteristic — they are a direct consequence of long periods of excessive strain. In other words, they belong to the large group of overuse injuries. It is our belief that the best term for this clinical entity is *runner's leg*.

Runner's leg is most commonly seen in runners and walkers, but can also be found in all other athletes (professional and recreational) who participate in athletic activities in which running plays an important part.[16,23,24] Even before the massive recreational jogging movement in the U.S., Slocum[25] attempted to describe terminologically and etiologically the term, shin splints. According to Slocum,[25] shin splints describe a complex clinical entity characterized by the appearance of pain and tenderness in the anterior part of the lower leg, which results as a consequence of repeated excessive strain procured while walking and/or running. With the advance of knowledge and the development of various diagnostic tools, specific diagnosis and treatment of shin splints are now possible.[3, 14,22] The term shin splints is, by itself, no more specific than "headache" or "chest pain". The physician must be able to distinguish the various pathological conditions which cause lower leg pain in the athlete.[6]

Benas and Jolk[2] cite three possible causes of runner's leg: (1) stress fracture of the tibia (osseous origin), (2) myositis, fascitis and tendinitis of the posterior tibial muscle (soft tissue origin), and (3) periositis of the tibia. This belief is shared by a majority of other authors,[4,9] so that nowadays the most common causes of runner's leg are thought to be

1. tibialis posterior syndrome
2. periostitis of the tibia
3. chronic (exertional) compartment syndrome
4. stress fracture of the tibia

Apart from the above-mentioned causative factors, other predisposing factors such as popliteal artery entrapment syndrome and soleus syndrome are mentioned in medical literature,[11,13,21] although it is our opinion that the latter represents a different clinical entity. Garrick and Webb,[15] when talking about chronic anterior leg pain, elaborate their opinion that nowadays there exist athletes suffering from symptoms characteristic for runner's leg in whom not even the most sophisticated and current diagnostic tools have been able to positively identify the causes leading to the development of this syndrome. Depending on the localization of the pain in the lower leg, Kulund[10] speaks of anterior shin splints and posteromedial shin splints. We feel, however, that for didactic and practical reasons (the possibility of prevention and therapy), it is more useful to describe the various causative factors leading to the development of runner's leg individually, as specific clinical entites of osseous, vascular, and soft tissue origin. This partially contradicts the standard nomenclature of the American Medical Association who attempts to make the term, shin splints, more precise. They use this term to describe the appearance of pain and tenderness in the lower leg resulting from repeated running on hard surfaces or from strong and excessive use of the dorsal flexors of the foot. The diagnosis in this case should be limited to musculotendinous inflammation and should not include stress fractures or ischemic changes. The term *medial tibial stress syndrome* is also encountered in medical literature (in the terminology selected by Drez[15]). Medial tibial stress syndrome has been reported to be either tibial stress fracture or microfracture, tibial periostitis, or distal deep posterior chronic compartment syndrome.[4] Three chronic types exist and may coexist:

- Type 1 — tibial microfracture, bone stress reaction, or cortical fracture
- Type 2 — periostalgia from chronic avulsion of the periosteum at the periosteal-fascial junction
- Type 3 — chronic compartment syndrome

However, in everyday clinical practice and in sports medicine literature, the term shin splints is deeply rooted together with the four most common causes of its development. From an etiological point of view, it is also correct to include all possible causative factors because according to *Webster's* dictionary the noun "shin" describes the anterior part of the leg (beneath the knee), the frontal edge of the tibia, and the lower part of the leg.

Disregarding the causes leading to runner's leg, prevention of this syndrome is based on avoiding errors in training, in the surface on which the runner habitually runs, in muscle dysfunction and inflexibility, in athletic footwear, and in the biomechanics of running. According to James et al.,[7] problems and pain can appear in runners as a consequence of training errors because of anatomical factors and inadequate athletic footwear and surfaces.

Disregarding the four main causes of runner's leg, the principal symptom is pain. In the early stages of the disease, the pain appears exclusively after running, while in later stages, tenderness and pain are present in the beginning, middle, and end of running and during normal everyday activities, including walking. Location of the pain is important and helps in differentiation between various syndromes. Pain in the medial area of the distal third of the leg suggests tibialis posterior syndrome. Pain along the anterolateral side of the leg indicates a chronic anterior compartment syndrome, while pain over the anterior surface of the tibia in the central (middle) leg is characteristic for tibial stress fracture. Pain that always occurs during a workout suggests a chronic (exertional) compartment syndrome, while pain that appears at the start of a workout and later disappears, only to reappear afterwards, indicates tibialis posterior syndrome. Tenderness, swelling, and other clinical indicators are characteristic of specific causes leading to runner's leg and as such will be described in the following.

A. Tibialis Posterior Syndrome

The tibialis posterior muscle begins at one end from the posterior plane of the tibia below the linea m. solei. Its muscle fibers converge distally and attach themselves to the aponeurosis that is located in the middle of the muscle and passes into the tendon in the distal part of the leg. The tendon passes behind the medial malleolus, below the calcaneonavicular ligament, and below the caput tali. It, to a large degree, holds up the caput tali and inserts itself to the navicular tuberosity, the cuneiform bones, the cuboid bone, and to the baseos of the first three metatarsal bones (Figure 1). The anatomical description of the muscle indicates, by itself, the importance of this muscle in maintaining the arch of the foot. With a pronated foot

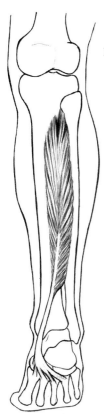

FIGURE 1. Muscles of the leg; tibialis posterior muscle.

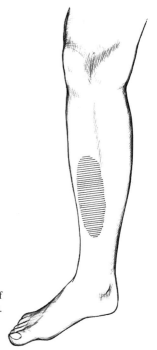

FIGURE 2. Characteristic area of pain/tenderness in cases of
tibialis posterior muscle.

and a lowered arch, overuse of the muscle, e.g., during, running, appears. This
excessive pressure leads gradually to a "separation" of the muscle fibers at the
insertion site of the muscle to the posterior side of the tibia. In other words, partial
ruptures appear. As this is a gradual process, the symptomatology of the syndrome
gradually develops. Tenderness felt along the medial side of the leg, behind the
medial edge of the tibia in the middle and distal thirds of the leg, are characteristic
for this syndrome (Figure 2). The diagnosis can be confirmed by palpation. Tenderness is limited to the localization of the pain, but a noteworthy characteristic of this
syndrome is that by pressing solely with the finger above the medial plane of the
tibia, one does not produce pain. To demonstrate tenderness by palpation, the
physician must "slip" his finger behind the medial edge of the tibia and continue
moving his finger from the proximal to the distal end of the tibia. Only by this method
will tenderness be produced — generally in the middle and distal thirds of the tibia
and in length from 8 to 12 cm. Pain will also be present during plantar flexion and
inversion of the foot against resistance. Radiographic and scintigraphic examination
will rule out the possibility of stress fracture of the tibia, while bone scanning
eliminates the possibility of tibial periostitis. The initial treatment of runner's leg, of
any etiology, is the cessation of painful activities. The treatment, among other things,
depends upon the stage of development of the syndrome. If for instance, pain is
present during everyday activities, the physician should recommend complete rest;
in other words, nonweight-bearing crutch ambulation is indicated.

Treatment of tibialis posterior syndrome in the beginning stages corresponds to
the standard treatment for all overuse injuries: nonsteroidal anti-inflammatory drugs
and other procedures such as ultrasound and high-intensity galvanic stimulation

performed with the aim of reducing pain. The most important part of the treatment is, however, performance of stretching and strengthening exercises for the muscles and correction of the static deformation of the foot with adequate arch supports and running shoes. Depending on the stage of the syndrome, cessation of athletic activities will last for a period of 1 to 2 weeks after which the athlete will be allowed to resume training, slowly increasing the speed of running and everyday mileage. With adequate stretching exercises and modification of footwear, tibialis posterior syndrome will not reoccur. Naturally, this implies that the patient should continue to act preventionally, avoiding the before-mentioned errors that lead to runner's leg. As a note of interest, we would like to mention that there has been an attempt, *per analogiam* with the treatment for tennis elbow, to treat runner's leg with the application of an adhesive tape or bandage that is wrapped firmly around the leg, 5 to 10 cm proximally from the malleolus.

B. Periostitis of the Tibia (Tibial Periostitis)

This term is often used by athletes and coaches when symptoms of runner's leg appear, regardless of the real cause of the syndrome. However, this term should only be used to describe periosteal changes on the anteromedial plane of the tibia, in the area approximately 10 cm above the ankle, and 5 to 10 cm in length. The appearance of pain and the development of the syndrome are similar to tibialis posterior muscle syndrome; it is most often encountered in long-distance runners and in runners who habitually run on hard, unyielding surfaces such as asphalt.[18]

During physical examination, tenderness immediately below the skin on the anterior side of the tibia is evident, while in some cases, a slight swelling and thickening above the bone can also be noticed. Tibial periostitis is approximately 10 times less frequently encountered than tibialis posterior syndrome. The correct etiopathogenetic explanation for its development is not yet known, although there are some indications that areas of micro bleeding immediately below the periosteum are connected with the development of this injury. Bone scan can help in differential diagnosis between periostitis and stress fracture (Figure 3). The typical picture of periostitis shows linear, vertically oriented increased uptake seen only on the delayed images.[5] When talking about tibial periostitis as one of the four most frequent causes of runner's leg, one is thinking about periostitis on the anterior plane of the tibia. Pathological changes on the periosteum, caused by excessive pulling of the muscle fibers of the tibialis posterior muscle, are part of the clinical picture of tibialis posterior syndrome. Periostitis at the insertion site of the medial half of the soleus muscle, on the posterior side of the tibia (soleus syndrome), is part of the clinical picture, and one of the causative factors of medial tibial stress syndrome.[13]

Treatment of tibial periostitis consists primarily of discontinuing symptomatic activities. Icing and nonsteroidal anti-inflammatory drugs usually produce good results. As soon as the symptoms disappear, the patient is encouraged to continue running on softer, more yielding surfaces — grass or athletic track made of synthetic materials. Strain (speed of running and daily mileage) should be increased gradually. Special consideration should be given to everyday and athletic footwear, particularly to the heel which must absorb impact from the surface.

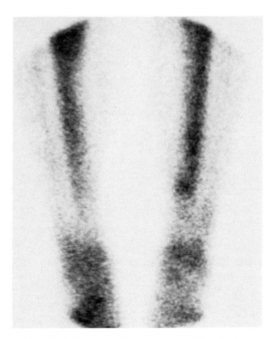

FIGURE 3. Bone scan demonstrating tibial periostitis.

C. Chronic (Exertional) Compartment Syndrome

The muscles of the lower leg are enveloped in the lower leg fascia (fascia cruris) from which extensions in the form of dividing walls (septa) extend deep into the leg and attach themselves to the anterior edge of the fibula — septum intermusculare cruris anterius and to the posterior edge of the fibula — septum intermusculare cruris posterius. This has the effect of dividing the muscle of the lower leg into three compartments: anterior, lateral, and posterior. Another fascia, situated between the posterior edge of the fibula and the medial edge of the tibia, divides the muscles of the posterior compartment into two layers, a deeper and shallower layer (Figure 4).

The etiology for chronic compartment syndrome relates in most instances to a limiting noncompliant fascia surrounding the affected muscle compartment. Sports activity leads to increased muscle volume, and if there is a noncompliant fascia, this will result in an excessive intracompartmental pressure which interferes with muscle blood flow. If local blood is reduced to the level where it no longer meets the metabolic demands of the tissue, functional abnormalities ensue, and an exercise ischemia or exertional compartment syndrome results.

Chronic (exertional) compartment syndrome causes lower leg pain and tightness, with muscle weakness and changes in nerve sensation amplified by physical exertion. Overuse injuries trigger muscular tissue damage, fluid leakage, and increased compartment pressure, as well as ischemic muscle and nerve dysfunction under exercise stress.[20] Rest and cessation of activities typically relieves the symptoms. However, exercise triggers the process at the next exposure and a chronic pattern is established. Some athletes experience the so-called "second day phenom-

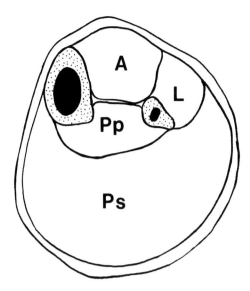

FIGURE 4. Schematic presentation of compartments (A) Anterior; (L) lateral; (Ps) posterior superficial; (Pp) posterior profundus.

enon" in which the amount of exercise that can be performed without pain in 1 d is less than the amount of exercise that could be painlessly performed on the previous day. The specific compartment involved determines the specific site of muscle weakness or paresthesia.

Lateral compartment syndrome is relatively infrequent. Analysis and measurement of intracompartmental pressure has failed to prove a significant increase in this pressure. Different opinions exist as to the importance of posterior compartment syndrome in the development of medial tibial stress syndrome. Eriksson and Wallensten have shown for instance that normal values for pressure in the posterior compartment are found in athletes with typical medial tibial stress syndrome symptomatology.[30] There is, however, no doubt that anterior compartment syndrome is a causative factor of runner's leg. When talking about this syndrome, one should differentiate between the acute type, characterized by a sudden development of ischemic changes, particularly in the tibialis anterior muscle (which is why it is called *tibialis anterior syndrome*), and the chronic type (chronic anterior exertional compartment syndrome), which develops gradually and belongs to the large group of overuse injuries.[18]

1. Chronic Anterior Exertional Compartment Syndrome

The etiopathogenesis and pathophysiological changes leading to the development of chronic anterior exertional compartment syndrome can best be described using the scheme compiled by Styf[26,27] (Table 1).

The main symptom indicating the existence of this syndrome is the appearance of pain felt during athletic activities, which is localized along the anterior side of the lower leg (Figure 5), along the lateral side of the tibia, and usually in the middle third or along the whole leg. The intensity of the pain increases with time. Another characteristic of this syndrome is that the pain appears after a certain amount of

TABLE 1
Development of the Chronic (Exertional) Compartment Syndrome
(Styf, 1990)

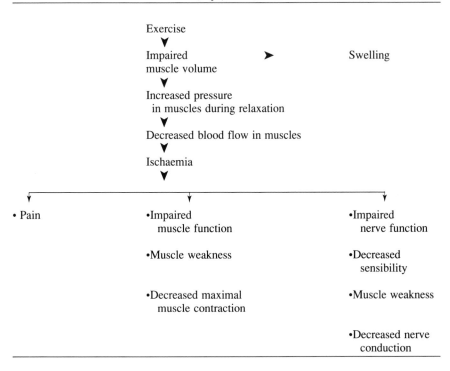

Exercise
▼
Impaired   ➤   Swelling
muscle volume
▼
Increased pressure
in muscles during relaxation
▼
Decreased blood flow in muscles
▼
Ischaemia
▼

• Pain	•Impaired muscle function	•Impaired nerve function
	•Muscle weakness	•Decreased sensibility
	•Decreased maximal muscle contraction	•Muscle weakness
		•Decreased nerve conduction

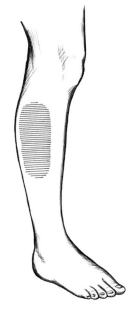

FIGURE 5. Characteristic area of pain in cases of chronic (exertional) anterior compartment syndrome.

time has elapsed, i.e., after a certain distance has been run. In the beginning stages of the syndrome, the athlete sometimes continues to run, disregarding the pain; he quickly worsens the symptoms. The appearance of a swelling, paresthesias in the area between the big toe and the second finger, loss of active muscle strength in the anterior compartment of the lower leg, as well as the appearance of pain during their passive stretching, confirm the diagnosis of this syndrome. Another characteristic of this syndrome is that during rest, the symptoms can completely disappear. An objective criteria for diagnosing this syndrome is measuring the intramuscular pressure, which can be accomplished by using various methods. The measurement can be made during physical activity, but is most commonly made during rest after physical exertion. Increased pressure after physical activity and a prolonged time for its return to normal values are considered to be positive indicators of the presence of chronic anterior compartment syndrome. Today, most authors agree that intramuscular pressure above 35 mmHg after physical activity and a return to normal time longer than 6 to 15 min positively confirm the diagnosis of this syndrome.

Nonoperative treatment for this syndrome includes icing after athletic activities and reducing the level of strain. As the latter is hard to accomplish in active athletes, most authors agree that surgical treatment (fasciotomy) is, in this case, the best solution.[1,5,10,12,17] The reasoning behind this is that 2 to 3 weeks after surgery, the athlete is able to continue training.[8] The fasciotomy is performed through two to three small skin incisions, through which the fascia is longitudinally cut. The whole procedure can be carried out under local anesthesia.

D. Stress Fractures of the Tibia

The most common localization of stress fractures of the tibia is in the area between the proximal and middle thirds of the bone. The symptoms include dull pain, localized in the same place and in a relatively small area (2 to 3 cm in circumference), and sometimes concomitant swelling. Palpation confirms the localization of the pain which is important in differential diagnosis. In stress fractures of the tibia, the pain, whether spontaneous or caused by palpation, is always strictly localized and never diffused, which serves to differentiate this syndrome from other possible causes leading to the development of runner's leg.

In the diagnostics of stress fractures of the tibia, important auxillary methods include radiographic examination and radionuclide scanning (Figure 6), with the provision that the latter can confirm the diagnosis of a stress fracture considerably earlier than the fracture becoming radiologically visible. Special emphasis must be placed on a specific type of tibial stress fracture — stress fractures of the anterior cortex of the mid-third of the tibia (Figure 7) — also known as anterior midshaft tibial stress fracture.[19] This fracture commonly progresses to delayed union or nonunion and frequently fractures completely.

Stress fracture of the fibula, which usually appears in the distal third of the fibula, is also considered by some authors to be a causative factor leading to the development of runner's leg.

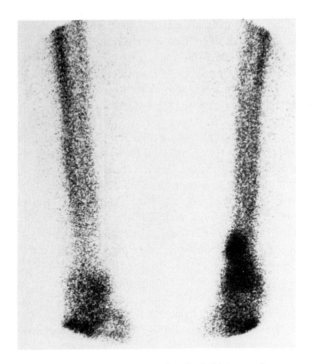

FIGURE 6. Bone scan demonstrating distal tibial stress fracture.

In conclusion, we feel safe in saying that runner's leg or shin splints in the past have been both a terminological and a diagnostic problem, which at present is no longer the case.

II. OVERUSE INJURIES OF THE ACHILLES TENDON

A. Achilles Tendinitis

The Achilles tendon is a common site for the development of overuse injuries. Depending on the localization of the inflammatory changes, either miotendinitis, tendinitis, peritendinitis, or enthesitis can be present. Achilles tendinitis is the most frequently encountered entity, affecting 11% of runners and having a high frequency of recurrence.[34,48,52,56,58,60,63,71,74] Apart from runners, Achilles tendinitis is also found in other athletes, primarily those who participate in sports activities where running and jumping represent the basic components of the sport. Typical examples of the latter include basketball, handball, soccer and tennis.

The Achilles tendon is the common tendon of the gastrocnemius and soleus muscles (Figure 8). It is the strongest tendon in the human body. It inserts on the lower half of the posterior side of the calcaneus. The insertion of the Achilles tendon is protected by two synovial bursae: (1) the subcutaneus bursa, located between the skin and the tendon, and (2) the retrocalcaneal bursa, lying between the tendon and the calcaneus. The tendon does not have a true synovial sheath (vagina synovialis), but is surrounded by a fine connective tissue sheath, the peritenon externum or the

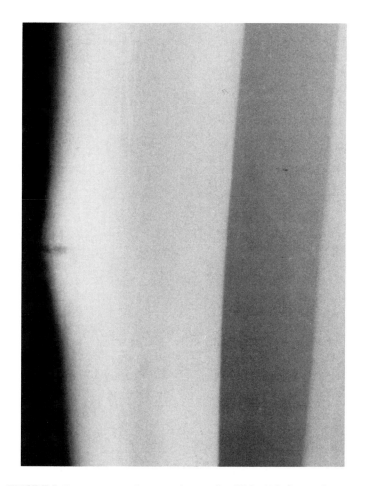

FIGURE 7. Roentgenogram demonstrating anterior tibial midshaft stress fracture.

epitenon, which is continuous on its inner surface with the endotenon. In the Achilles tendon, the epitenon is surrounded by a thin filmy layer of transparent areolar tissue, the paratenon. The paratenon functions as an elastic sleeve, permitting force movement against the surrounding tissue while maintaining continuity with adjacent structures. The epitenon and paratenon are collectively referred to as the *peritendon.*

1. Etiopathogenesis

The development of Achilles tendinitis is correlated, according to most authors, with excessive force being placed on the Achilles tendon during walking and/or running. The force placed on the tendon can be of different types, including stretching force (contraction of the triceps surae muscle); compression force (the reactive force of the surface), and torsion force (walking on uneven terrain).[44,48,52,56,58,60,63,68,71,74] Due to some predisposing factors (flat or pronated foot, high-arched foot, "tight" Achilles tendon, etc.), the effects of these forces can, either individually or collectively, be increased.

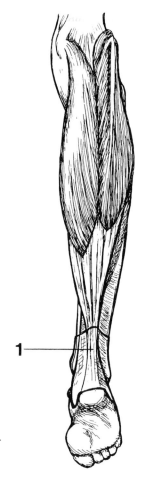

FIGURE 8. Muscles of the leg; triceps surae with Achilles tendon (1).

The etiology of Achilles tendinitis is multifactorial. Numerous internal and external predisposing factors, acting synchronistically, lead to the development of this syndrome.[37,41,58,63,71,72,75] Among the many internal predisposing factors, the most frequently cited are anatomical deviations of the lower extremity, which lead to excessive and/or prolonged pronation of the foot. These include a forefoot varus, flat foot, and high-arched foot (pes cavus). Another frequently cited predisposing factor is excessive tightness of the Achilles tendon, i.e., imbalance between the strength and flexibility of the muscles which form the Achilles tendon. Vascularization of the tendon is another predisposing factor that can lead to the development of Achilles tendinitis.[36,57] The reason for this is that the tendon is supplied with blood at the musculotendinous junction, the bone-tendon junction, and along its length through the paratenon (small vessels from branches of the posterior tibial and peroneal arteries). Microangiographic investigations have shown that blood supply is decreased in the middle third of the tendon (2 to 6 cm above its insertion on the calcaneus). In recent times, this finding has been confirmed by quantitative analysis of the number of blood vessels in the tendon.[55,57] According to many authors, this explains why the tendon is particularly prone to injury (development of tendinitis), and, likewise, why the tendon ruptures (which represents the final stage of Achilles tendinitis) in this area. Degeneration of the fat pad below the calcaneus is another frequently cited predisposing factor.[37,50] In this case, because of lessened impact absorption when the heel hits the surface during running, excessive force is placed upon the Achilles tendon. Increased Achilles tendon strain has also been proven in individuals with unstable ankle joints. Age is another factor that plays a role in the development of overuse injury of the Achilles tendon. The reason for this is that with aging, the elasticity of the tendon decreases, which increases the possibility of injury.

In general, the most common cause leading to the development of overuse injuries in runners, including the development of Achilles tendinitis, is training errors. These include sudden increases in training intensity, sudden changes in the duration and/or frequency of training, and an excessively quick return to full athletic activities after a prolonged break in training. Running on steeply inclined or uneven terrain/hard surface also have implications in Achilles tendinitis. According to Clement et al.,[37] these causes lead to the development of Achilles tendinitis in 75% of the cases they have investigated, while Nelen et al.[63] have reported an incidence of 63% for their patients suffering from Achilles tendinitis. Inadequate running surfaces, such as hard (e.g., asphalt) or uneven, and frequent changes of running surfaces, as well as old or inadequate running shoes, also significantly increase the risk of injury.

2. Clinical Picture and Diagnostics

Achilles tendinitis can develop either suddenly, as the so-called acute form, or gradually, as the so-called chronic form (which occurs more frequently). Inflammatory changes in the tendon and/or paratenon are situated 2 to 6 cm above its insertion on the calcaneus. The main symptom is the appearance of localized pain in this area, which is typically felt during athletic activities in such a manner that it appears at the beginning, decreases or disappears during, and increases after athletic activities. Another characteristic symptom is the appearance of pain and stiffness in the ankle joint when the patient gets out of bed in the morning; this pain subsides after the first few steps. In later stages, pain impedes normal walking. Patients frequently complain that they cannot walk barefoot and feel most comfortable in shoes with higher heels. In some cases, particularly in those that develop suddenly, patients complain of "creaking" along the length of the tendon, an auditory phenomenon which they describe as being similar to the sound produced when walking on freshly fallen snow.

Physical examination reveals local tenderness directly on the Achilles tendon and a local or diffuse swelling around the tendon. In some acute cases, crepitus may be felt. Detailed palpation along the tendon, performed by squeezing the tendon between thumb and index finger, usually reveals one small segment that is considerably more tender than the surrounding area. Pain can also be produced by passive dorsiflexion of the ankle with the knee extended. Pain appears even more frequently during active plantar flexion against resistance. This is tested by having the patient stand on tiptoe. Pain typically appears when the patient tries to stand on tiptoe of the injured leg. Less frequently, pain appears when the physician applies resistance (by pressing down on the patient's shoulders) while the patient attempts to stand on tiptoe. In acute cases of Achilles tendinitis, a localized swelling around the tendon is frequently found, while chronic cases are characterized by the presence of diffuse swelling, which is felt during palpation as a thickening around the tendon. The latter are in fact fibrous extensions, which are, according to Pećina, [43] called *tendon scarf*. Palpable and visible masses within the tendon (nodular swelling), representing swollen, poorly healed partial ruptures, can occasionally be observed.

Physical examination should also be directed toward identifying anatomical deviations of the foot and/or ankle. These include a forefoot varus, a varus position of the heel, a valgus position of the heel, flat foot (pes planovalgus), and high-arched foot (pes cavus). For these reasons, adequate footwear is of the utmost importance — old and worn-out running shoes, especially those with worn-out soles, negatively affect the biomechanics of walking and/or running.[34,35,38] An excessively worn-out outer heel edge, for instance, indicates a varus position of the heel.

Radiographic analysis of the foot and distal part of the lower leg can reveal an abnormally shaped calcaneus, bony spurs on the calcaneus, and ossification of the Achilles tendon. Nowadays, however, a complete physical examination of the Achilles tendon must also include ultrasound examination.[41,43,62,65] A detailed ultrasound examination of the Achilles tendon, in both the longitudinal and perpendicular direction, can reveal details in the tendon structure (Figure 9) and the shape of the tendon sheath, while a dynamic examination (one carried out during passive and active movements of the ankle) enables the physician to precisely diagnose possible tendon damage. Besides its use in diagnostics, thermography is also useful in monitoring the success of the prescribed treatment. In recent times, MRI has also been used to evaluate damage and/or changes to the Achilles tendon.[66]

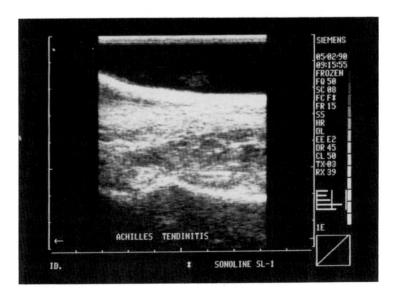

FIGURE 9. Sonogram of the Achilles tendon demonstrating Achilles tendinitis.

3. Treatment

Treatment of Achilles tendinitis is directed towards lessening or eliminating pain, controlling the inflammatory reaction, facilitating the healing process, controlling the biomechanical parameters, and completely rehabilitating the tendon as well as preventing it from further injury. Treatment is nonoperative in the vast majority of cases; surgical treatment is indicated only in exceptional cases.[32,37,42,53–56,58,59,63,69,70,71] It is of the utmost importance that treatment begins as soon as possible — ideally as soon as the first symptoms appear.

a. Nonoperative Treatment

The program for nonoperative treatment includes the following:

- short-term cessation or modification of athletic activities
- lifting the heel 1 to 2 cm by inserting a heel wedge
- ice massage of the tender area
- application of nonsteroidal anti-inflammatory drugs
- stretching exercises and strengthening the triceps surae muscle and Achilles tendon
- correcting predisposing factors.

In the beginning stages of Achilles tendinitis, a complete cessation of athletic activities is not mandatory. Reducing the intensity of training, principally running, along with the application of other nonoperative procedures is sufficient. In later stages of the syndrome, a complete rest from athletic activities, lasting at least 1 month, is mandatory. During this interval, the functional capabilities of the athlete can be kept up with alternative training — swimming freestyle and backstroke and running in deep water without touching the bottom.

Relaxing the Achilles tendon is accomplished by inserting a heel wedge and lifting the heel for a height of 1 to 2 cm. The patient must be made aware that heel wedges should be worn in all footwear; in other words, the heel must be lifted in "everyday" activities as well as in athletic ones. After treatment is completed, the height of the heel wedge is gradually decreased.

Cryotherapy is recommended in the beginning stages of Achilles tendinitis. Ice massages of the tender area should be carried out after athletic activities. In later stages of the injury, cryotherapy is performed 2 to 3 times daily during the first week of therapy, while after this interval, various physical procedures are used (laser or ultrasound) to increase the temperature of the injured tendon. Nonsteroidal anti-inflammatory drugs, taken in maximal daily dosages, are recommended during the first 10 d of therapy.

The principal component of nonoperative Achilles tendinitis therapy consists of stretching exercises. Passive stretching exercises should begin at once and (equally important) the patient must be taught how to perform them correctly (Figure 10). Starting with the seventh day of therapy, the patient should begin strengthening exercises for the lower leg muscles, particularly the gastrocnemius-soleus complex.

Recognizing and correcting predisposing factors plays an important part in the treatment, as well as in prevention of Achilles tendinitis. Achilles tendinitis is an

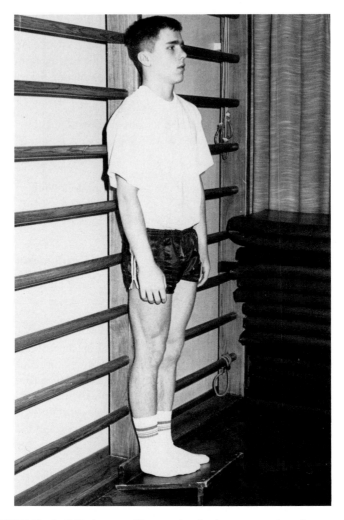

FIGURE 10. (A-C) Various stretching exercises for the gastrocnemius-soleus complex.

excellent example of how correctly carried out prevention, targeting predisposing factors, can significantly decrease the frequency of an overuse injury in athletes. Prevention carried out with the aim of avoiding mistakes in training (i.e., sudden increases in the intensity of training), in the choice of running surface (i.e., running on uneven and hard terrains), and in the choice of athletic footwear (i.e., wearing adequate running shoes), as well as orthotic correction of biomechanical irregularities, which lead to excessive and/or prolonged pronation of the foot during running, has, during the past 10 years, decreased the frequency of Achilles tendinitis by more than 50%. To illustrate this, we will cite the results of investigations performed by James et al.[48] and Krissoff and Ferris[52] who reported an overall frequency of Achilles tendinitis in athletes suffering from sports-related injuries of, in the former investi-

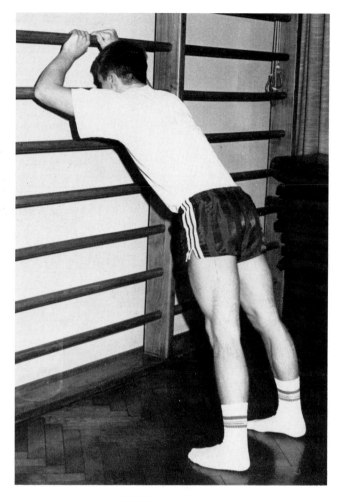

FIGURE 10 (continued).

gation, 11%, and in the later investigation, 18%. Recent frequencies, as reported by Taunton et al.[72] and Nelen et al.[63], comprise significantly less, around 6% of all sports-related injuries.

Corticosteroid injections into and around the Achilles tendon are contraindicated because of the risk of tendon rupture. Only in some cases of peritenonitis are these injections allowed, but only in the area around the Achilles tendon or in its sheath and never in the tendon itself.

An important point to stress is that nonoperative treatment should be carried out persistently, during the course of at least a couple of months, and that surgical treatment is recommended only in resistant cases in which the symptoms fail to disappear after a long-term application of correctly applied nonsurgical therapy.

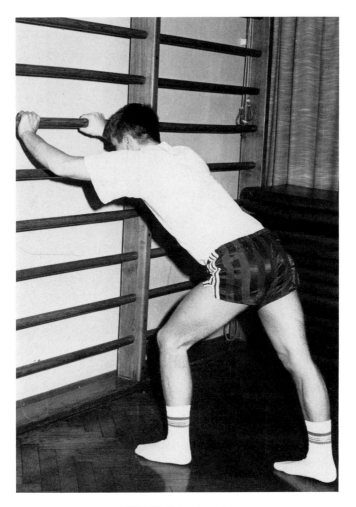

FIGURE 10 (continued).

b. Surgical Treatment

Surgical treatment of Achilles tendinitis is based on the localization of the pathological changes and on intraoperatively found changes in and on the tendon and tendon sheath.[32,37,42,53–56,58,59,63,69,70,71] If only the tendon sheath (peritendon) exhibits pathological changes, which is often the case, an adhesiolysis of the tendon is performed; the peritendon, in its entire length and circumference, is completely removed (Figure 11). On one hand this has the effect of removing the injured tendon sheath, and on the other hand, of creating a new tendon sheath, which is not pathologicaly changed. With regards to the latter, postoperative rehabilitation plays an important role and must strive, by means of functional adaptation, to form a new tendon sheath, while at the same time taking care not to cause irritation of the newly formed peritendon. Postoperative rehabilitation should immediately begin with the

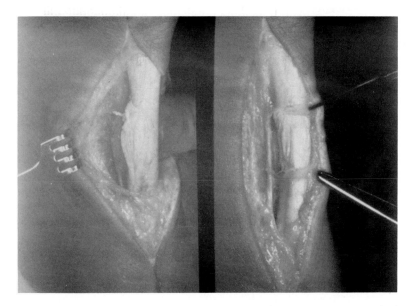

FIGURE 11. Intraoperative finding of inflamed peritendon "sheath".

functional animation necessary for the formation of the new tendon sheath, the so-called neoperitendon of the Achilles tendon.

If the physician, during surgery, palpates degeneratively changed areas in the Achilles tendon (which could also have been discovered preoperatively, e.g., by ultrasound examination), these parts of the tendon are excised. Some authors recommend an "untangling" of that area of the tendon into fascicles which, besides performing excision of the degeneratively changed part of the tendon, has the side-effect of effecting an intratendon decompression. The same procedure applies to calcificates in the tendon (Figure 12). However, if the calcificates are large, or if they infiltrate the tendon to such a degree that their excision will result in a significant loss of strength in the tendon, the tendon should be reinforced with tendon flaps.

In cases with partial tendon ruptures (which can also develop as an iatrogenous consequence of corticosteroid injections into the tendon) (Figure 13), excision of the injured area of the tendon is effected, as well as, depending on the size of the newly developed defect, reinforcing that part with tendon flaps should be performed. Total ruptures of the Achilles tendon, which are the result of the final stage of Achilles tendinitis, are treated surgically.

B. Enthesitis of the Achilles Tendon

Unlike Achilles tendinitis, enthesitis of the Achilles tendon is characterized by pathological changes in the tendon-bone junction. For this reason, Achilles enthesitis is regarded as belonging to the group of insertion tendinopathies.[35,42,58,71] As with other insertion tendinopathies, a change in the tendon-bone junction zones is evident, i.e., the border between the mineralized and nonmineralized adhesive cartilage is

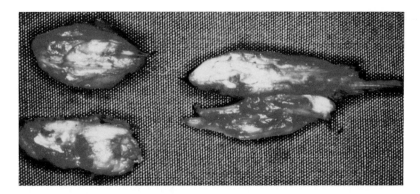

FIGURE 12. Calcificates removed from the Achilles tendon.

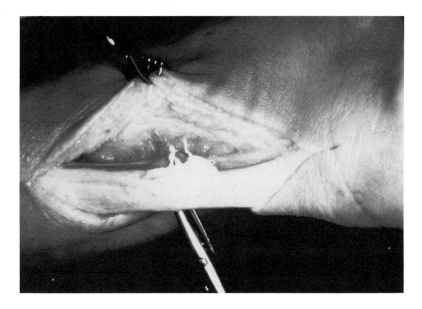

FIGURE 13. Intraoperative finding of iatrogenic partial rupture of Achilles tendon.

missing (Figure 14) and cystic formations frequently develop. Clinically, enthesitis is differentiated from Achilles tendinitis solely by the localization of the pain; the tenderness is localized in the tendon-bone junction area. Treatment involves the same principles as in Achilles tendinitis; the only difference is that enthesitis is generally more resistant and necessitates surgical treatment more frequently. Depending on the stage of the enthesitis, various types of surgical procedures are recommended. In long-term cases with radiologically visible changes on the bone insertion site (de-mineralization), drilling of the bone insertion site and longitudinal cutting into the tendon at the tendon-bone junction are recommended. The aim of this procedure is to effect decompression of the tendon and to initiate the healing process. In cases

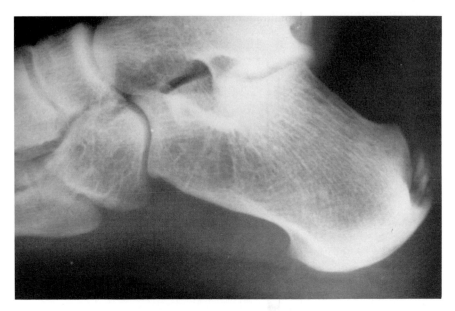

FIGURE 14. Ossification of the Achilles tendon.

where, as a consequence of long-term enthesitis, complete tendon rupture has occurred in the tendon-bone junction area, reinsertion of the tendon through a drilled canal in the calcaneus is indicated.

C. Retrocalcaneal Bursitis

Retrocalcaneal bursitis is a term used to describe an inflammation of the bursa between the Achilles tendon and the calcaneus. It can develop either as a consequence of irritation caused by inadequate footwear or of a calcaneus with prominent superior and inferior ends. Calcaneus shaped in this manner are called *Haglund's heel* and are easily visible on lateral roentgenograms.[44-47,64,67,74] If retrocalcaneal bursitis is accompanied by enthesitis of the Achilles tendon (this combination is known as Haglund's syndrome), tenderness is localized somewhat proximally from the insertion site of the tendon to bone, and unlike tendinitis, increases when pressure is applied. Along with all the other methods of nonoperative treatment that are applied in cases with tendinitis, corticosteroid injections directly into the bursa are also recommended. Occasionally, surgical treatment is indicated, in which case it consists of removing the bursa and performing an osteotomy (Figure 15) of the prominent superior pole of the calcaneus.[44,46,74]

D. Rupture of the Achilles Tendon

Achilles tendon is characterized by the last stage of overuse injuries — total rupture of the tendon.[31,33,40,51,73] Most often, this occurs in middle-age (30 to 50 years)

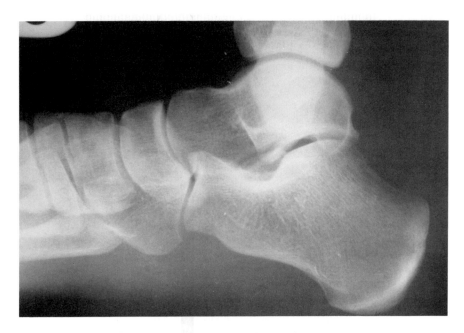

FIGURE 15. Haglund's disease. (A) Preoperative roentgenogram.

males during recreational sports activities such as soccer, basketball, or jogging. A positive diagnosis is made on the basis of history, physical examination, and recently, ultrasound examination[41,43,62,65] (Figures 16 and 17). During rupture, the patient, besides feeling intense pain, feels "as if a stone has hit him" in the heel area. In some cases, an audible snapping sound is also heard.

Clinical signs include a painful, palpable "depression" in the Achilles tendon and a partial or complete loss of plantar flexion. In some cases, active plantar flexion of the foot is possible, but the patient is always incapable of walking and standing on tiptoe on the injured leg. A positive Thompson "squeeze" test (loss of plantar flexion of the foot during manual compression of the lower leg muscles) is a certain indicator of tendon rupture. In our opinion, which is shared by a majority of other authors, the best results in treating Achilles tendon rupture are achieved by surgical treatment.

E. Sever's Disease (Ccacaneal Apophysitis)

Calcaneal apophysitis (Sever's disease) is a common cause of heel pain, particularly in the athletically active child. Symptoms of pain in the region of the heel, local tenderness at the posteroinferior or inferior surface of the heel, and roentgenographic evidence of disordered ossification of the calcaneal apophysis are the classical criteria for the diagnosis of Sever's disease.[78-80] Tenderness over the os calcis apophysis at the insertion of the Achilles tendon along with a tight gastrosoleus mechanism are usually sufficient to make the diagnosis of os calcis

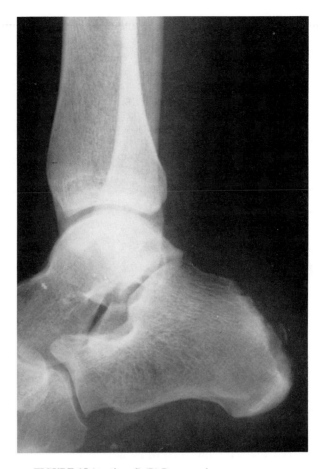

FIGURE 15 (continued) (B) Postoperative roentgenogram.

apophysitis. This condition can frequently be bilateral. The syndrome of heel pain and tenderness localized to the os calcis apophysis in children and adolescents was first described in 1912 by Sever.[80] Sever, in his original paper, hypothetized that this heel pain was due to an inflammatory apophysitis associated with increased muscular activity in the growing child and he believed it was traumatic in origin. Roentgenograms of the feet usually show some type of disorderly ossification of the calcaneal apophysis, either as fragmentation, incomplete appearance, or complete formation but with increased sclerosis (Figure 18). The natural history of calcaneal apophysitis is spontaneous recovery and remodeling of an irregular apophysis and its normal fusion with the main mass of os calcis. Treatment is based on the hypothesis that the etiology of this condition is related to overgrowth. The relative increased tightness of the gastrosoleus mechanism and weakness of the dorsiflexors, when associated with repetitive microtraumas, initiate the occurrence of tiny microfractures at the junction of the apophysis with the bone.[81] Treatment

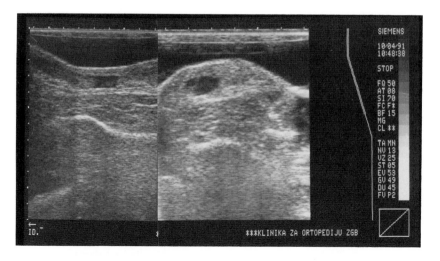

FIGURE 16. Sonogram of the Achilles tendon demonstrating acute rupture.

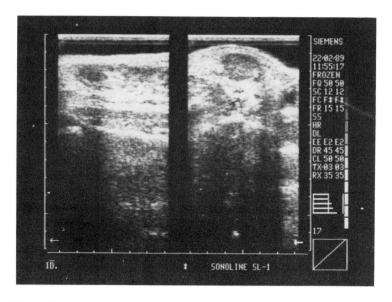

FIGURE 17. Sonogram of the Achilles tendon demonstrating an old rupture of the tendon.

serves exclusively to modify discomfort and restore function and does not influence the natural history of spontaneous full recovery.[76,77] All children are managed with supervised therapeutic exercises, which include lower extremity flexibility and dorsiflexion strengthening, as well as the prescription of heel cups or total foot orthotics. Total foot orthotics are prescribed in children with associated biomechanical abnormalities of the foot or lower extremities, such as pronation or

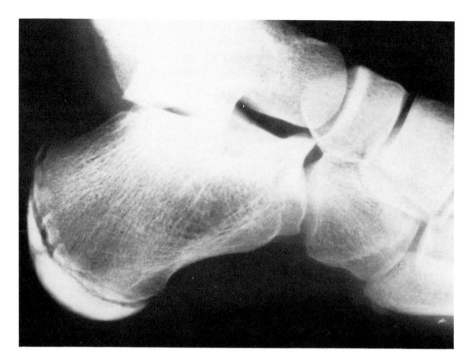

FIGURE 18. Typical roentgenologic findings of Sever's disease.

forefoot supination; heel cups or lifts are used in children with normal alignment and discontinued when the child becomes asymptomatic.

REFERENCES

Shin Splints (Runner's Leg)

1. **Andrish, J. T., Bergfeld, J. A., and Walheim, J.** A prospective study on the management of shin splints. *J. Bone Joint Surg.*, 1974; 56(A):1697–1700.
2. **Benas, D. and Jolk, P.** Shin splints. *Am. Correct. Ther. J.*, 1978; 32:53–57.
3. **Clement, D. B.** Tibial stress syndrome in athletes. *J. Sports Med.*, 1974; 2:81–85.
4. **Detmer, D. E.** Chronic shin splints. Classification and management of medial tibial stress syndrome. *Sports Med.*, 1986; 3:436–446.
5. **Garrick, J. G. and Webb, D. R.** *Sports Injuries: Diagnosis and Management.* Philadelphia: W. B. Saunders 1990.
6. **Jackson, R., Fitch, K., and O'Brien, M.,** Eds. *Sport Medicine Manual.* Lausanne: International Olympic Committee, 1990.

7. **James, S. L., Bates, B. T., and Ostering, L. R.** Injuries to runners. *Am. J. Sports Med.,* 1978; 6:40–49.

8. **Jarviennen, M., Aho, H., and Nuttymaki, S.** Results of the surgical treatment of the medial tibial syndrome in athletes. *Int. J. Sports Med.,* 1989; 10:55–57.

9. **Jones, D. C. and James, S. L.** Overuse injuries of the lower extremity. *Clin. Sports Med.,* 1987; 6:273–290.

10. **Kulund, N. D.** *The Injured Athlete,* 2nd ed. Philadelphia: J. B. Lippincott, 1988.

11. **Lysens, R. J.** Intermittent claudication in young athletes: popliteal artery entrapment syndrome. *Am. J. Sports Med.,* 1983; 11:177–179.

12. **Martens, M. A. and Moeyersoons, J. P.** Acute and recurrent effort-related compartment syndrome in sports. *Sports Med.,* 1990; 9:62–68.

13. **Michael, R. H. and Holder, L. E.** The soleus syndrome. A cause of medial tibial stress (shin splints). *Am. J. Sports Med.,* 1985; 13:87–94.

14. **Milgrom, C., Giladi, M., Stein, M., et al.** Medial tibial pain. *Clin. Orthop.,* 1986; 213:167–171.

15. **Mubarak, S. J., Gould, R. N., Lee, Y. F., et al.** The medial tibial stress syndrome. A cause of shin splints. *Am. J. Sports Med.,* 1982; 10:201–205.

16. **Murtagh, J.** Pain in the leg. *Aust. Fam. Phys.,* 1991; 20:670–673.

17. **Orava, S. and Puranen, J.** Athletes' leg pain. *Br. J. Sports Med.,* 1979; 13:92–97.

18. **Pećina, M. and Bojanić, I.** Overuse injuries in track and field athletes. *Croat. Sports Med. J.,* 1991; 6:24–37.

19. **Pećina, M. and Bojanić, I.** Compressive osteosynthesis in the treatment of tibial midshaft stress fracture. *Arch. Orthop. Trauma Surg.,* 1993; in press.

20. **Pećina, M., Bojanić, I., and Markiewitz, A. D.** Nerve entrapment syndromes in athletes. *Clin. J. Sports Med.,* 1993; 3:36–43.

21. **Pećina, M., Krmpotić-Nemanić, J., and Markiewitz, A. D.** *Tunnel Syndromes.* Boca Raton: CRC Press, 1991.

22. **Puranen, J.** The medial tibial syndrome. *Ann. Chir. Gynaecol.,* 1991; 80:215–218.

23. **Rudt, R.** What is your diagnosis? Shin Splints. *Schweiz. Rundsch. Med. Prax.,* 1991; 80:281–282.

24. **Sepulchre, P., Blaimont, P., and Pasteels, J. L.** Douleurs tibiales interenes chez les coureurs a pied. *Int. Orthop. (SICOT),* 1988; 12:217–221.

25. **Slocum, D. B.** The shin splint syndrome. Medical aspects and differential diagnosis. *Am. J. Surg.,* 1967; 114:875–881.

26. **Styf, J.** Diagnosis of exercise — induced pain in the anterior aspect of the lower leg. *Am. J. Sports Med.,* 1988; 16:165–169.

27. **Styf, J.** Chronic exercise-induced pain in the anterior aspect of the lower leg. An overview of diagnosis. *Sports Med.,* 1989; 7:331–339.

28. **Taunton, J. E., McKenzie, D. C., and Clement, D. B.** The role of biomechanics in the epidemiology of injuries. *Sports Med.,* 1988; 6:107–120.

29. **Viitasalo, J. T. and Kvist, M.** Some biomechanical aspects of the foot and ankle in athletes with and without shin splints. *Am. J. Sports Med.,* 1983; 11:125–130.

30. **Wallensten, R.** Results of fasciotomy in patients with medial tibial syndrome or chronic anterior-compartment syndrome. *J. Bone Joint Surg.,* 1983; 65(A):1252–125.

Overuse Injuries of the Achilles Tendon

31. **Aldam, C. H.** Repair of calcaneal tendon ruptures. A safe technique. *J. Bone Joint Surg.,* 1989; 71(B):486–488.

32. **Anderson, D. L., Taunton, J. E., and Davidson, R. G.** Surgical management of chronic Achilles tendinitis. *Clin. J. Sport Med.,* 1992; 2:38–42.

33. **Beskin, J. L., Sanders, R. A., Hunter, S. C., and Hughston, J. C.** Surgical repair of Achilles tendon ruptures. *Am. J. Sports Med.,* 1987; 15:1–8.

34. **Bordelon, R. L.** Orthotic, shoes and braces. *Orthop. Clin. N. Am.,* 1989; 20:751–757.

35. **Brody, D. M.** Running injuries. *Clin. Symp.,* 1980; 39:1–36.

36. **Carr, A. J. and Norris, S. H.** The blood supply of the calcaneal tendon. *J. Bone Joint Surg.,* 1989; 71(B):100–101.

37. **Clement, D. B., Taunton, J. E., and Smart, G. W.** Achilles tendinitis and peritendinitis: etiology and treatment. *Am. J. Sports Med.,* 1984; 12:179–184.

38. **Cook, S. D., Brinker, M. R., and Poche, M.** *Sports Med.,* 1990; 10:1–8.

39. **Davidson, R. G. and Taunton, J. E.** Achilles tendinitis. *Med. Sport Sci.,* 1987; 23:71–79.

40. **De Tullio, B., Guaganini, M., Orsi, R., and Sarda, G. Rottura** sottocutanea del tendine di Achille: trattamento chirurgico e recupero funzionale. *Riv. Patol. Appar. Locom.,* 1988; 8:203–206.

41. **Fornage, B. D.** Achilles tendon: U.S. examination. *Radiology,* 1986; 159:759–764.

42. **Frey, C. C. and Shereff, M. J.** Tendon injuries about ankle in athletes. *Clin. Sports Med.,* 1988; 7:103–118.

43. **Hašpl, M. and Pećina, M.** Ultrazvučna dijagnostika koljena i potkoljenice. U: Matasović, T. (urednik). Ultrazvučna dijagnostika sustava za kretanje. Zagreb: Skolska Knjiga, 1988; 71–98.

44. **Heneghan, M. A. and Pavlov, H.** The Haglund painful heel syndrome. *Clin. Orthop.,* 1984; 187:228–234.

45. **Hintermann, B. and Holzach, P.** Die Bursitis subachilla - eine biomechanische Analyse und klinische Studie. *Z. Orthop.,* 1992; 130:114–119.

46. **Huber, H. and Waldis, M.** Die Haglund Exostose — Eine Operations — indikation und ein kleiner Eingriff? *Z. Orthop.,* 1989; 127:286–290.

47. **Ippolito, E. and Ricciardi - Pollini, P. T.** Invasive retrocalcaneal bursitis: a report of three cases. *Foot Ankle,* 1984; 4:204–208.

48. **James, S. L., Bates, B. T., and Ostering, L. R.** Injuries to runners. *Am. J. Sports Med.,* 1978; 6:40–50.

49. **Jones, D. C. and James, S. L.** Partial calcaneal osteotomy for retrocalcaneal bursitis. *Am. J. Sports Med.,* 1984; 12:72–73.

50. **Jorgensen, U.** Achillodinya and loss of heel pad shock absorbency. *Am. J. Sports Med.,* 1984; 13:128–132.

51. **Jozsa, L., Kvist, M., Balint, B. J., et al.** The role of recreational sport activity in Achilles tendon rupture. *Am. J. Sports Med.,* 1989; 17:338–343.

52. **Krissoff, W. B. and Ferris, W. D.** Runners injuries. *Phys. Sportsmed.,* 1979; 7:55–64.

53. **Kvist, H. and Kvist, M.** The operative treatment of chronic calcaneal paratenonitis. *J. Bone Joint Surg.,* 1980; 62(B):353–357.

54. **Kvist, M., Lehto, M. K., Jozsa, L., Jarvinen, M., and Kvist, H. T.** Chronic Achilles paratenonitis — an immunohistologic study of fibronectiin and fibrinogen. *Am. J. Sports Med.,* 1988; 16:616–623.

55. **Kvist, M., Jozsa, L., Jarvinen, M., et al.** Chronic Achilles paratenonitis in athletes — histological and histochemical study. *J. Pathol.,* 1987; 19:1–11.

56. **Kvist, M.** Achilles tendon injuries in athletes. *Ann. Chir. Gynecol.,* 1991; 80:188–201.

57. **Lagergen, C. and Lindholm, A.** Vascular distribution in the Achilles tendon — an angiographic and microangiographic study. *Acta Chir. Scand.,* 1958/59; 116:491–495.

58. **Leach, R. E., James, S., and Wasilewski, S.** Achilles tendinitis. *Am. J. Sports Med.,* 1981; 9:93–98.
59. **Leach, R. E.** Leg and foot injuries in racquet sports. *Clin. Sports Med.,* 1988; 7:359–370.
60. **Leppilahati, J., Orava, S., Karpakla, J., and Takala, T.** Overuse injuries of the Achilles tendon. *Ann. Chir. Gynaecol.,* 1991; 80:202–207.
61. **Lysholm, J. and Wiklander, J.** Injuries in runners. *Am. J. Sports Med.,* 1987; 15:168–171.
62. **Milbradt, H., Reiner, P., and Thermann, H.** Die Sonomorphologie der normalen Achillessehne und Muster pathologischer Veranderungen. *Radiologe,* 1988; 28:330–333.
63. **Nelen, G., Martens, M., and Burssens, A.** Surgical treatment of chronic Achilles tendinitis. *Am. J. Sports Med.,* 1989; 17:754–759.
64. **Pavlov, H., Heneghan, M., Hersh, A., Goldmann, A., and Vigorita, V.** The Haglund syndrome: initial and differential diagnosis. *Radiology,* 1982; 144:83–88.
65. **Pfister, A.** Experimentelle und klinische Ergebnisse der Ultraschallsonographie bei sportorthopadischen Weichteilerkrankungen. *Sportverletzung — Sportschaden,* 1987; 3:130–141.
66. **Quinn, S. F., Murray, W. T., Clark, R. A., et al.** Achilles tendon: MR imaging at 1.5 T. *Radiology,* 1987; 164:767–770.
67. **Rossi, F., La Cava, F., Amato, F., and Pincelli, G.** The Haglund Syndrome: clinical and radiological features and sports medicine aspects. *J. Sports Med.,* 1987; 27:258–265.
68. **Saillant, G., Radinean, J., Thoraeux, P., and Roy-Camille, R.** La tendinite d'Achille. *Rev. Prat.,* 1991; 41:1644–1649.
69. **Santilli, G.** Achilles tendinopathies and paratendinopathies. *J. Sports Med.,* 1979; 19:245–259.
70. **Schepsis, A. A. and Leach, R. E.** Surgical management of Achilles tendinitis. *Am. J. Sports Med.,* 1987; 15:308–315.
71. **Smart, G. W., Taunton, J. E., and Clement, D. B.** Achilles tendon disorders in runners — a review. *Med. Sci. Sports Exercise,* 1980; 12:231–243.
72. **Taunton, J. E., McKenzie, D. C., and Clement, D. B.** The role of biomechanics in the epidemiology of injuries. *Sports Med.,* 1988; 6:107–120.
73. **Thermann, H. and Zwipp, H.** Achillessehnenruptur. *Orthopade,* 1989; 18:321–335.
74. **Torg, J. S., Pavlov, H., and Torg, E.** Overuse injuries in sport: the foot. *Clin. Sports Med.,* 1987; 6:291–320.
75. **Williams, J. G. P.** Achilles tendon lesion in sport. *Sports Med.,* 1986; 3:114–135.

Sever's Disease (Calcaneal Apophysitis)

76. **Clain, R. M. and Hershman, E. B.** Overuse injuries in children and adolescents. *Phys. Sportsmed.,* 1989; 17:111–123.
77. **Katz, J. F.** Nonarticular osteochondroses. *Clin. Orthop.,* 1981; 158:70–76.
78. **Micheli, L. J.** The traction apophysities. *Clin. Sports Med.,* 1987; 6:389–404.
79. **Micheli, L. J. and Ireland, M. L.** Prevention and management of calcaneal apophysitis in children: an overuse syndrome. *J. Pediatr. Orthop.,* 1987; 7:34–38.
80. **Sever, J. W.** Apophysitis of the os calcis. *N.Y. Med. J.,* 1912; 95:1025–1029.
81. **Stanitski, C. L.** Management of sports injuries in children and adolescents. *Orthop. Clin. N. Am.,* 1988; 19:689–697.

Chapter

9

Foot and Ankle

I. PLANTAR FASCIITIS

Plantar fasciitis is an overuse injury manifested by pain at the medial tubercle of the calcaneus and/or along the medial longitudinal arch. It usually develops when repetitive and prolonged stress is placed on the plantar fascia, which may cause microtears and inflammation in the fascia at or near its insertion on the calcaneus, i.e., when the activity of mechanical force outbalances the healing capacity of the tissue. Plantar fasciitis was first described by Wood in 1812, and its development was erroneously attributed to complications of tuberculosis.[9]

Plantar fasciitis occurs most commonly in runners, especially in long-distance runners, but may also be seen in basketball players, tennis players, and dancers. In various studies, the incidence of plantar fasciitis is about 5% of running injuries seen.[15,16,28]

A. Etiopathogenesis

Originating as a thick, fibrous band of connective tissue attached to the medial tubercle of the calcaneus, the plantar fascia (Figure 1) spreads distally in a fan-like manner.[7,10,15,19] It forms three slips (medial, central, and lateral), which proceed toward the toes where it inserts on the base of each of the proximal phalanx of the toes. In histology, fascia and fibroblasts are arranged in layers and usually classified in the group of differentiated connective tissue.[15,28]

The analysis of biomechanical events taking place in the foot during walking has made it clear that the role of the plantar fascia is twohold.[6,7,14,18] When the foot touches the ground, the plantar fascia extends because of plantar dorsiflexion at the ankle joint and simultaneous dorsiflexion of proximal phalanxes of the toes.[7,14] By its extension, the plantar fascia stabilizes metatarsal joints, thus enabling the foot to be prepared for accommodation of the reactive force of the ground. (Figure 2) The cushioning role of the plantar fascia is called a *mechanical shock absorbing effect*.[7,14,15] At the same time, it is an active load placed upon the plantar fascia since it is caused by contraction of extensor muscles of the foot (dorsiflexion of the toes). The second role of the plantar fascia is displayed during the take-off phase. On account of inertia, the body weight is transferred to the anterior region of the foot, causing the take-off of the heel and extension of the toes. The movement leads to passive stretching of

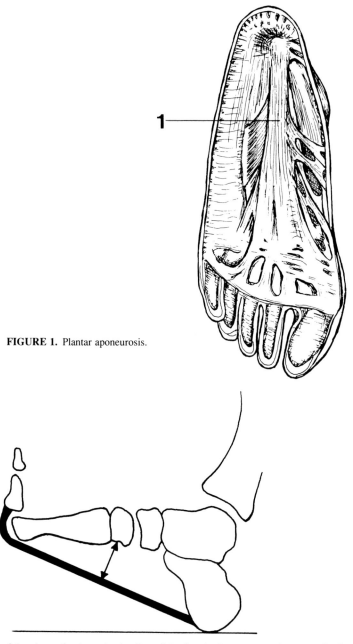

FIGURE 1. Plantar aponeurosis.

FIGURE 2. Action of the plantar fascia: active loading of the foot in the prestance phase as a shock-absorbing mechanism.

the fascia, resulting in its lifting the longitudinal foot arch to prepare it for take-off (Figure 3). This function of the fascia is called the *windlass effect*.[7,12,14,15] The static qualities of plantar fascia were identified by mechanical analysis.[18] Longitudinal 90-kp extension force load upon the plantar fascia in postmortem specimens yielded the

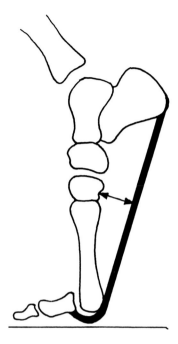

FIGURE 3. Action of plantar fascia: passive action in late stance as a foot — stabilizing mechanism.

value of 4% of the normal fascial length as the maximum ability of adjustment to stretching without tearing the fascial tissue.[18] However, *in vivo* studies have shown that the ability of fascia to adjust to stretching is smaller than in postmortem specimens, i.e., only 1.7% of its normal length.[18] Along the lines of these findings, it has also been observed that the fascia is relatively nonresistant to strong stretching force, which is probably why during the activity of greater mechanical force, overuse injury develops in the plantar fascia.[7,25] The actions of supination and pronation are essential for the normal functioning of the foot. Different anatomical and functional alterations in the foot may result in excessive pronation. This causes the normal force of mechanical load acting upon the foot to be not supported by basic structures, i.e., bones and ligaments, but rather by joint capsules and plantar fascia, thus enabling easy damage of these structures.[12,15,19,20,27,28]

Other commonly stated predisposing conditions of plantar fasciitis are a rigid cavus foot, flat feet, and tight Achilles tendon.[10,12,14,15,28] The majority of cases of plantar fasciitis are associated with training errors.[27,28] Occasionally, plantar fasciitis signifies an underlying systemic disorder, e.g., rheumatoid arthritis, systemic lupus erythematosus, gout, ankylosing spondylitis, or Reiter's syndrome.[7,17,19]

B. Clinical Picture and Diagnostics

Clinical manifestation of plantar fasciitis is painful heel, or more specifically, painful sensation in the bottom of the heel bone. Various terms and expressions have been used to describe painful heel syndrome, such as subcalcaneal pain, stone bruise, medial arch sprain, calcaneal periostitis, and calcaneodynia.[2,3,8,10,25] Different causes of this clinical syndrome have also been identified, like entrapment of the medial calcaneal branch of the posterior tibial nerve or entrapment of the nerve to abductor digiti quinti.[7,19] Painful heel syndrome is also often described as an inflammation of common origin of plantar fascia and smaller foot muscles or as a consequence of certain systemic diseases. It has been reported that the calcaneal stress fracture and calcaneal periostitis may easily be mistaken for plantar fasciitis.[25,30] For these reasons, it is very important to find out the exact cause of painful heel syndrome (Table 1). The site and quality of pain are essential to differentiate plantar fasciitis from other possible causes of painful heel syndrome.

The pinpoint, knife-like pain of plantar fasciitis is localized specifically at the medial tubercle of the calcaneus, i.e., at the site of the medial plantar fascia origin. There are cases when pain radiates along the medial longitudinal arch of the foot, but swelling occurs quite rarely. Swelling is usually localized to the area just anterior to the calcaneus (Figure 4).

TABLE 1
Possible Causes of Calcaneodynia[7]

Inflammatory
    Juvenile rheumatoid arthritis
    Rheumatoid arthritis
    Ankylosing spondylitis
    Reiter's syndrome
    Gout
Metabolic
    Migratory osteoporosis
    Osteomalacia
Degenerative
    Osteoarthritis
    Atrophy of the heel fat pad
Nerve entrapment
    Tarsal tunnel syndrome
    Entrapment of the medial calcaneal branch of the posterior tibial
        nerve
    Entrapment of the nerve to abductor digiti quinti
Traumatic
    Calcaneal fractures
    Calcaneal malunions
    Traumatic arthritis
    Rupture of the fibrous septae of the fat pad
    Puncture of the fat pad
Overuse injuries
    Plantar fasciitis
    Stenosing tenosynovitis of the flexor digitorum longus and flexor
        hallucis longus
    Calcaneal apophysitis (Sever's disease)
    Subcalcaneal bursitis
    Periostitis
    Calcaneal stress fractures
    Achilles tendinitis and peritendinitis
    Haglund's deformity.

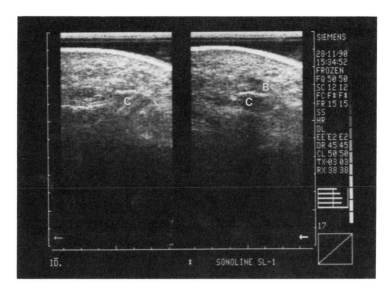

FIGURE 4. Sonogram of the sole of the foot showing bursa at the origin of the plantar fascia. (C) Calcaneus; (B) bursa.

Similar to other overuse injuries, pain is usually of gradual onset. Initially, the symptoms are noticed only with athletic activity. Pain is present at the beginning of an activity, becomes bearable after a few minutes, and will recur with increased severity toward the end of the activity. As the condition progresses, pain may be present with all activities of daily living. Most patients have severe pain in the morning upon getting up, which disappears after a few dozen steps. On physical examination, the patient feels tenderness on firm palpation at the medial tubercle of the calcaneus, as well as diffuse tenderness along the medial longitudinal arch. Passive dorsiflexion of the great toe (with or without simultaneous dorsiflexion of the foot) increases the pain because of the stretching of the plantar fascia.[24]

The usual X-ray findings in plantar fasciitis are more or less reduced to noticing bone spur on the calcaneus, which is more common in patients with plantar fasciitis, although it was observed in about 15% of patients without symptoms of the disease.[3,8,21] The spur is thought to be the result, not the cause, of chronic fascial inflammation. The most recent research has shown that on 45° medial oblique X-ray examination, changes in the cortex and/or trabecular pattern in 85% of the patients with painful heel syndrome may be seen, while on lateral roentgenograms, the majority of them demonstrated thickening of heel fat pad and subfascial area.[2]

Bone scan is used to differentiate calcaneal stress fractures from calcaneal periostitis and plantar fasciitis. In patients with plantar fasciitis, there is an early increase in the flow of blood through the damaged area of the fascia, but there is no late accumulation of radionuclides in the calcaneus, otherwise a characteristic feature in stress fracture or calcaneal periostitis.[26,30]

Plantar fasciitis may occur unilaterally or bilaterally. The majority of patients with plantar fasciitis are middle-aged males.[14] Higher tendency toward plantar fasciitis has been observed in those patients who have engaged in activities often requiring maximum plantar flexion with simultaneous metatarsophalangeal dorsiflexion.[7,14] Thus, plantar fasciitis occurs much more frequently in runners and ballet dancers.

C. Treatment

1. Nonoperative Treatment

Treatment of plantar fasciitis is directed at relieving the inflammatory process of the fascia and correcting predisposing factors. Initial management should include local application of ice, administration of nonsteroidal anti-inflammatory drugs, and cessation of athletic activities. A 15 to 20-min ice massage applied several times daily is recommended for quickly relieving pain. However, it has been noticed that when cryotherapy is applied for a longer period of time, the results are less satisfactory.[14,25] Anti-inflammatory drugs are quite effective in relieving inflammatory alterations of the fascia, regardless whether they are used as nonsteroidal anti-inflammatory agents or as steroid injections into the calcaneal attachment of the plantar fascia. During the application of steroid injections, caution is necessary for possible adverse reactions so that no more than three injections should be given in any one series. Atrophy of calcaneal fat tissue, affected nerves, or resistance to applied treatment may accompany repeated application of steroid injection.[7,15,20,25] Although there have been reports of dramatic improvements in plantar fasciitis by athletes given steroid injections, these are temporary improvements which must be connected along with correction of training errors, running on appropriate surfaces, orthotic treatment, and flexibility and strength exercises. To provide immediate relief from plantar fasciitis symptoms, reduced physical activity or even complete rest are often very useful.

Ultrasound, high-voltage galvanic stimulation and deep transverse friction massage are used additionally with treatment of plantar fasciitis.[14,15,28] Besides, alternating use of ultrasound and ice, or contrast bath has shown beneficial effects upon the course of plantar fasciitis.[10,25]

Despite its being useful, quick alleviation of symptoms only has temporary effects in the treatment of plantar fasciitis unless it is used in combination with orthotic therapy.[19,24] The purpose of orthotic therapy is to decrease the stretching of plantar fascia caused by excessive and/or prolonged foot pronation. The improvement in abnormal pronation is achieved by supporting the longitudinal arch, precisely positioning the calcaneus, supporting the head of the first metatarsal bone, and providing adequate heel support in shoes. The use of UCBL (University of California Biomechanical Laboratory) device is recommended and so is the use of specially designed shoes that assume the role of the plantar fascia in stabilizating the foot during an activity.[4] The correction of biomechanical foot abnormalities may also be achieved by special technique of fixation of the foot with an adhesive strapping, the so-called low Dye strapping technique.[25] In the treatment of plantar fasciitis, a variety of orthotic devices may be used, such as heel lifts or ready-made arch supports (rigid, semirigid, and flexible). In order to improve the range of movement in the ankle following plantar fasciitis, stretching exercises for plantar fascia, Achilles tendon, gastrocnemius-soleus complex, and foot muscles are recommended as a part of the rehabilitation program.[7,14,19,23,24,25]

2. Surgical Treatment

Although there are many nonoperative therapeutic measures used for the treatment of plantar fasciitis, a minor number of patients do not exhibit satisfactory improvement. The majority of these patients are competitive athletes. Surgical treatment of plantar fasciitis is recommended when symptoms last longer than 1 year and do not recede in spite of nonoperative treatment measures and complete rest.[9,15,24]

Several procedures are employed for surgical treatment of plantar fasciitis.[9,13,22,29] Most of them entail removing the bone spur, if it exists at all. It is a well-established fact that the results of this operation are not satisfactory (although they may be in a very small number of patients) since the bone spur is most often not the cause but rather the consequence of plantar fasciitis. Surgical revision and suturing of the torn plantar fascia have provided satisfactory outcome in a certain number of patients.[1,5,11]

It should be pointed out that the best results in the treatment of plantar fasciitis have been obtained by releasing the plantar fascia from its origin.[9,22] This release has a beneficial effect upon the inflammation of plantar fascia, probably because afterwards the fascia assumes the position at which it possesses weaker internal tension, and at the same time the natural healing process of the fascia is stimulated. Recovery time after surgery is about 2 months.

II. ANTERIOR IMPINGEMENT SYNDROME OF THE ANKLE

Repeated maximal dorsal flexion of the foot leads to the development of bony growths (exostoses) on the anterior edge of the tibia, the neck of the talus, and occasionally the navicular bone. This is caused by the repetitive collisions of the anterior edge of the tibia against the neck of the talus. The newly developed bony exostosis incapacitate maximal dorsal flexion of the foot in the ankle, and repeated efforts to perform this movement lead to pain and swelling limited to the anterior side of the ankle, i.e., anterior impingement syndrome of the ankle.[16,20,34] This syndrome is most often encountered in soccer players, especially older soccer players. For this reason, some authors refer to this syndrome as soccer players exostosis on the neck of the talus (Figure 5). In soccer players, the development of this syndrome is linked with, besides the previously mentioned causes, repeated maximal plantar flexion movements of the foot performed while kicking the ball. This is explained by the fact that during these movements, the joint capsule is subjected to stress localized at its insertion points. The development of bony exostosis in the anterior ankle area is also described in other athletes, most frequently in ballet dancers. Besides limited dorsiflexion which reduces the depth obtained while performing the plié, the patient complains of pain, swelling, and localized tenderness during palpation of the area between the medial malleolus and the tibialis anterior muscle tendon, and between the lateral malleolus and the extensor digitorum longus muscle tendon. Symptoms of anterior impingement syndrome of the ankle increase in severity during maximal dorsal flexion of the foot and decrease during the performing of plantar flexion. The limited dorsal flexion characteristic for this syndrome is often incorrectly attributed to an excessively "tight" Achilles tendon; this results in the unsuccessful application

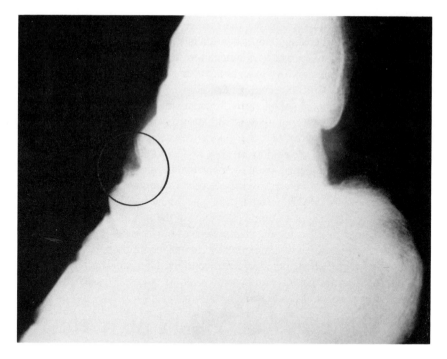

FIGURE 5. Soccer player's exostosis on the neck of the talus.

of stretching exercises which are generally extremely painful to the patient. Lateral roentgenograms of the foot taken in a maximally dorsally flexed position reveal contact between the anterior edge of the tibia and the talus.

Basic treatment for anterior impingement syndrome of the ankle consists of avoiding maximal dorsal flexion of the foot. Raising the heels of the shoes for 1 to 2 cm, bandaging the lower leg and foot with adhesive tape, and strengthening the muscles on the posterior side of the lower leg usually prove helpful. Physical therapy, use of nonsteroid anti-inflammatory drugs, and in severe cases, local application of corticosteorids and anesthetics usually releaves the symptoms. The best results, however, are obtained by causative treatment, i.e., by removing the bony exostosis surgically. The surgery can be performed arthroscopically.[5,6,16] Surgical excision does not prevent the future development of bony exostosis, and the patient should be advised of this before surgery.[10]

III. POSTERIOR IMPINGEMENT SYNDROME OF THE ANKLE

Repeated maximal plantar flexion may lead to posterior impingement syndrome of the ankle due to the existence of os trigonum or Stieda's process on the talus.[1,19,20,24,28] This syndrome can also be caused by an exceptionally developed posterior process of the calcaneus, by the existence of an ankle meniscus, or by the thickening of soft tissues resulting from repeated injuries sustained during maximal plantar flexion of the foot. The posterior aspect of the talus is grooved by the tendon of flexor hallucis longus, producing the medial and lateral tubercles. The lateral tubercle is either short or long. If it is long, it is called *Stieda's process.* Instead of the process, there may be an ossicle attached to the body of the talus by a fibrous tissue. This accessory ossicle is known as the os trigonum and is present in 5 to 20% of individuals, appearing unilaterally in two thirds.[1,24]

Since most individuals who have an os trigonum are not aware of its presence, it is accidentally spotted while radiographing the ankle. Nevertheless, os trigonum or Stieda's process may cause trouble. During extreme plantar flexion, Stieda's process is trapped between the calcaneus and tibia like "a nut in a nutcracker", limiting extreme plantar flexion (Figure 6). Its trapping causes compression and irritation of the adjacent synovial and capsular tissue. With repeated entrapment and irritation, the soft tissue undergoes inflammatory changes and eventually thickens, preventing already reduced plantar flexion from flexing any further (Figure 7). The pain located on the posterior side of the ankle is caused by trying to force the foot further down than it can go. This syndrome, commonly seen in ballet dancers and therefore called *dancer's heel,* is also encountered in soccer players, high jumpers, and pole vaulters.[13,14,15,18,30,31]

In differential diagnosis, posterior impingement syndrome must be distinguished from other conditions that can produce similar posterior ankle pain, especially Achilles tendinitis and peroneal and flexor hallucis longus tendinitis. These conditions are also common in ballet dancers.[9,20,33] The symptoms of Achilles tendinitis occur 2 to 6 cm above the insertion of the tendon into the calcaneus, or in the tendon-bone junction when referring to the insertional Achilles tendinitis or enthesitis.[11] Symptoms and signs of peroneal tendinitis include pain, swelling, and tenderness in the posterior lateral malleolar area.[9,33] The most difficult differential diagnosis is the

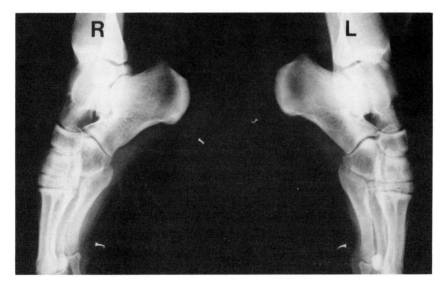

FIGURE 6. Lateral roentgenogram of both ankles taken in a plantar flexed position. Note the limitation in plantar flexion of the right ankle (R) when compared to the left (L).

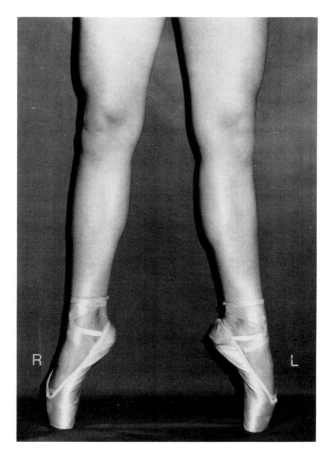

FIGURE 7. Lack of maximal plantar flexion in the right ankle (R) during pointe position.

flexor hallucis longus tendinitis whose symptoms include pain, swelling, and tenderness localized in the posterior medial malleolar region; its most significant finding on physical examination is the functional (pseudo) hallux valgus.[7,12,22,35] In some patients, the flexor hallucis longus tendinitis may coexist with posterior impingement syndrome.[1,7,14,15,28,31] The initial treatment of posterior impingement syndrome of the ankle involves cessation or moderation of activities that provoke entrapment and irritation of the tissue, physical therapy to increase the flexibility of the ankle, and application of nonsteroidal anti-inflammatory drugs. In cases in which this therapy does not produce the expected results, infiltration of the tender area with corticosteroids and anesthetics may be performed. In resistent cases, surgical treatment — excision of the os trigonum along with the surrounding thickened fibrous tissue — comes into consideration.[1,19,20,28] If symptoms of tendinitis of the flexor hallucis longus muscle are also present, tenolysis, which requires the opening of the ankle, is indicated. The results of surgical treatment confirm the opinion held by many authors that too much time should not be wasted on nonoperative treatment especially when dealing with professional dancers and athletes.

IV. FLEXOR HALLUCIS LONGUS TENDINITIS

Tendinitis of the flexor hallucis longus muscle is a common entity in ballet dancers; therefore, it is known as dancer's tendinitis.[37,42–45,48,52,60,61,65] Dancers, especially ballerinas, are constantly stressing the flexor hallucis longus tendon in pointe work, dancing on the tips of their toes in hyperplantar flexion of the ankle and hallux. The main dynamic stabilizing factor of the medial region of the foot in this position is the flexor hallucis longus muscle. Because of its functional importance, the flexor hallucis longus muscle has been referred to as the "Achilles tendon of the foot".

The flexor hallucis longus tendon is formed above the ankle, crosses behind the medial malleolus traveling through a groove in the talus, and goes under the sustentaculum tali as it passes in to the foot (Figure 8). The tendon encased in the synovial sheath (vagina synovialis) courses through the tarsal tunnel as it passes into the foot and than goes along the lower medial side of the foot to its origin on the base of the distal phalanx of the great toe. Repeated overuse of the foot may lead to degenerative changes within the tendon, ranging from characteristic inflammatory changes to formation of a knot, thickening of the tendon, development of cysts in the

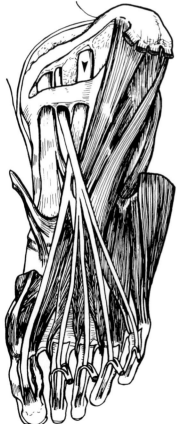

FIGURE 8. The flexor hallucis longus muscle (arrowhead).

tendon, and even partial rupture of the collagen fibers in the tendon (Figure 9). Thickening of the tendon usually develops in the lacuna tendinum, below and behind the medial malleolus, and in rare cases, at the exit of the lacuna tendinum. Development of this thickening can lead to stenosing tenosynovitis of the flexor hallucis longus muscle with a clinical picture similar to trigger finger.[52,65] Functional hallux rigidus also develops because of the barrier effect of the thickened tendon. This disables flexion of the great toe during dorsiflexion of the foot until the resistance of the thickened tendon passing through the lacuna tendinum is overcome, either passively or actively.

Clinical findings include pain and swelling in the medial aspect of the ankle, behind the medial malleolar region. In some cases, during passive movements of the thumb, crepitations are felt in the same region, and sometimes the trigger finger phenomenon is also felt. Flexion of the great toe against resistance will produce pain in the area posterior to the medial malleolus. The pain is blunt and increases in severity during physical activity while disappearing after rest, depending, of course, on the stage and severity of the tendinitis. In diagnosing this symptom, tenography used to be frequently employed, but nowadays, ultrasound examination is generally used. Differential diagnostics include ruling out Achilles tendon overuse syndrome (tendinitis and enthesitis). Posterior impingement syndrome of the ankle, however, is the most difficult clinical entity to differentiate, especially since both syndromes may be present.[37,58]

The basic nonoperative treatment for tendinitis of the flexor hallucis longus muscle consists of cessation or reduction of athletic activities (especially those

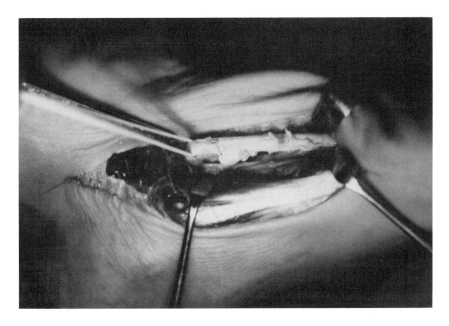

FIGURE 9. Intraoperative finding of partial rupture of the flexor hallucis longus muscle in a long-distance runner.

involving standing on the toes), physical therapy (stretching exercises), and use of nonsteroidal anti-inflammatory drugs. Dancers are encouraged to exercise in a pool since this enables them to imitate exercises done on dry land but with considerably less pressure. Local applications of corticosteroids with anesthetics are also suggested in some cases. Surgical treatment should remain as the last option and consists of tenolysis while in cases of stenosing tenosynovitis, freeing of the tendon in the tarsal canal is indicated.[47,52,65] We successfully treated tendinitis of the flexor hallucis longus muscle in one long-distance runner by tenolysis and debridement of the plantar part of the tendon.

V. TENDINITIS OF THE COMMON EXTENSOR MUSCLE

The tendons of the long and short extensors of the toes and the long extensor of the great toe stretch along the dorsal side of the foot (Figure 10). Excessive pressure from footwear or too tightly laced shoestrings can lead to overstimulation of these tendons and/or their enveloping synovial sheaths, resulting in tendinitis or tendovaginitis.[33,34,39,51,59] In most cases, the symptoms of tendinitis gradually increase while cases of tendinitis resulting from one episode of excessive irritation are rare. Pain located on the dorsal side of the foot which increases during running is the most common and indicative sign of tendinitis. Another very characteristic symptom is the appearance of a localized swelling on the dorsal side of the foot, which can best be noticed by comparing the affected foot with the other unaffected foot (bilateral tendinitis of the toe extensors of the foot is rare). Tendinitis of the extensors of the toes is characterized by pain and tenderness felt when moving the toes. Later stages of the syndrome are characterized by painful limping during running and, in long standing cases, by the inability to walk without a limp. Differential diagnosis should take into account the possibility of stress fractures of the metatarsal bones of the foot (marching fracture) which manifest themselves with similar symptoms.

Treatment of tendinitis of the toe extensors is carried out according to the principles that apply to all overuse syndromes of the musculoskeletal system. Athletic activities should be stopped for a period of at least 7 d, nonsteroidal anti-inflammatory drugs and local cryotherapy should be applied (2 times per day for a period of 20 min), and the way that the shoelaces are laced should be corrected. The shoelaces should be laced in a step-like manner (not criss-crossed), and in some cases, the tongue of the shoe should be thickened with a sponge or some other similar substance. In cases where this therapy does not produce results, local infiltration of corticosteroids and anesthetics is recommended.

VI. TENDINITIS OF THE POSTERIOR TIBIALIS MUSCLE

The contribution of the posterior tibialis muscle to forming the arch of the foot is of paramont importance. For this reason, the exertion of that muscle during athletic activities in individuals with lowered arches is considerable. Excessive exertion of this muscle can manifest itself either by the appearance of pain in the region of its origin on the posterior side of the tibia (runner's leg or shin splint), or by the development of an overuse syndrome in the region of the muscle tendon and its origin

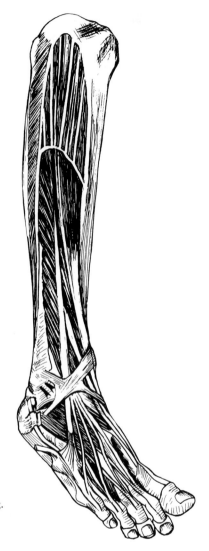

FIGURE 10. Anterior muscles of the leg.

on the navicular bone, in which case the term *tendinitis of the posterior tibial muscle* is applied.[39,63] This tendinitis can develop in athletes who participate in various athletic activities, but is most common in athletes who habitually run for long periods of time. The most characteristic symptom of tendinitis of the posterior tibial muscle is a gradually increasing pain localized on the central and medial part of the sole of the foot, i.e., in the area of insertion of the tendon. Tenderness along the tendon, in the area behind the posterior part of the medial malleolus is also common. The appearance of pain and/or the increasing of this pain while jumping and landing is also characteristic for this syndrome. During physical examination, swelling of the tendon's sheath is also fairly frequently noticed (Figure 11). Differential diagnostics includes ruling out stress fractures.

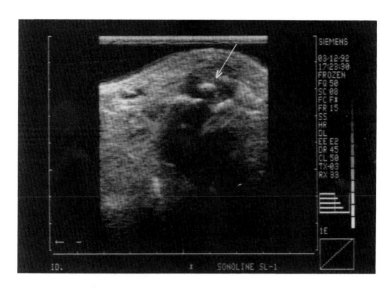

FIGURE 11. Sonogram of the leg showing tibialis posterior tendovaginitis (arrow).

Treatment of this syndrome is carried out according to the principles that apply to treatment of all tendinitises, with special emphasis on the static correction of the sole of the foot by using semirigid orthopedic implants. In resistant cases, local infiltration of corticosteroids and anesthetics often produces good results. Surgical treatment (tenolysis and decompression) is rarely needed.[39,63]

VII. DISLOCATION OF THE PERONEAL TENDONS

The tendons of the long and short peroneal muscle pass behind the lateral malleolus in a variably deep groove which, together with the retinaculum mm. peroneorum proximale et distale, forms a channel (Figure 12). During complete dorsiflexion of the sole of the foot, e.g., when a skier falls forward over the tips of his skies, these retinaculs can snap (sometimes audibly), while the muscle tendons can dislocate. This is accompanied with intense pain and rapid swelling while physical examination reveals tenderness to palpation localized in the area behind the lateral malleolus. After several hours, subcutaneous bleeding appears while the pain diffusely spreads, which often leads to incorrect diagnosis of dislocation of the ankle. In some cases, the dislocated peroneal tendons can be palpated. In clinical diagnostics, the eversion and dorsiflexion test for the sole of the foot is helpful (Figure 13). In this test, eversion and dorsiflexion of the sole of the foot against resistance produces pain in the retromalleolar region if dislocation of the peroneal tendons is present. These symptoms can be mistaken for anterior impingement syndrome of the ankle. In cases of acute dislocation of the peroneal tendons, surgical treatment is indicated although some authors recommend immobilization and refrain from surgery except in cases where repeated dislocations of the peroneal tendons develop.[39,55,56,62,63,67] In those cases of repeated dislocations, the peroneal tendons are

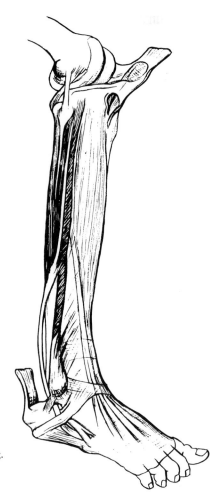

FIGURE 12. Peroneal group of muscles of the leg.

placed retromalleolarly during plantar flexion of the sole of the foot, while during dorsal flexion, they dislocate. These repeated dislocations are extremely unpleasant and lead to instability of the ankle.

VIII. SESAMOIDITIS

Two small sesamoid bones, medial and lateral, exist in the flexor hallucis brevis muscle tendon below the head of the first metatarsal bone. Their function is to distribute and ease the pressure produced during walking on the head of the first metatarsal bone. The term *sesamoiditis* applies to acute and chronic injuries of these bones.[53] Acute injuries consist of fractures that are very difficult to diagnose due to the high frequency of bipartite sesamoid bones often seen on lateral and axial roentgenographs. Chondromalacia of the sesamoid bones is also described while degenerative changes and stress fractures are likewise fairly frequent.[38,50,53,66] The mechanism leading to injury of the sesamoid bones is related to overuse of the

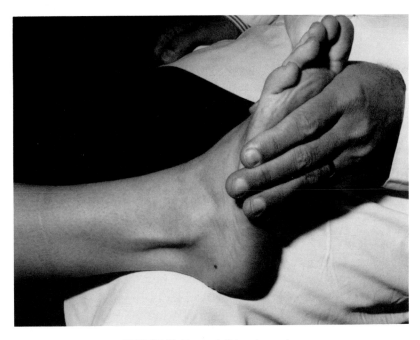

FIGURE 13. Peroneal dislocation testing.

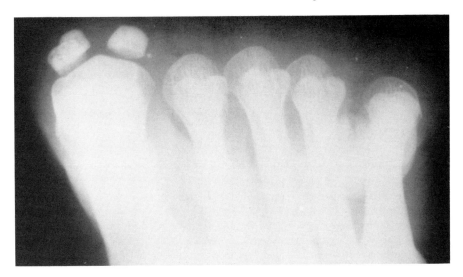

FIGURE 14. Axial roentgenogram of the foot demonstrating great toe sesamoids.

anterior part of the sole of the foot accompanied by excessive dorsiflexion of the great toe. Sesamoiditis is most commonly caused by running and jumping, especially when beginning to run and during sprints. In dancers, it results when the sole of the foot is in the relevé position, which creates maximal loading of the head of the first metatarsal bone.[43-45] The development of sesamoiditis is fascilitated by pes cavus and a rigid sole. The most characteristic symptoms are pain and localized swelling. Standing on the tip of the toes is painful while running is impeded. In later stages of the disease, pain appears on the lateral side of the sole of the foot because the patient walks with inverted feet to ease the pressure on his great toe. Clinical examination reveals localized tenderness. During dorsal flexion of the great toe, the sesamoid bones move distally, which also moves the area of greatest tenderness. Swelling is hard to notice because of the present adipose tissue. Ultrasound examination is generally helpful in determining the potential presence of swelling. Radiological diagnostics (Figure 14) and scintigraphy are also useful, especially when diagnosing stress fractures and degenerative changes of the sesamoid bones.[32] Treatment of sesamoiditis is hard to implement, primarily because it is hard to avoid putting pressure on the sesamoid bones when walking. To decrease the pressure, we recommend placing a small sponge, or some other soft material (material from which hats are made of is particularly good) cut out in the shape of a crescent below the head of the first metatarsal bone. A hard shoe sole beneath the great toe of the foot is also recommended. Nonsteroid anti-inflammatory drugs can also be applied. Orthopedic implants can correct the biomechanics of the sole of the foot, thus eliminating the cause of the sesamoiditis. In long standing cases of degenerative changes of the sesamoid bone, surgical excision can be performed. However, because of the concomitant degenerative changes in the cartilage of the head of the first metatarsal bone, this procedure can be unsuccessful.

REFERENCES

Plantar Fasciitis

1. **Ahstrom, J. P.** Spontaneous rupture of the plantar fascia. *Am. J. Sports Med.,* 1988; 16; 306–307.
2. **Amis, J., Jennings, L., Graham, D., and Graham, C. E.** Painful heel syndrome: radiographic and treatment assessment. *Foot Ankle,* 1988; 9:91–95.
3. **Bordelon, R. L.** Subcalcaneal pain. A method of evaluation and plan for treatment. *Clin. Orthop.,* 1983; 177:49–53.
4. **Campbell, J. W. and Inmann, V. T.** Treatment of plantar fasciitis and calcaneal spurs with the UCBL shoe insert. *Clin. Orthop.,* 1974; 103:57–62.
5. **Herrick, R. T. and Herrick, S.** Rupture of the plantar fascia in a middle-aged tennis player. *Am. J. Sports Med.,* 1983; 11:95.
6. **Kibler, W. B., Goldberg, C., and Chandler, T. J.** Functional biomechanical deficits in running athletes with plantar fasciitis. *Am. J. Sports Med.,* 1991; 19:66–71.
7. **Kwong, P. K., Kay, D., Voner, R. T., et al.** Plantar fasciitis: mechanics and patomechanics of treatment. *Clin. Sports Med.,* 1988; 7:119–127.

8. **Lapidus, P. W. and Guidotti, F. P.** Painful heel: reports of 323 patients with 364 painful heels. *Clin. Orthop.*, 1965; 39:178–186.

9. **Leach, R. E., Seavey, M. S., and Salter, D. K.** Results of surgery in athletes with plantar fasciitis. *Foot Ankle*, 1986; 7:156–161.

10. **Leach, R. E., Dilorio, E., and Harney, R. A.** Pathologic hindfoot condition in the athlete. *Clin. Orthop.*, 1982; 177:116–119.

11. **Leach, R. E., Jones, R., and Silva, T.** Rupture of the plantar fascia in athlete. *J. Bone Joint Surg.*, 1978; 60(A):537–539.

12. **Leach, R. E.** Leg and foot injuries in racquet sports. *Clin. Sports Med.*, 1988; 7:359–370.

13. **Lester, K. D. and Buchanan, J. R.** Surgical treatment of plantar fasciitis. *Clin. Orthop.*, 1984; 186:202–204.

14. **Marshall, P.** Overuse foot injuries in athletes and dancers. *Clin. Sports Med.*, 1988; 7:175–191.

15. **McBryde, A. M.** Plantar fasciitis. *AAOS Instr. Course Lect.*, 1984; 33:278–282.

16. **Macintyre, J. G., Taunton, J. E., Clement, D. B., et al.** Running injuries. A clinical study of 4173 cases. *Clin. J. Sports Med.*, 1991; 1:81–87.

17. **Paice, E. W. and Hoffbrand, B. I.** Nutritional osteomalacia presenting with plantar fasciitis. *J. Bone Joint Surg.*, 1987; 69(B):38–40.

18. **Perry, J.** Anatomy and biomechanics of the hindfoot. *Clin. Orthop.*, 1983; 177:9–15.

19. **Ribarić, G., Pećina, M., and Bojanić, I.** Plantarni fascitis. *Acta Orthop. Iugosl.*, 1989; 20:18–22.

20. **Roy, S.** How I manage plantar fasciitis. *Phys. Sportsmed.*, 1983; 11:27–31.

21. **Shereff, M. J. and Johnson, K. A.** Radiographic anatomy of the hindfoot. *Clin. Orthop.*, 1983; 177:16–22.

22. **Snider, M. P., Clancy, W. G., and McBeath, A. A.** Plantar fascia release for chronic plantar fasciitis in runners. *Am. J. Sports Med.*, 1983; 11:215–219.

23. **Stanish, W. D., Rubinovich, R. M., and Curwin, S.** Eccentric exercise in chronic tendinitis. *Clin. Orthop.*, 1986; 208:65–68.

24. **Tanner, S. M. and Harvey, J. S.** How we manage plantar fasciitis. *Phys. Sportsmed.*, 1988; 16:39–47.

25. **Torg, J. S., Pavlov, H., and Torg, E.** Overuse injuries in sport: the foot. *Clin. Sports Med.*, 1987; 6:291–320.

26. **Vasavada, P. J., DeVries, D. F., and Nishiyama, H.** Plantar fasciitis — early blood pool images in the diagnosis of inflammatory process. *Foot Ankle*, 1984; 5:74–76.

27. **Warren, B. L. and Jones, C. J.** Predicting plantar fasciitis in runners. *Med. Sci. Sports Exercise*, 1987; 19:71–73.

28. **Warren, B. L.** Plantar fasciitis in runners. *Sports Med.*, 1990; 338–345.

29. **Ward, W. G. and Clippinger, F. W.** Proximal medial longitudinal arch incision for plantar fascia release. *Foot Ankle*, 1987; 8:152–155.

30. **Williams, P. L., Smibert, J. G., Cox, R., et al.** Imaging study of the painful heel syndrome. *Foot Ankle*, 1987; 7:345–9.

Anterior Impingement Syndrome and Other Subchapters (III., IV., V., VI., VII., and VIII.)

31. **Brodsky, A. E., Khall, M. A.** Talar compression syndrome. *Foot Ankle*, 1987; 7:338–344.

32. **Chung, Y., Rosenberg, Z. S., Mogee, T., and Chinitz, L.** Normal anatomy and pathologic conditions of ankle tendons: current imaging techniques. *Radiographics*, 1992; 12:429–444.

33. **Coughlin, R. R.** Common injuries of the foot. *Postgrad. Med.*, 1989; 86:175–85.
34. **Duddy, R. K., Meredith, R., Visser, J., and Brooks, J. S.** Tendon sheath injuries of the foot and ankle. *J. Foot Surg.*, 1991; 30:179–186.
35. **Ewing, J. W.** Arthroscopic management of transchondral talar-dome fractures (osteochondritis dissecans) and anterior impingement lesions of the ankle joint. *Clin. Sport Med.*, 1991; 10:677–687.
36. **Ferkel, R. D., Karzel, R. P., Del Pizzo, W., Friedman, M. J., and Fischer, S. P.** Arthroscopic treatment of anterolateral impingement of the ankle. *Am. J. Sports Med.*, 1991; 19:440–446.
37. **Fond, D.** Flexor hallucis longus tendinitis — a case of mistaken identity and posterior impingement syndrome in dancers: evaluation and management. *J. Orthop. Sports Phys. Ther.*, 1984; 5:204–206.
38. **Frankel, J. P. and Harrington, J.** Symptomatic bipartite sesamoids. *J. Foot Surg.*, 1990; 29:318–323.
39. **Frey, C. C. and Shereff, M. J.** Tendon injuries about the ankle in athletes. *Clin. Sports Med.*, 1988; 7:103–118.
40. **Fricker, P. A. and Williams, J. G. P.** Surgical management of os trigonum and talar spur in sportsmen. *Br. J. Sports Med.*, 1979; 13:55–57.
41. **Garrick, J. G. and Webb, D. R.** *Sports Injuries: Diagnosis and Management.* Philadelphia: W. B. Saunders, 1990.
42. **Garth, W. P.** Flexor hallucis tendinitis in a ballet dancer. A case report. *J. Bone Joint Surg.*, 1981; 63A:1489.
43. **Hamilton, W. G.** Foot and ankle injuries in dancers. *Clin. Sports Med.*, 1988; 7:143–173.
44. **Hardaker, W. T., Jr., Margello, S., and Goldner, J. L.** Foot and ankle injuries in the artical dancers. *Foot Ankle,* 1985; 6:59–69.
45. **Hardaker, W. T., Jr.** Foot and ankle injuries in classical ballet dancers. *Orthop. Clin. Am.,* 1989; 20:621–627.
46. **Hawkins, R. B.** Arthroscopic treatment of sports - related anterior osteophytes in the ankle. *Foot Ankle,* 1988; 9:87–90.
47. **Holt, K. W. G. and Cross, M. J.** Isolated rupture of the flexor hallucis longus tendon. A case report. *Am. J. Sports Med.*, 1990; 18:645–646.
48. **Howse, A. J. G.** Orthopedists aid ballet. *Clin. Orthop.*, 1972; 89:52–63.
49. **Johnson, R. P., Collier, D. B., and Carrera, G. F.** The os trigonum syndrome: use of bone scan in the diagnosis. *J. Trauma,* 1984; 24:761–764.
50. **Keene, J. S. and Lange, R. H.** Diagnostic dilemmas in foot and ankle injuries. *JAMA,* 1986; 256:247–251.
51. **Lillich, J. S. and Baxter, D. E.** Common forefoot problems in runners. *Foot Ankle,* 1986; 7:145–151.
52. **Lynch, T. and Pupp, G. R.** Stenosing tenosynovitis of the flexor hallucis longus at the ankle joint. *J. Foot Surg.*, 1990; 29:345–352.
53. **McBryde, A. M. and Anderson, R. B.** Sesamoid foot problems in the athlete. *Clin. Sports Med.*, 1988; 7:51–60.
54. **McDougall, A.** The os trigonum. *J. Bone Joint Surg.*, 1955; 37(B):257–265.
55. **McLennan, J. G.** Treatment of acute and chronic luxations of the peroneal tendons. *Am. J. Sports Med.*, 1980; 8:432–436.
56. **Micheli, L. J., Waters, M. P., and Sanders, D. P.** Sliding fibular graft repair for chronic dislocation of the peroneal tendons. *Am. J. Sports Med.*, 1989; 17:68–71.
57. **Paulos, L. E., Johnson, C. L., and Noyes, F. R.** Posterior compartment fractures of the ankle. *Am. J. Sports Med.*, 1983; 11:439–443.

58. **Pećina, M. and Bojanić, I.** Posterior impingement syndrome of the ankle. *Acta Orthop. Iugosl.,* 1989; 20:120–123.
59. **Plattner, P. F.** Tendon problems of the foot and ankle. *Postgrad. Med.,* 1989; 86:155–170.
60. **Sammarco, G. J.** The foot and ankle in classical ballet and modern dance. In: *Disorders of the Foot,* Jahss M. H., Ed. Philadelphia: W. B. Saunders, 1982; 1626–1659.
61. **Sammarco, G. J.** Diagnosis and treatment in dancers. *Clin. Orthop.,* 1984; 187:176–187.
62. **Sarmiento, A. and Wolf, M.** Subluxation of the peroneal tendons. *J. Bone Joint Surg.,* 1975; 57(A):115–116.
63. **Scheller, A. D., Kasser, J. R., and Quigley, T. B.** Tendon injuries about the ankle. *Orthop. Clin. N. Am.,* 1980; 11:801–811.
64. **Stoller, S. M., Hekmat, F., and Kleiger, B.** A comparative study of the frequency of anterior impingement exostoses of the ankle in dancers and nondancers. *Foot Ankle,* 1984; 4:201–203.
65. **Tudisco, C. and Puddu, G.** Stenosing tenosynovitis of the flexor hallucis longus tendon in a classical ballet dancer. A case report. *Am. J. Sports Med.,* 1984; 12:403–404.
66. **Van Hal, M. E., Keene, J. S., and Lange, T. A.,** Stress fractures of the great toe sesamoids. *Am. J. Sports Med.,* 1982; 10:122–128.
67. **Zoellner, G. and Clancy, W, Jr.** Recurrent dislocation of the peroneal tendon. *J. Bone Joint Surg.,* 1979; 61(A):292–294.

Other Overuse Injuries

Chapter
10

Bursitis

Synovial bursae make an integral part of the bone-tendon-joint complex. They are particularly susceptible to injuries and damages in athletes. Direct acute trauma leads to bleeding into the bursal space, causing acute swelling and pain with limited motion; this is usually called *acute hemorrhagic bursitis*. Repetitive microtraumas, such as permanently increased friction of tendon over the bursa or constant outer pressure upon bursa (ill-fitting shoes or athletic equipment), bring about chronic inflammation clinically referred to as *chronic bursitis*. Bursitis may be infected either primarily or secondarily, and these cases are referred to as *septic bursitis*. Overuse injuries comprise chronic bursitis as well.[1,5,11,12,19]

I. ANATOMY

Synovial bursae are either small or large closed sac-like structures that lie in continuity with, but not normally in communication with, a joint. They are found between individual muscles and their tendons, at sites of tendinous or muscular attachment to a hard base, and as subcutaneous localized mucous sacs.

The structure of the mucous sac membranous wall is similar to that of the joint capsule synovial membrane; it normally secretes a small amount of fluid, which acts as a lubricant, enabling the two bursal surfaces to glide easily over one another. The basic function of mucous sacs is to improve the gliding motion of two adjoining structures by dissipating friction.

More than 150 synovial sacs are found in a human body, and each of them may show clinical symptoms. Our aim is to emphasize only a few, specifically those most commonly affected in athletes. Even if in the shoulder area there are eight synovial sacs (Figure 1), only the subacromial bursa is of greater clinical significance.[7,16] The subacromial bursa is located between the acromion, coracoacromial ligament, and deltoid muscle on one side, and joint capsule with coracohumeral ligament and rotator cuff tendons of the shoulder on the other side (Figure 2). Several bursae are found in the elbow region — the olecranon bursa, the radial and ulnar epicondylar bursae, the radiohumeral bursa, the supinator bursa, and the bicipital radial bursa. Only the olecranon bursa (Figure 3) is of practical clinical significance.[2,24]

The wrist region is characterized by frequent synovial herniation or synovial cyst at the volar or dorsal side of the joint. Due to weak membrane of the joint capsule,

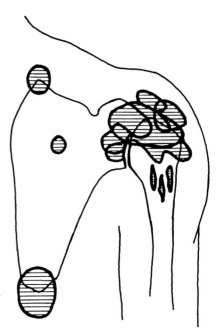

FIGURE 1. Bursae in the shoulder region.

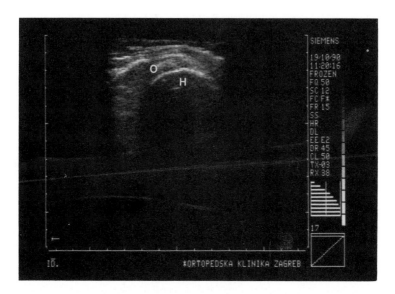

FIGURE 2. Sonogram showing ossification in the subacromial bursa. (H) Humeral head; (O) ossification.

usually resulting from long-term and chronic overuse, part of the synovial membrane herniates under the skin, forming a relatively hard node that may be either large or small in size. The lesion is known as *ganglion cyst* and is not to be confused with bursitis.[22]

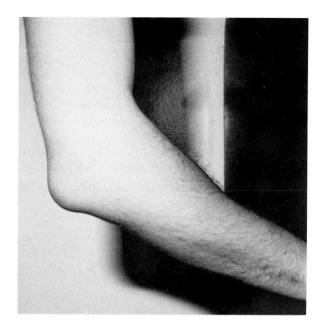

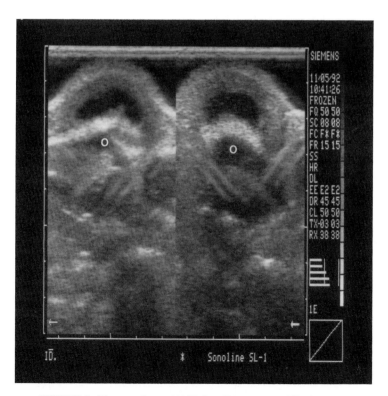

FIGURE 3. Olecranon bursa. (A) Native; (B) sonogram; (O) olecranon.

The hip region is known for many synovial sacs. Specific mention should be made of the great trochanter bursa, the subgluteal, ischiogluteal, and iliopectineal bursae, and the iliopsoas tendon attachment bursa. The trochanteric bursa is the most important one from the practical and clinical viewpoint (Figure 4). A lot of synovial sacs are found in the knee region (Figure 5): prepatellar bursa, infrapatellar bursa, suprapatellar bursa, semimembranosus bursa, pes anserina bursa, bursa between the fibular collateral ligament and popliteal tendon, bursa between popliteal tendon and lateral femoral condyle, bursa of the lateral head of the gastrocnemius, bursa between the fibular collateral ligament and biceps tendon, medial collateral ligament bursa, and medial head of the gastrocnemius muscle bursa.[8,20] Some of the bursae communicate with the joint space (articular cavity). For example, the bursa between the medial head of the gastrocnemius and the semimembranous muscle communicates through the posterior joint capsule with the knee joint (Figure 6). Frequent swelling of the bursa results in the formation of popliteal cyst (Baker's cyst).[5]

In regards to the ankle and the foot, the bursae located in the region of the heel bone and Achilles tendon attachment are of greater clinical significance, as are those in the region of the metatarsophalangeal joint of the big toe. The retrocalcaneal bursa is located between the posterior plane of the heel bone and the anterior aspect of the Achilles tendon (Figure 7), while the superficial Achilles tendon bursa is located between the posterior aspect of the tendon and the skin.[14,6,21] As a result of long-term pressure upon the foot caused by ill-fitting shoes, bursitis may occur in different sites, while septic bursitis commonly develops in the big toe region.[19]

II. ETIOPATHOGENESIS

Direct blow as in collision either with an athletic competitor or through contact with a hard surface may cause an acute hemorrhagic bursitis.[1,5,11,12,14,19] A direct

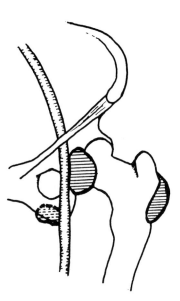

FIGURE 4. Bursae in the hip region.

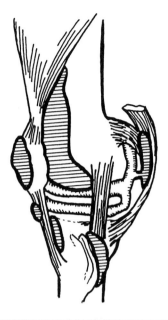

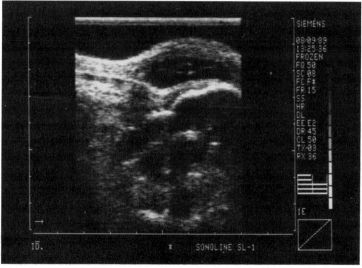

FIGURE 5. (A) Bursae in the knee region. (B) Sonogram demonstrating prepatellar bursitis.

trauma causes bleeding into the bursal space which results in acute swelling, pain, and limited mobility.

Bursae may be injured by a less violent but constant repetitive stress, usually occurring during athletic or some other professional activities.[1,5,11,12,19] The repetitive stress in sports may be caused by artificial surfaces, wrestling mats, and gymnastic floor exercise mats.[9,19] However, repetitive joint motion is the most common cause. The most characteristic example is the development of chronic bursitis of the shoulder joint in throwers because of their repetitive swinging motions of the arm.[7,19]

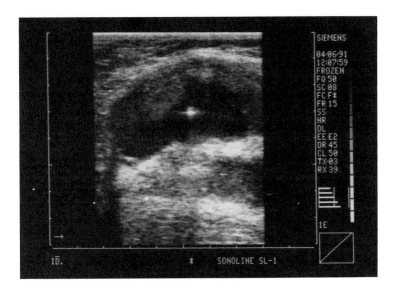

FIGURE 6. Sonogram of the posterior part of the knee, demonstrating a large Baker's cyst.

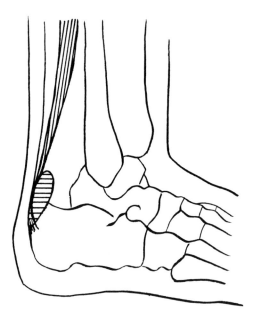

FIGURE 7. Retrocalcaneal bursa.

The initial physiologic reaction to repetitive stress is vasodilation resulting from the increased blood flow into the injured area. The bursa becomes warm and sometimes erythematous. Changes take place in the permeability of the capillary wall, and extracellular fluid and serum protein accumulate in the bursa. These processes are clinically manifested as swelling. If the condition persists, the bursal wall thickens and calcium may be deposited, causing the bursal fluid to acquire consistency similar to toothpaste.[15] The condition is referred to as *chemical bursitis*. This type of bursitis causes degeneration and calcification of tendons, very much like calcification of the supraspinatus tendon. The direct cause of calcification in tendon and bursa has not yet been fully explained. According to Reilly and Nicholas,[9] changes in the collagen structure of the bursa and its neighboring tendons result in increased affinity for calcium salts, possibly with a local increase in the hydrogen ion concentration.

Chronic subacromial bursitis is caused by repetitive motions in sports requiring a significant amount of overhead throwing-type motions, such as swimming, gymnastics, baseball, tennis, and weight lifting.[7,16,19] Bursitis may precede rotator cuff tendinitis, although in most cases it is a secondary sign.[7] Bursal reaction and swelling result from the need to decrease friction, i.e., an effort to create a soft cushion in the area of tendinous lesions.

Acute olecranon bursa injuries have often been noticed in athletes participating in sport activities like football, hockey, handball, and basketball.[2,24] Weight lifters and gymnasts often suffer from chronic inflammation of this bursa.[24] A specific feature of this lesion is the so-called *student's elbow*. It is marked by inflammation of the olecranon bursa caused by long-term pressure upon the bursa as a result of a characteristic position when studying (leaning upon elbows on the table).[19]

According to the findings of some authors,[10,18] bursitis in the hip region may develop as a result of abductor tendinitis, i.e., dancing activities or gymnastics (bursitis of the medial gluteal muscle and the piriformis muscle). The best illustration of bursitis resulting from repetitive friction of an anatomic structure over the bursa is trochanteric bursitis. In cases when the iliotibial band is excessively tight, during flexion and extension in the hip joint, the friction of the iliotibial band against the greater trochanter of the femur and the underlying bursa leads to chronic bursitis.[17]

Bursitis in the knee region most commonly develops as a consequence of overuse. Anatomical malalignment of the lower leg is often mentioned as a predisposing factor to bursitis. For instance, lower leg valgum alignment predisposes to anserine bursitis, while the increased Q-angle predisposes to the prepatellar and infrapatellar bursitis.[8,14]

Bursitis in the ankle (retrocalcaneal and superficial Achilles tendon bursitis) are common in runners and walkers.[21] Anatomical malalignment of the lower leg, such as tibia vara, equinus or cavus feet, and tight calf muscles predispose the athlete to the development of these types of bursitis. The retrocalcaneal bursitis caused by prominence of the posterior superior portion of the calcaneus ("hatchet" sign) are considered separate entity. This type of bursitis is usually accompanied by insertional tendinitis (enthesitis) of the Achilles tendon, commonly referred to as Haglund's syndrome or disease.[4,6,19,21]

III. CLINICAL PICTURE AND DIAGNOSTICS

In trying to identify the cause of pain in athletes and in treatment and prevention of injuries occurring in sports or recreation, bursae are rarely taken into account, although their acute or chronic injuries may significantly diminish the abilities of an athlete. Swelling and pain with a limited motion are signs of acute bursitis. The major symptoms of chronic bursitis comprise of dull pain in the bursal region during certain motions of the joint. Clinical examination reveals pain when pressure is applied either upon the affected bursa or upon the pathologically altered tendon that is the underlying cause of bursitis.

Clinical finding greatly depends upon the location of bursitis. Subacromial bursitis is characterized by pain in the position of the arm above the head and in its abduction above the auxillary line. The impingement sign and test are positive in subacromial bursitis.[7] Chronic olecranon bursitis causes no pain; the patient complains of swelling in the elbow region as a major clinical symptom and difficulty in the elbow flexion above 90°.[19] Contrary to the chronic olecranon bursitis, trochanteris bursitis is usually rather painful and often will cause the patient to limp.[17] The patients complain of their inability to put on their shoes because of severe pain. Clinical examination shows localized tenderness on the lateral aspect of the great trochanter and antalgic gait. Straight leg raising and quadriceps stretching will elicit pain, as will the Ober's test. Passive range of hip motion is normal but often weakness is detected in the hip abductors and flexors.[10,17,18] Prepatellar bursitis is characterized by gradual swelling and pain in the anterior aspect of the knee and slightly limited terminal knee flexion.[8,14] Beside antalgic gait, clinical examination also shows quadriceps hypotrophy and tightness of hamstrings. As opposed to prepatellar bursitis, in the case of intra-articular effusion, pain is present and range of motion is markedly decreased. Pes anserine bursitis is manifested by tenderness in the anteromedial aspect of the proximal tibia (just below the joint line).[8,19] The tenderness may also extend proximally along the pes anserine tendons to the posteromedial corner of the knee. Pes anserine bursitis has been encountered more often in athletes with tight hamstrings, lower limb valgus alignment, increased external tibial torsion, and increased femoral anteversion. Semimembranous bursitis causes tenderness at the posteromedial corner of the knee. The pain may be elicited by passive knee extension and resisted active flexion.[8] In retrocalcaneal bursitis, the patient usually complains of pain in the morning when getting out of bed and when getting out of a chair after a shorter period of sitting. Swelling prominence is noticed on both sides of the Achilles tendon, although thickened areas or nodes do not appear and cannot be palpated on the tendon itself. Clinical examination provokes pain by placing the thumb and index fingers in the space behind the tendon and in front of the talus. Crepitation may also be noticed in this region. No limping is seen during normal walking, but it may be clearly noticed during running.[19,21]

In addition to clinical findings, X-ray diagnosis is also necessary. Radiographic finding shows that certain osseous alterations may cause bursitis — enlarged prominence of the posterior superior portion of the calcaneus, changes in the acromion, and intratendinous and intrabursal calcifications. By introducing noninvasive ultrasonographic diagnostic procedures, bursography (the injection of contrast media into the bursal space) is no longer of prime importance. Ultrasonography has proved to be of great help in the diagnosis of acute and chronic bursitis.[3,13] Diagnostic ultrasound not only enables the evaluation of density and amount of bursal content but also alterations in bursal walls. Arthroscopy has recently been used more extensively both for the diagnosis and treatment of some types of bursitis, e.g., subacromial bursitis.[16] CT and scintigraphy are also used, although MRI is the diagnostic method of choice in the future. Laboratory analysis of bursal aspirate is performed whenever nontraumatic etiology of bursitis is suspected e.g., when bursitis could be of septic, tuberculous, rheumatoid, or gouty origin.

It is always important to bear in mind that when diagnosing sports injuries, one should always consider the possibility of bursitis.

IV. TREATMENT

Nonoperative treatment is the method of choice in acute and chronic bursitis; it entails rest, reduction of activity that provokes pain, administration of nonsteroid anti-inflammatory medication, and aspiration of bursal content with compression dressing. In chronic bursitis, water-soluble steroid injections are applied directly into the bursa. It has been noticed that in chronic bursitis, the mere aspiration of the bursal content is not sufficient since effusion tends to recur. Physical therapy of chronic bursitis is based upon stretching exercises with the purpose of increasing muscle flexibility, thus reducing pressure upon bursa and achieving painless motion.

Nonoperative treatment procedures depend upon the underlying cause and site of bursitis. It has been observed that in chronic trochanteric bursitis, good treatment outcome is achieved by corticosteroid injections. Orthotic foot corrections are essential in the treatment of retrocalcaneal bursitis.[10,19] The introduction of angiocatheter into the bursa followed by compressive dressing of the elbow for 3 d is the procedure proposed for the treatment of chronic olecranon bursitis.[2]

Surgical treatment is indicated when adequate nonoperative treatment fails. Operative treatment comprises of removing the bursa but only in terms of space decompression (resection of coracoacromial ligament or acromioplasty) or in terms of bursectomy (arthroscopic technique being possible for subacromial bursitis).[4,16,19,23] The cause of bursitis should also be removed surgically — resection of the prominence of the posterior superior portion of the calcaneus or removal of the tip of the olecranon.[4,10,24] Following operative treatment, progressive physical therapy is always prescribed, consisting primarily of stretching exercises in order to achieve and even increase the active range of painless motion. After that, and depending upon the site of bursitis and type of athletic activity, the patient engages in gradual exercises to strengthen the affected muscles.

REFERENCES

1. **Brody, D. M.** Running injuries. *Clin. Symp.*, 1987; 39:1–36.
2. **Fisher, R. H.** Conservative treatment of distended patellar and olecranon bursae. *Clin. Orthop.*, 1977; 123:98–99.
3. **Fornage, B. D. and Rifkin, M. D.** Ultrasound examination of tendons. *Radiol. Clin. N. Am.*, 1988; 26:87–107.

4. **Heneghan, M. A. and Pavlov, H.** The Haglund painful heel syndrome. *Clin. Orthop.,* 1984; 187:228–234.
5. **Herring, S. A. and Nilson, K. L.** Introduction to overuse injuries. *Clin. Sports Med.,* 1987; 6:225–239.
6. **Hintermann, B. and Holzach, P.** Die Bursitis subachillea — eine biomechanische Analyse und klinische Studie. *Z. Orthop.,* 1992; 130:114–119.
7. **Jobe, F. W. and Bradley, J. P.** Diagnosis of shoulder injuries. *Clin. Sports Med.,* 1989; 8:419–438.
8. **Kujala, U. M., Kvist, M., and Osterman, K.** Knee injuries in athletes. *Sports Med.,* 1986; 3:447–460.
9. **Larson, R. L. and Ostering, L. R.** Traumatic bursitis and artificial turf. *Am. J. Sports Med.,* 1974; 2:183–188.
10. **Lloyd-Smith, R., Clement, D. B., McKenzie, D. C., and Taunton, J. E.** A survey of overuse and traumatic hip and pelvic injuries in athletes. *Phys. Sportsmed.,* 1985; 12:131–141.
11. **Mattalino, A. J., Deese, J. M., Jr., and Campbell, E. D., Jr.** Office evaluation and treatment of lower extremity injuries in the runner. *Clin. Sports Med.,* 1989; 8:461–475.
12. **McCarthy, P.** Managing bursitis in the athlete: an overview. *Phys. Sportsmed.,* 1989; 17:115–123.
13. **Mellerowicz, H., Stelling, E., and Kefenbaum, A.** Diagnostic ultrasound in the athlete's locomotor system. *Br. J. Sports Med.,* 1990; 24:31–39.
14. **Mysyk, M. C., Wroble, R. R., and Foster, D. T.** Prepatellar bursitis in wrestlers, *Am. J. Sport Med.,* 1986; 14:46–54.
15. **Newman, R. J., Curtis, G. D. W., and Slack, M. P. E.** Bursal fluid lactate determination and the diagnosis of bursitis. *Br. Med. J.,* 1983; 286:2022–2023.
16. **Ogilvie-Harris, D. J. and D'Angelo, G.** Arthroscopic surgery of the shoulder. *Sports Med.,* 1990; 9:120–128.
17. **Pećina, M. and Bojanić, I.** The snapping hip syndrome. *Croat. Sports Med. J.,* 1992; 7:28–32.
18. **Reid, D. C.** Prevention of hip and knee injuries in ballet dancers. *Sports Med.,* 1988; 6:295–307.
19. **Reilly, J. P. and Nicholas, J. A.** The chronically inflamed bursa. *Clin. Sports Med.,* 1987; 6:345–370.
20. **Roland, G. C., Beagley, M. J., and Cawley, P. W.** Conservative treatment of inflamed knee bursitis. *Phys. Sportsmed.,* 1992; 20:67–77.
21. **Rossi, F., La Cava, F., Amato, F., and Pincelli, G.** The Haglund syndrome: clinical and radiological features and sports medicine aspects. *J. Sports Med.,* 1987; 27:238–265.
22. **Wood, M. B. and Dobyns, J. H.** Sports-related extraarticular wrist syndromes. *Clin. Orthop.,* 1986; 202:93–102.
23. **Zoltan, D. J., Clancy, W. G., and Keene, J. S.** A new operative approach to snapping hip and refractory trochanteric bursitis in athletes. *Am. J. Sports Med.,* 1986; 14:201–204.
24. **Yocum, L. A.** The diagnosis and nonoperative treatment of elbow problems in the athlete. *Clin. Sports Med.,* 1989; 8:439–451.

Chapter

11

Stress Fractures

Biomechanical laws according to which the strength of bone depends on the force acting upon it have indeed been well known for quite a long time. Bone may bear the load produced by the forces of tension, compression, bending, pulling, and torsion, while in everyday life, these forces act upon a bone in a combined manner. The size and form of bone largely affect its resistance to the activity of these forces. Also, bones are generally known as being highly capable of repair.

A break in a bone may result from the activity of either a single strong force or multiple repetitive weak forces. Stress fractures are classified in the latter category, i.e., in the group of overuse injuries. Repetitive forces acting on a bone cause remodeling of the bone, with the strength of the bone increasing in the direction of force activity. The remodeling process in the bone starts with osteoclastic activity and bone resorption followed by osteoblastic activity and formation of new bone tissue. The ability of bone to bear repetitive load depends on the extent of the load, number of repetitions, and frequency of the load. Stress fractures usually occurs when the load, i.e., the strain, overpowers the reparative ability of the bone.

There are two theories explaining stress fractures. Nordin and Frankel[39] reported that the repetitive load results in overuse of muscles; in this way, the muscles lose their capacity of absorption and even distribution of stressful forces acting on a bone, thus leading to the situation in which abnormally strong forces act upon single bone areas. Stanitski et al.[70] state that mere muscle force acts upon a bone in a way that results in stress fracture.

Most common stress fractures occur on all bones of lower extremities, followed by lumbar spine interarticular segments stress fractures, and then on some bones of the upper extremities, especially those not bearing a static load. This favors the opinion that both theories of stress fracture occurrence might be correct.

The first clinical description of stress fracture is credited to Breithaupt, a Prussian military physician. In 1855, he described clinical picture and symptoms of metatarsal bone stress fractures in soldiers. Since then, this very fracture site has been commonly called a *march fracture* or *Deutschlander fracture*.[8]

Only about 40 years later, in 1897, the radiographic identification of these injuries was first delineated by Strechow.[31] The first stress fracture in an athlete was reported in 1934 by Pirker; it was a transverse stress fracture of the femoral shaft in an 18-year-old athlete actively involved in skiing, swimming, and handball.[31] The so-called runner's fracture, i.e., stress fracture of the distal fibula, was reported for the first time in 1940.[31]

Since that time, more cases of stress fractures in athletes are being reported, and the first large series of stress fracture in athletes is owed to Devas. In 1975, he published a monograph series on stress fractures, the first of its kind in medical literature.[13–15] In a certain way, stress fractures in athletes may be assumed as professional injuries or diseases. Since sports are getting more popular, both as a profession and as recreation, the number of overuse injuries is increasing and so is the number of medical publications discussing these issues. Running, either as an activity per se, or as an essential part of sports such as football, basketball, handball, etc. or also as part of preparatory training for almost all athletic activities, contributes to the development of overuse injuries more than any other physical activity.

I. AGE, SEX, AND TYPE OF ACTIVITY

Stress fractures are common problems in sports medicine, comprising between 1.1 to 3.7% of all athletic injuries, while in the population of runners, they account for 15% of all injuries (although the data may vary from one medical institution to another).[4,27,36,46,48,72] The average age of patients ranges from 19 to 30 years. Considering the present-day tendency of including children and adolescents in top athletic activities, the number of overuse injuries in children and adolescents are increasing.[13,55] The so-called epiphyseal stress fractures have been reported on the humerus, olecranon, distal radius, distal femur, and proximal tibia, although when compared to apophyseal overuse injuries (Osgood-Schlatter's disease, Haglund's disease, etc.), they occur much more rarely.[31,55]

For a long time, stress fractures have been considered a rare case in females. However, identical military conditions and physical training have shown that women are 3 to 12 times more often affected by stress fractures than men. Likewise, a rapid increase in female participants in athletic and recreational activities, especially as active runners, is accompanied by a similarly rapid increase in the number of stress fractures among women. With stress fractures in women, it is necessary to consider the regularity of their menstrual cycles. Barrow and Saha[3] have reported higher incidence of stress fractures in female athletes with irregular menstrual cycles. Therefore, the regulation of menstrual cycle seems to be an essential part of treatment of stress fractures in women.

The site and frequency of stress fractures in athletes depend to a large extent on the type of activity. Evidence shows that certain stress fracture sites are reported more often in some athletes than in others, e.g., tarsal navicular stress fracture in basketball players.[19,24,34,38,60,74] Nevertheless, authorities almost invariably agree that running ranks highest as a contributive factor in the event of stress fractures; runners account for 67 to 85%, followed by high and long jumpers, basketball players, volleyball players, football players, tennis players, baseball players, and gymnasts.[36,46] As has already been pointed out, it is possible to identify typical fracture sites for a given athletic activity. In runners, the most typical stress fracture sites are tibia, fibula, tarsal and metatarsal bones, and femoral neck; in jumpers, these are tarsal navicular, patella, and metatarsal bones.[36] Tennis players most often suffer from stress fracture of the fibula, tarsal navicular, humerus, and ulna, while basketball players are known for stress fractures occurring most often on the tibia, fibula, tarsal navicular, base of the fifth metatarsal bone (Jones' fracture), and sesamoid bones of the great toe.[36]

II. PREDISPOSING FACTORS

A. Biomechanical Factors

Research evidence shows that certain anatomical deviations on lower extremities, e.g., genu varum, tibia vara, forefoot varus, flat feet, and cavus feet, by altering the distribution of load, contribute to the development of stress fracture.[46] For example, cavus feet is found more often in athletes with stress fracture of the metatarsal bones and the femur, while flat feet with excessive pronation significantly contributes to the development of stress fractures of the tibia, fibula, and tarsal bones. The difference in the length of the legs is also an important factor. For instance, stress fractures of the femur, tibia, and metatarsal bones occur more often in longer legs, while stress fractures of the fibula are more common in shorter legs. Besides these factors, it is important to point out the mediolateral width of the tibia, which Gilaldi et al.[22] have reported, is linked to tibial stress fracture in soldiers.

B. Muscles

The condition and tone of muscles, i.e., their strength, are directly related to stress fracture. During a rapid increase of physical activity, the muscular tone also increases, resulting in rather strong stress forces acting on a bone. Muscular weakness may be a predisposing factor to the development of stress fracture. Clement et al.[11] reported about the triceps surae muscle weakness in 40 to 56% of patients with tibial stress fracture. Tired muscles, to a sufficient degree, cannot absorb the stresses, which, i.e., in runners, leads to an increased lowering and pronation of the foot; this results in a new distribution of stress forces, compression of the bone, and its pulling that might eventually cause a stress fracture. Increased muscular tension and decreased flexibility, including tendons, cause the action of chronic stress forces on a bone. This is precisely why stretching and strengthening exercises of muscles are essential.

C. Training Errors

There is wide research evidence showing that training errors cause stress fractures in as many as 22 to 75% of cases.[46,48,72] They are characterized by "mileage mania" (excessive mileage), extremely intensive training, or too rapid changes in both the qualitative and quantitative aspects of training. In this way, runners will be more exposed to the possibility of developing a stress fracture if during a 3-month period, their mileage is rapidly increased, they run too much uphill and downhill, their running surface is changed too often, and they change their running shoes too much.[72]

D. Surface

The type of ground for running (tartan, asphalt, grass, etc.), i.e., the surface quality of a playground (parquet, concrete, asphalt, etc.), is extremely important in the event of stress fracture.[48] The harder the ground, the greater the shocks to the foot, lower leg, and back, and therefore the greater the possibility for stress fracture. During the assessment of two groups of runners having stress fractures, it has been found that 50% of them were running on a hard surface.[15,72] Running along the margin of the road, i.e., on a sloped surface, leads to the so-called *short-long leg syndrome,* which may cause stress fracture, especially proximal tibial stress fracture.[36]

E. Footwear

Sports shoes are nowadays an essential factor in the prevention of stress fractures since they absorb shocks on the foot, lower leg, and back.

III. PREVENTION

To prevent stress fractures and other overuse injuries, it is of utmost importance that the athlete, the coach, and the physician cooperate. It is essential to identify the group at higher risk of stress fracture; most commonly, athletes with biomechanical irregularities in lower extremities are classified into such a group.

These athletes should be kept under constant surveillance and provided with various orthotic devices. In extreme cases, surgery may be required to correct biomechanical disorders. Furthermore, athletic and training activities should be adapted to age and abilities of individual athletes, i.e., maximum load should be achieved gradually and restful and active periods should be alternated at regular intervals. Athletic requisites are very important for the prevention of stress fractures, especially the shoes and quality of playground surface.

A tennis racket may be taken as an example of how a requisite is important to stress fracture prevention. A highly elastic racket creates quite stressful forces to act upon the forearm of the player, whereas the change in racket network tension and the use of a less elastic racket diminish these stressors on the forearm.

An important preventive measure also entails stretching and strengthening exercises, which also diminish stressful forces on the bone.

IV. DIAGNOSTICS

Similar to other overuse injuries, when attempting to diagnose a stress fracture, it is essential to have the possibility of such a condition constantly in mind. Thus, clinical diagnosis represents basic procedure followed later on by other diagnostic methods — first by radiologic examination and then scintigraphy. At times, ultrasound, thermography, CT, or MRI may be used.

A. Clinical Diagnosis

The main symptom of stress fracture is pain. Initially, it appears during the activity and usually at the end of it. Then it disappears during a resting period. Later on, the pain appears earlier at an increasing intensity so that the athlete is compelled to discontinue the activity, i.e., the pain makes it impossible to engage actively in sports. At times, the pain persists even when resting.

The most common physical signs of stress fracture are local tenderness and swelling, although swelling has been observed in a smaller number of cases. As reported in literature, local tenderness has been observed in 66 to 88%, local swelling in 25 to 50%, while limping has been found in 45% of cases with stress fracture.[46,72] Local tenderness may best be provoked over bones that can be easily palpated, such as the metatarsal bones or fibula. Pain can irradiate from the fracture site, which is a situation characteristic for pubic bone stress fracture, and stress fracture in the femoral neck and its diaphysis.

B. Radiologic Diagnosis

Standard X-ray imaging may well show bone lesions in 50 to 70% of stress fracture cases.[31,46] It has also been found that from the onset of pain to the moment when alterations become visible on a standard X-ray film, it takes from 2 weeks to even 3 months, depending upon the fracture site. For certain locations, e.g., tarsal bones, femur, or spine, it is often not possible to identify any changes whatsoever, even if followed up for a longer period of time.

The first noticeable change resulting from stress fracture localized on a cortical bone segment is characterized by decrease of calcium deposit and diminished sharpness of the outline of the affected bone. Such a fracture usually affects only one cortex and only later on (2 to 4 weeks following the onset of symptoms), it may be seen as an oblique or transverse fissure, or even as endosteal or periosteal callus. These changes are not so easily recognized, i.e., they can be identified with greater certainty only on tangenital radiographs or tomograms. Blickenstaff and Morris[6] and Hallel et al.[28] have classified these types of stress fractures with regard to radiologic finding into the following three groups:

1. stress fractures in which endosteal or periosteal callus is visible only on one side of the bone and without an evert fracture line
2. stress fractures with a fracture line through one cortex or across the bone and where circumferential periosteal reaction is present
3. stress fractures with displacement, i.e., fractures with dislocation of the segments

Stress fractures in the spongious bone area (e.g., calcaneus, medial tibial plateau) are known as trabecular fractures and occur more often in soldiers than in athletes.[25] In the population of athletes, these fractures are most common in runners. To identify the trabecular stress fracture by standard radiography, an approximately 50% change in bone density is necessary. The initial changes are characterized by hardly noticeable flake-like patches of new bone that may be seen 10 to 21 d following the onset of symptoms.[25] Later, the patches transform into wider cloud-like areas of mineralized bone, and then a sclerotic line, being among the most characteristic signs of trabecular fracture, appears within the bone.

CT may sometimes be helpful to make diagnosis in individual cases; however, it is much more important as a diagnostic procedure that enables differentiating between stress fracture and bone tumor.

C. Scintigraphy

Bone scintigraphy is a method of choice in early diagnosis of stress fracture (Figure 1). At the same time, it is the most sensitive method since the accumulation of radionuclides, usually technetium 99 m diphosphate, occurs 6 to 72 h following the appearance of initial symptoms.[67] A typical scintigraphic finding (imaging) of a stress fracture is characterized by an oval or spindle, sharply bordered focus of

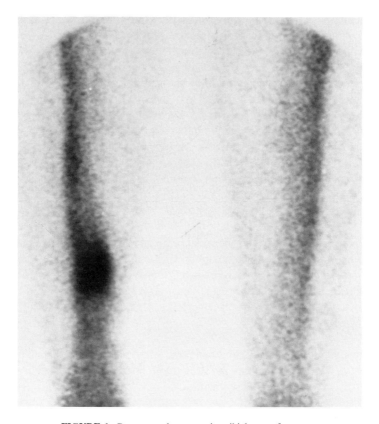

FIGURE 1. Bone scan demonstrating tibial stress fracture.

increased activity.[47] False-positive results are found only in about 5% of cases, while false-negative findings are extremely rare.[46]

Nevertheless, on account of higher specificity of X-ray findings, scintigraphy is recommended only when radiograph seems negative in spite of reasonable doubt that stress fracture might be the issue. Also, stress fracture can be diagnosed only on the basis of scintigraphic finding, especially in cases where localized increased accumulation of radionuclides corresponds to the site of pain.

Routine scintigraphy of the pelvis and lower extremities often shows multiple focuses of increased activity that remain silent, i.e., are not manifested either clinically (as pain) or radiographically.[45] The asymptomatic accumulation of radionuclides, the so-called stress reaction, only indicates remodeling of bone caused by a physical stress.[45,47] As scintigraphic finding may remain positive for several years, clinical and radiographic findings are used as discriminative ones for the follow-up of stress fracture treatment.

Quite a number of scintigraphic classifications of stress fractures have been reported in reference literature, the most common is that of Zwas et al.[79] identifying four grades:

- Grade 1 — a small, ill-defined lesion with mildly increased activity in the cortical region
- Grade 2 — larger then grade 1; well-defined, elongated lesion with moderately increased activity in the cortical region
- Grade 3 — a wide fusiform lesion with markedly increased activity in the corticomedullary region
- Grade 4 — wide extensive lesion with intensely increased activity in the transcorticomedullary region

Ultrasound and thermography have recently been used to diagnose stress fracture, especially in bones located near the surface (metatarsal bones or the fibula).[16,23,51] Intentions have also been reported to use the therapeutic ultrasound as a diagnostic test. Moss and Mowat[51] have found that when applied to the fracture site, the diagnostic ultrasound causes pain. However, the test is of questionable reliability.

Already initial research[69] has shown the true value and great importance of MRI in diagnosing stress fractures; it is considered an invaluable tool in the differential diagnosis of stress fracture.

V. DIFFERENTIAL DIAGNOSIS

In children and adolescents, it is of utmost importance to differentiate stress fracture from osteogenic sarcoma and Ewing's tumor. A follow-up roentgenogram, repeated after 2 to 3 weeks, usually solves the problem of diagnosis.[18,48,71] Osteoid osteoma, osteomalacia, Paget's disease, osteitis, and osteomyelitis may cause difficulties in differential diagnosis.[18,44]

Differential diagnosis of stress fracture and overuse injuries of soft tissue cannot be based solely on clinical findings and radiologic diagnosis; it also requires scintigraphy.[47] The differential diagnosis between shin splints and tibial stress fracture shown by triple-phase bone scan may serve as a very good example. The fact is that the difference may be noticed only at a delayed image of scintigraphic examination. The delayed image of a stress fracture is intense, solitary, and focal, while in shin splints, it is less intense, linear, and longitudinal.

VI. DISTRIBUTION OF STRESS FRACTURE

Stress fractures account for about 5% of all injuries in athletes. The most recent research has shown that tibia is the fracture site in 35 to 54% of all stress fractures, followed by fibula (7 to 24%), and metatarsal bones (9 to 20%).

A. Upper Extremities

1. Scapula

Stress fracture of the coracoid process has been reported in trapshooters.[7] The development of this type of fracture is linked to repeated hitting of a gunstock on the coracoid process during shooting. Physical examination reveals tenderness on the coracoid process, and pain may also be provoked by adduction and anteflexion of the arm against resistance. The fracture fissure occurs in the mid-third or on the base of the coracoid process and may best be seen on axillary view radiograph of the shoulder. Treatment consists of rest with elimination of trapshooting until the patient is asymptomatic (4 to 6 weeks). Healing is noted on subsequent axillary radiographs.

Stress fracture of the superiormedial border of the scapula has been reported in a recreational runner who was jogging with weights in his hands, and stress fracture of the lateral border of the scapula (teres minor muscle attachment) in a treadmill worker.

2. Humerus

Stress fractures of humeral diaphysis have been reported in tennis players, shot putters, and cricket players.[2,65] The fracture line is either transverse or spiral. Signs that should alert the physician to the presence of a humeral stress fracture include deep aching within the mid-arm during activity and at rest. If not attended to, these symptoms may progress to an evert fracture. A period of rest resolves this problem if identified early. Delayed union may occur, and return to athletic activity should not be permitted until the athlete is asymptomatic.

Stress fracture of the proximal humeral epiphysis is called *Little League shoulder* because it most often occurs in children and adolescents, especially in baseball throwers, i.e., the pitchers.[31] This type of fracture is caused by strong rotational forces during the cocking phase and acceleration phase of pitching. With rest from throwing, this type of stress fracture heals without complications.

3. Ulna

Ulnar stress fractures may be located either on the olecranon or diaphysis. Stress fracture of the olecranon has been reported in javelin throwers and baseball pitchers.[35,54,73] The fracture is caused by strong muscle forces applied to the olecranon during the act of throwing (final phase of delivery); when this occurs, there is impingement of the olecranon against the medial and upper border of the olecranon fossa on the humerus. The fracture fissure is located either at the tip or in the mid-portion of the olecranon. The fracture occurring at the tip (apex) is treated nonoperatively, i.e., by refraining from throwing activities. When a persistent pain makes engagement in throwing activity impossible, surgical treatment is recommended (excision of the tip). Since the stress fracture of the mid-portion of the olecranon is characterized by delayed union or nonunion, surgical treatment is commonly recommended (insertion of bone graft or tension band plus two Kirschner wires).[35]

Stress fractures of ulnar diaphysis are located at the mid-third or junction of the middle and distal third and are reported for tennis players, volleyball players, softball pitchers, and bodybuilders.[52,64] Athletes often complain of pain over the ulna shaft. If symptoms have been noted for some time, early callus may be palpable along the subcutaneous ulna shaft. Complete rest from athletic activities for 4 to 6 weeks is sufficient for healing.

4. Radius

The most common stress fracture affecting the radial bone is that of its distal epiphysis found in young gymnasts.[10] The main symptom is pain, occurring during or after athletic activity and relieved by rest. With wrist pain, it is localized mainly to the dorsal aspect of the distal radius and carpal area. Clinical findings include painful limitation at the extreme of forced active and passive dorsiflexion of the wrist. The fracture is also characterized by the following radiological changes: widening of the growth plate of the distal, radial epiphysis, fragmentation, irregularity of the metaphyseal margin, and cystic alterations. When a fracture shows no visible radiological changes, rest from athletic activity from 2 to 4 weeks usually suffices, while in fractures with visible radiological alterations, athletic activity should be discontinued for several months, sometimes even 1 year.

Stress fracture of the distal radial metaphysis in gymnasts has also been recently reported.[10]

5. Carpal Bones

Stress fracture of the pisiform bone has been reported in volleyball players. It seems to be caused by repetitive trauma of the bone occurring during hitting and blocking the ball with the base of their palm. Stress fractures of the lunate and scaphoid are more common in gymnasts.[30] The principal symptom of scaphoid stress fracture is pain within the wrist, appearing in the course of the activity and disappearing during rest, without any history of a wrist trauma. Radiographic examination usually shows a transverse fracture fissure with rather sclerotic margins. The method of choice in the treatment of this type of stress fracture is immobilization in a thumb-spica cast that should be worn for a minimum of 10 weeks.

6. Ribs

Stress fracture of the first rib is located on its thinnest and weakest segment, i.e., between the attachments of the anterior scalenus muscle and the medial scalenus muscle. Fractures have been reported in tennis players, basketball players, volleyball players, dancers, golfers, and baseball pitchers.[32] The pain is rarely local but more often radiating along the arm, into the anterior part of the neck, and sometimes even into the sternum and the pectoral region. Usually, these fractures heal with an adequate period of rest. Rarely do first rib fractures become nonunions.

Stress fractures of other ribs are rare and have been described in female rowers, especially those rowing in pairs (scullers), and also in golfers, tennis players, and gymnasts.[28,45] These fractures usually occur in the posterolateral segment of the rib. The main symptom is pain spreading from the medial scapular border to the mid-axillary line at the level of the affected rib.

McKenzie[50] has reported a stress fracture of the ninth rib in the anterolateral portion of the rib in an elite oarsman. Stress fractures of the ribs are treated nonoperatively, and discontinuation from the activity is recommended for 4 to 8 weeks, together with correction of the rowing technique.

7. Sternum

Stress fracture of the sternum has been reported in a wrestler.[42] The fracture fissure is located 2 cm distally from the sternal angle and is usually clearly seen on the lateral radiograph of the sternum. Discontinuation of wrestling activities from 6 to 8 weeks is a sufficient measure for the fracture to heal.

8. Lumbar Spine

Stress fractures of the lumbar spine are most commonly located in the interarticular parts of the fourth and fifth lumbar vertebrae, although they may also occur in the laminae and pedicles.[1] Stress fracture of the pars interarticularis has been reported in gymnasts, hockey players, weight lifters, football players, and runners. The basic signs of pars interarticularis stress fracture comprise of absence of periosteal reaction and great possibility of refracturing, i.e., development of spondylolysis and sometimes even spondylolysthesis. Early recognition of the fracture, and rest from athletic activities together with thoracolumbar orthosis are essential to good treatment outcome.

It should repeatedly be pointed out, as already stated in Chapter 5, that adolescent athletes engaging in activities requiring repetitive flexion and extension motions of the lumbar spine are at increased risk of getting a stress fracture; therefore, each complaint of low back pain should be taken seriously, with doubt of pars interarticularis stress fracture.

9. Sacrum

Stress fracture of the sacrum has been reported in soldiers, runners, and gymnasts.[77] This type of stress fracture, or stress reaction in the region of the sacroiliac joint, is manifested by pain in the sacral region.

B. Lower Extremities

1. Pelvis

When discussing stress fractures of the pelvis, it has been noticed that they most often occur in the lower branch of the pubic bone (ramus inferior ossis pubis). The fracture is usually located in the inferior ischiopubic junction between the origin of adductor muscles and hamstring muscles. It is the type of stress fracture that has often been reported in soldiers; with regard to the population of athletes, it has been described for the first time in a fencer. However, it most frequently affects the long-distance and marathon runners and joggers; also, the incidence of this type of fracture is very high in women.[53,59] The leading symptom is pain in the groin, and sometimes in the buttocks or upper leg. The pain appears during running, and after a while, it becomes so severe that the activity must be discontinued. Physical examination reveals strictly limited painful tenderness of the affected pubic bone to deep palpation. Noakes[53] has also reported that the patients cannot stand on the foot of the affected side on account of sharp pain in the groin and has called this clinical sign *a positive standing sign*. Radiologically, the fracture is initially manifested as a transverse fissure or a small cloud-like callus in the upper border of the obturator forearm. If, in spite of the pain, the activity is continued, a massive callus will develop. When reasonable clinical suspicion exists of a pubic bone stress fracture and X-ray finding is negative, scintigraphy should be performed. A positive scintigraphic finding confirms the diagnosis.

Since this type of fracture shows a tendency toward a delayed and prolonged union, athletic activity should be discontinued, especially running, for several weeks, usually from 10 to 16 weeks. The patient is free to walk although in the case of pain and/or limping during normal walking, crutches should be used in the first few weeks of treatment. Athletic activity may be resumed only following a sufficiently long period of rest, i.e., when there is no more pain upon pressure and when radiographic finding shows that the healing process of the fracture is about to end.

2. Femur

The most common stress fracture of the femur is that of its neck, but not for its frequency as much as for the resulting complications: delayed union, nonunion, dislocation of fragments, and avascular femoral head necrosis.[19] It most often occurs in soldiers who are on military exercise and in long-distance runners. However, it has also been reported in basketball players and gymnasts.[20,21,44] The initial symptom is groin pain radiating into the hip and along the thigh toward the knee. Pain appears only with weight bearing and is accompanied by an antalgic gait. During physical examination, the pain appears when hip joint flexibility is examined; during this procedure, limited internal rotation is often found. Treatment largely depends upon changes that are visible on radiographs. Having in mind the mechanism of its development and position of the fracture line, Fullerton and Snowdy[20] have proposed the following classification of the fracture: (1) compression-side fracture (located on the compression side of the femoral neck), (2) tension-side fracture (located on the tension side of the femoral neck), and (3) displaced fracture of the femoral neck. When radiographs show sclerosis without overt fracture line, as well as in the case of positive scintigraphy with normal radiograph, nonoperative treatment will suffice for both the "compression" and "tension" type of femoral neck stress fracture; this is comprised of absolute bed rest until the pain resolves. The patient is then advanced from partial to full weight bearing on crutches as symptoms permit. Once the patient is free of pain, he is allowed to progress to a cane and then to unprotected weight bearing. Athletic activity may be resumed only after a period of a minimum 6 to 8 weeks. When radiographs show an undisplaced cortical crack on either the tension or compression side of the femoral neck, the treatment is nonoperative (hospitalization and bed rest). Surgical treatment is indicated if there is any widening of the fracture, if both cortices develop a defect, if bed rest is not feasible, or if the patient is not reliable and cooperative. In those patients who have any widening or defect in both cortices, as well as in patients with a displaced femoral neck stress fracture, immediate surgical treatment is recommended.

Stress fractures of the femoral shaft (Figure 2) have also been reported, especially medial subtrochanteric region (in long and middle-distance runners, hurdlers, basketball players), central third (long-distance runners, baseball players), and epiphyseal fracture in the distal femoral shaft segment in adolescents (basketball players, runners).[4,9,31,36,63,72] It should be pointed out that diagnosis is often delayed due to scarce clinical signs. In the majority of cases, the only symptom is pain in the upper leg. A

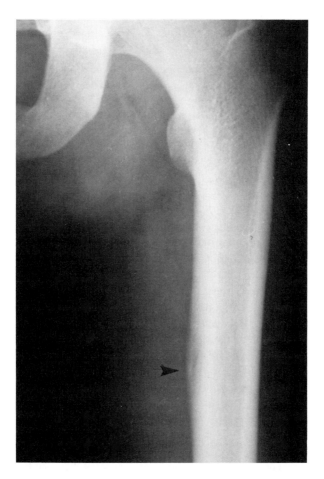

FIGURE 2. (A) Stress fracture in the proximal third of the femoral shaft.

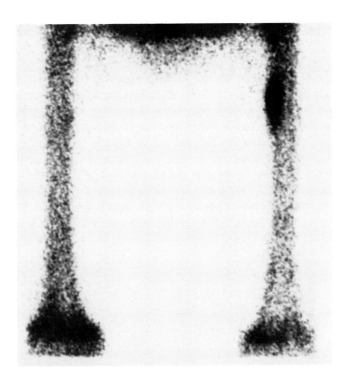

FIGURE 2 (continued) (B) Bone scan.

full range of motion in the hip and knee is usually present. Occasionally, an antalgic gait is present. The treatment is usually nonoperative and entails rest from athletic activity from 8 to 14 weeks. In extreme cases (severe pain, limping), walking with crutches is indicated during the first 2 or 3 weeks of treatment. Orava[56] has observed three distal femoral shaft stress fractures that required open treatment with AO plate fixation after complete fractures went on to displacement. Provost and Morris[56] also reported displacement of distal third stress fracture in nine military recruits.

3. Patella

It is an uncommon location for a stress fracture and has been reported in child or adolescent athletes.[13,14,39,55] The fracture line may be either transverse or longitudinal. The transverse fracture is the consequence of muscular traction stresses, while the longitudinal fracture results from compression forces which compress the patella against the femoral condyles. Treatment of the so-called longitudinal patellar stress fracture is nonoperative, i.e., rest from athletic activities for 8 to 12 weeks. For nondisplaced transverse stress fracture, immobilization is indicated, while displaced transverse stress fracture requires surgical treatment for reduction and internal fixation.

4. Tibia

Tibial stress fracture is the most common site of stress fractures among athletes and may be located on the posteromedial aspect of the diaphysis either at its proximal (more often) or distal end, on the anterior tibial midshaft, and on the proximal epiphyseal-metaphyseal area. Stress fracture of the medial malleolus also has been reported.[22,26,31,36,37,46,48,49,56,66,68]

Stress fracture of the tibial shaft on the posteromedial aspect is most common in runners, although it may occur in basketball players, football players, gymnasts, figure skaters, and dancers[4,31,46,48,62,72] (Figure 3). The main symptom is pain appearing during activity and disappearing when resting. Physical examination reveals painful tenderness to palpation and percussion at the fracture site, while at a later stage, callus may be palpated. Occasionally, swelling is present.

Radiologic diagnosis is possible only 2 to 5 weeks following the appearance of pain, when callus as well as the fracture line may be seen (usually oblique radiographs are also required).[43] Besides for early diagnosis, scintigraphy helps to differentiate stress fracture from the posterior tibialis muscle syndrome, tibial periostitis, and external chronic compartment syndrome. Treatment is rest and a graduated

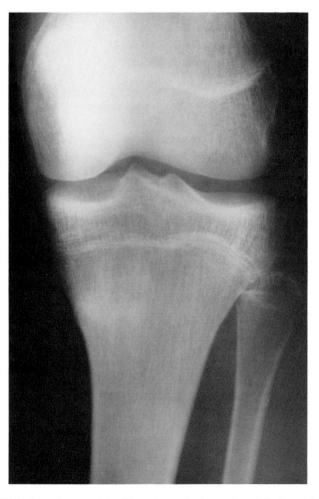

FIGURE 3. Stress fracture of the tibia at the proximal metaphyseal-diaphyseal junction.

return to sports 4 to 6 weeks from the time of cessation of activity, at which time the athlete should be pain free.

Anterior midshaft tibial stress fracture is characterized by one or more transverse fissures of the cortex and its thickening (Figure 4). This type of fracture tends to occur in basketball players, runners, pole vaulters, handball players, figure skaters, and ballet dancers.[25,56-58,62,66] Healing of these fractures is quite poor. It is quite common for these stress fractures to develop delayed union or nonunion. They even fracture completely, and serial radiographs may remain unchanged for years. The recommended treatment modalities vary from prolonged immobilization and/or rest, pulsating electromagnetic field therapy, biopsy and drilling of the fracture site, to excision of the lesion and bone grafting.[25,56-58,66] In one patient, we performed successfully a compressive osteosynthesis in the treatment of tibial midshaft stress fracture.

5. Fibula

Stress fracture of the fibula occurs most commonly in the lower third, approximately 3 to 8 cm proximal to the lateral malleolus. In sports medicine, it is commonly called *runner's fracture*[15] (Figure 5). However, volleyball players, football players, gymnasts, figure skaters, and squash players are also known to be affected by this

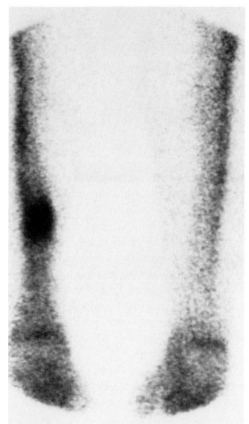

FIGURE 4. Anterior tibial midshaft stress fracture. (A) Bone scan.

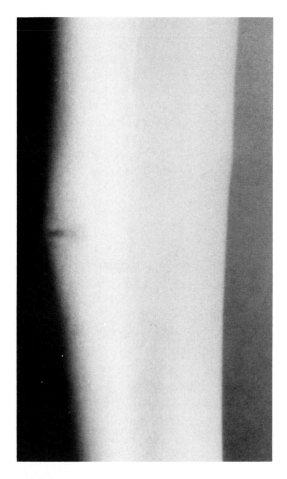

FIGURE 4 (continued). (B) Lateral roentgenogram.

type of stress fracture.[15,18,48,62] It has been suggested that fibular stress fractures are caused either by a combination of compression and torsion forces against the lateral malleolus or by the rhythmic contractions of flexor muscles of the foot. Pain is usually localized along the affected area, and the swelling is often apparent. An antalgic gait is also common. Tenderness is found at the fracture site. Radiologic changes are visible only after 3 or 4 weeks following the onset of symptoms. Initially, only an oblique or transverse fissure may be seen on radiographs, but later, callus appears. Discontinuation of the activity for 6 weeks is sufficient for the fracture to heal. These fractures are present with lateral leg pain. Healing is generally uneventful, with 6 weeks as the average length of time to return to sport activity.

Gymnasts and volleyball players have also been reported with fibular stress fracture, occurring in the proximal (upper) third of the bone.[27]

It is interesting also to mention spontaneous proximal third fibular stress fracture in athletes, i.e., the fracture that occurs in the course of an athletic activity but without any trauma or visible signs of stress fracture on the radiologic image.

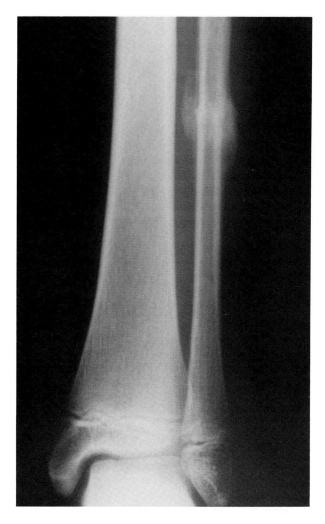

FIGURE 5. Stress fracture of the fibula.

6. Tarsal Bones

The most recent research on the incidence of tarsal bone stress fractures, specifically the tarsal navicular bone, shows that the number of cases is increasing and so is the number of reports discussing the possibilities and results of treatment (Figure 6).

Stress fracture of the tarsal navicular bone is most common in sprinters, basketball players, high and long jumpers, and obstacle racers.[19,24,34,40,60,74] The athlete usually complains of a vague pain along the dorsum of the foot which increases during jumping (usually the take-off foot is affected) and sudden starts persists for a longer period of time (according to reference literature, the time span between the onset of symptoms and the diagnosis is rather long — 4.5 months on the average). Physical examination shows that the lateral half of the tarsal navicular bone is extremely painful on palpation; swelling in that area occurs quite rarely. Two tests

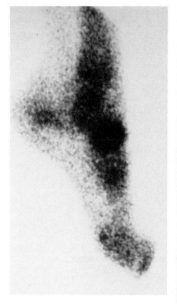
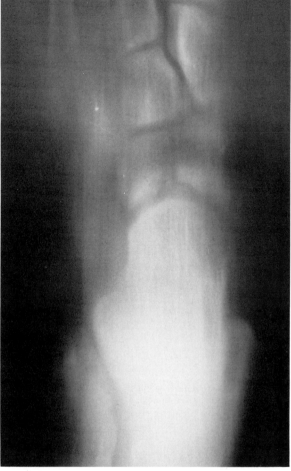

FIGURE 6. Navicular tarsal stress fracture. (A) Bone scan; (B) tomogram in the true anteroposterior position.

are helpful in the diagnosis: (1) tiptoeing on the affected leg, and (2) an attempt at jumping from this position, which causes sever pain, thus indicating the probability of the tarsal navicular bone stress fracture. The fracture line is almost always in the central third of the bone, and on account of reduced blood supply to the area, healing is rather difficult. Therefore, the tendency of this type of fracture to delay union or nonunion and to refracture is high.

Uncomplicated, partial stress fractures and nondisplaced complete stress fractures should be treated by cast immobilization and nonweight bearing for 6 to 8 weeks. In the case of displaced complete fracture, delayed union, nonunion, and refracture, surgery is indicated — multiple drilling, compression screws, and bone grafting is necessary — followed by immobilization and nonweight bearing until union has occurred.

Calcaneal bone stress fracture is common in soldiers and quite rare among athletes.[31,36,63] Still, it has been reported in joggers. In more recent times, stress fractures of the talus, cuboid, and cuneiform bones have been reported.[46,48] These fractures are characterized by a negative X-ray image so that diagnosis is made solely on the basis of positive scintigraphy. They are treated nonoperatively; however, it is not yet quite clear whether it suffices to refrain from athletic activities for 6 to 8 weeks or whether to immobilize in a cast with nonweight bearing or any other load.

7. Metatarsal Bones

Although both physicians and laymen seem to be best acquainted with stress fractures of the metatarsal bones, either as stress fractures primarily affecting soldiers or as march fractures, these fractures rank third among athletes, being preceded by tibial and fibular fractures. In more than 80% of metatarsal bone stress fractures, the shaft of the third and second metatarsal bone is affected[17] (Figure 7). They are typical

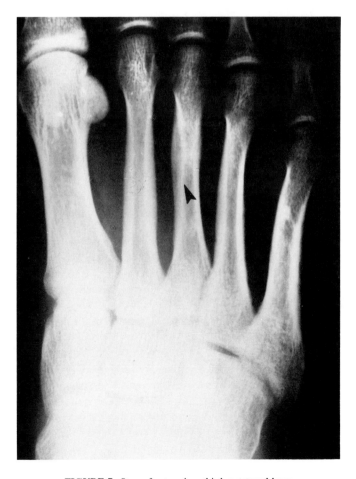

FIGURE 7. Stress fracture in a third metatarsal bone.

in long-distance runners, high and long jumpers, basketball players, volleyball players, football players, figure skaters, and gymnasts.[4,31,36,46,48,49,56,62] Diagnosis is a very simple one once the stress fracture is suspected. Physical examination reveals tenderness over the involved bone and radiological evidence periosteal callus in the shaft region. Rest from athletic activities for 1 month and immobilization in a boot cast with a heel for walking (2 to 4 weeks) yield good results, i.e., complete bone healing. Stress fracture of the first metatarsal bone is located at its base, and the radiography shows intraosseal reaction sclerosis without periosteal reaction.

a. The base of the fifth metatarsal bone (Jones' Fracture)

Stress fracture of the base of the fifth metatarsal bone, Jones' fracture, should be pointed out as a separate entity, especially since it tends toward delayed union, nonunion, and refracture (Figure 8). The Jones' fracture is most common in basketball players, football players, runners, and throwers (javelin, hammer).[12,33,41,61,78] The main symptom is pain in the lateral foot region. Physical examination shows pain on palpation in the proximal end of the fifth metatarsal (about 1.5 cm distally from the tuberosity). Based on radiography, Pećina and co-workers[61] divide Jones' fracture into three types, and according to the type, suggest treatment. If the X-ray shows an evident narrow fissure of the cortex and a passable medullar cavity (type 1), immobilization in a plaster cast boot with nonweight bearing for 6 to 8 weeks is suggested. When there is a fissure with an evident sclerosing of its edges (type 2), they suggest the same treatment with the exception of active athletes, in which case they suggest surgery. If X-ray demonstrates that the sclerosing completely obliterates medullar cavity (type 3), they suggest that both athletes and nonathletes undergo surgery. The following surgical methods are proposed: (1) intramedullary fixation with AO-malleolar screw performed under radiographic control, (2) curettage of the medullary cavity bone grafting, and (3) tension band.

8. Sesamoid Bones

Sesamoid bones of the great toe located within the tendon of the short flexor of the great toe beneath the head of the first metatarsal bone may be sites for stress fractures; equally often are the medial one (larger bone) and lateral one (smaller bone). These fractures have been reported in runners, basketball players, gymnasts, and dancers.[48,49,76]

The principal clinical symptom is pain in the region of the metatarsophalangeal joint of the great toe, characteristically accompanying the activity (e.g., running) and disappearing upon resting. Physical examination reveals painful tenderness of the plantar side of the metatarsophalangeal joint of the big toe, and the mere passive dorsiflexion of the great toe provokes pain. Anteroposterior, lateral, and axial foot X-ray is made; stress fracture is characterized by a specific fissure form, i.e., the indented line with sharp angles, sometimes comprising even two such lines. If the line is straight and smooth, a bipartite sesamoid bone should be considered. It should be further pointed out that multipartite sesamoid bone may be found in a large number of asymptomatic individuals. According to some research results, a multipartite medial sesamoid bone may be found in 5 to 30% of people while a multipartite lateral sesamoid bone may be found in 0.6 to 2.4% of people.[48] When stress fracture of the sesamoid bone is only clinically suspected but not seen on an X-ray image, bone scintigraphy should be made and X-ray repeated in 3 weeks. In differential diagnosis of the sesamoid bone stress fracture, the following conditions should be taken into account: congenital variations and anomalies of the sesamoid bones, sesamoiditis, osteochondritis, nonunion of previous fractures, metatarsalgia, podagra (gout), and

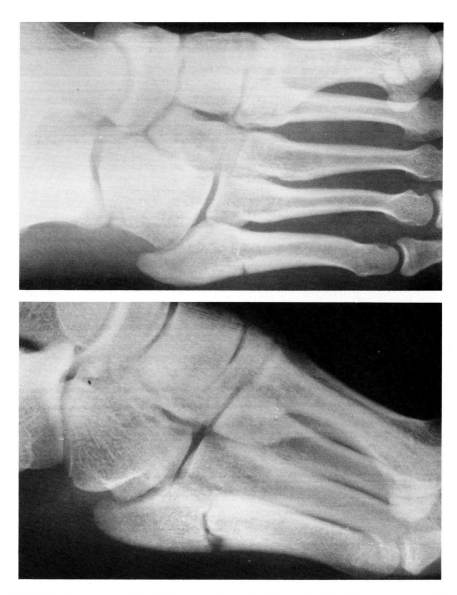

FIGURE 8. Stress fracture of the fifth metatarsal bone (Jones' fracture). (A) Initial roentgenogram; (B) roentgenogram preceding surgery.

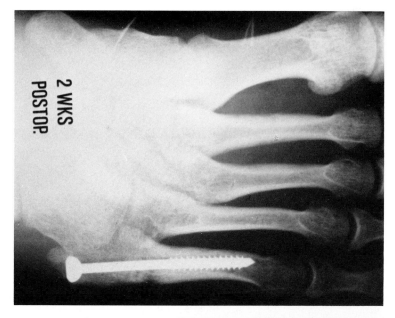

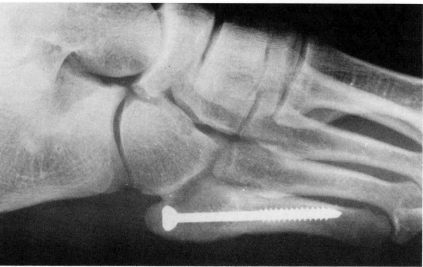

FIGURE 8 (continued). (C) 2 weeks after surgery; (D) 8 weeks after surgery when the athlete resumed full sports activities.

arthrosis of the metatarsophalangeal joint of the toe. The initial treatment of sesamoid bone stress fracture is invariably nonoperative. As these fractures show the tendency of delayed union and nonunion, surgery may often be necessary during which the sesamoid bone is removed (extirpated).

REFERENCES

1. **Abel, M. S.** Jogger's fracture and other stress fractures of the lumbosacral spine. *Skeletal Radiol.,* 1985; 13:221–227.
2. **Allen, M. E.** Stress fracture of the humerus: a case study. *Am. J. Sports Med.,* 1974; 12:244–245.
3. **Barrow, G. W. and Saha, S.** Menstrual irregularility and stress fractures in collegiate female distance runners. *Am. J. Sports Med.,* 1988; 16:209–216.
4. **Belkin, S. C.** Stress fractures in athletes. *Orthop. Clin. Am.,* 1980; 11:735–742.
5. **Blank, S.** Transverse tibial stress fractures. A special problem. *Am. J. Sports Med.,* 1987; 15:597–602.
6. **Blickenstaff, L. D. and Morris, J. M.** Fatique fracture of the femoral neck. *J. Bone Joint Surg.,* 1966; 48(A):1031–1047.
7. **Boyer, D. W.** Trapshooter's shoulder — stress fracture of the coracoid process: case report. *J. Bone Joint Surg.,* 1975; 57(A):562.
8. **Briethaupt, M. D.** Zur pathologie des menschlichen Fusses. *Med. Zeitung.,* 1855; 24:169.
9. **Butler, J. E., Brown, S. L., and McConnell, B. G.** Subtrochanteric stress fractures in runners. *Am. J. Sports Med.,* 1982; 10:228–232.
10. **Carter, S. R., Aldridge, M. J., Fitzgerald, R., et al.** Stress changes of the wrist in adolescent gymnasts. *Br. J. Radiol.,* 1988; 61:109–112.
11. **Clement, D. B., Taunton, J. E., Smart, G. W., and McNicol, K. L.** A survey of overuse running injuries. *Phys. Sportsmed.,* 1981; 9:47–58.
12. **De Lee, J. C., Evans, J. P., and Julian, J.** Stress fracture of the fifth metatarsal. *Am. J. Sports Med.,* 1983; 11:349–353.
13. **Devas, M. B.** Stress fractures in children. *J. Bone Joint Surg.,* 1963; 45(B):528–541.
14. **Devas, M. B.** Stress fractures of the patella. *J. Bone Joint Surg.,* 1960; 42(B):71–74.
15. **Devas, M. B. and Sweetnam, R.** Stress fractures of the fibula: a review of fifty cases in athletes. *J. Bone Joint Surg.,* 1956; 38(B):818–829.
16. **Deveraux, M. D., Parr, G. R., Lachmann, S. M., et al.** The diagnosis of stress fractures in athletes. *JAMA,* 1984; 252:531–533.
17. **Drez, D., Young, J. C., Johnson, R. D., et al.** Metatarsal stress fractures. *Am. J. Sports Med.,* 1980; 8:12–25.
18. **Fitch, K. D.** Stress fractures of the lower limbs in runners. *Aust. Fam. Phys.,* 1984; 13:511–515.
19. **Fitch, K. D., Blakwell, J. B., and Gilmour, W. N.** Operation for nonunion of stress fracture of the tarsal navicular. *J. Bone Joint Surg.,* 1989; 71(B):105–110.
20. **Fullerton, L. R., Jr. and Snowdy, H. A.** Femoral neck stress fractures. *Am. J. Sports Med.,* 1988; 16:365–377.
21. **Fullerton, L. R., Jr.** Femoral neck stress fractures. *Sports Med.,* 1990; 192–197.
22. **Giladi, M., Milgrom, C., Simkin, A., et al.** Stress fractures and tibial bone width: a risk factor. *J. Bone Joint Surg.,* 1987; 69(B):326–329.
23. **Goodman, P. H., Heaslet, M. W., Pagliano, J. W., et al.** Stress fracture diagnosis by computer-assisted thermography. *Phys. Sportsmed.,* 1985; 13:114–132.
24. **Graff, K. H., Krahl, H., and Kirschberger, R.** Stressfrakturen des os naviculare pedis. *Z. Orthop.,* 1986; 124:228–237.
25. **Greaney, R. B., Gerber, F. H., and Laughlin, R. L.** Distribution and natural history of stress fracture in U.S. Marine recruits. *Radiology,* 1983; 146:338–346.

26. **Green, N. E., Rogers, R. A., and Lipscomb, A. B.** Nonunion of stress fractures of the tibia. *Am. J. Sports Med.,* 1985; 13:171–176.

27. **Ha, K., Hahu, S. H., Chung, M. Y., Yang, B. K., and Yi, S. R.** A clinical study of stress fractures in sports activities. *Orthopedics,* 1991; 14:1088–1095.

28. **Hallel, T., Amit, S., and Segal, D.** Fatique fractures of tibial and femoral shaft in soldiers. *Clin. Orthop.,* 1976; 118:35–43.

29. **Hamilton, H. K.** Stress fracture of the diaphysis of the ulna in a body builder. *Am. J. Sports Med.,* 1984; 12:405–406.

30. **Hanks, G. A., Kalenak, A., Bowman, L. S., et al.** Stress fracture of the carpal scaphoid. *J. Bone Joint Surg.,* 1989; 71(A):938–941.

31. **Hershman, E. B. and Mailly, T.** Stress fractures. *Clin. Sports Med.,* 1990; 9:183–214.

32. **Holden, D. L. and Jackson, D. W.** Stress fractures of the ribs in female rowers. *Am. J. Sports Med.,* 1985; 13:342–348.

33. **Hulkko, A., Orava, S., and Nikula, P.** Stress fracture of the fifth metatarsal in athletes. *Ann. Chir. Gynaecol.,* 1985; 74:233–238.

34. **Hulkko, A., Orava, S., Peltokallio, P., et al.** Stress fracture of the navicular bone: nine cases in athletes. *Acta Orthop. Scand.,* 1985; 56:503–505.

35. **Hulkko, A., Orava, S., and Nikula, P.** Stress fractures of the olecranon in javelin throwers. *Int. J. Sports Med.,* 1986; 210–213.

36. **Hulkko, A. and Orava, S.** Stress fractures in athletes. *Int. J. Sports Med.,* 1987; 8:221–226.

37. **Hulkko, A. and Orava, S.** Diagnosis and treatment of delayed and non-union stress fractures in athletes. *Ann. Chir. Gynecol.,* 1991; 80:177–184.

38. **Hunter, L. Y.** Stress fracture of the tarsal navicular: more frequent than we realize? *Am. J. Sports Med.,* 1981; 9:217–218.

39. **Jerosch, J. G., Castro, W. H. M., and Jantea, C.** Stress fracture of the patella. *Am. J. Sports Med.,* 1989; 17:579–586.

40. **Johansson, C., Ekenman, I., Tornkvist, H., et al.** Stress fracture of the femoral neck in athletes. *Am. J. Sports Med.,* 1990; 18:524–528.

41. **Kavanaugh, J. H., Browe, T. D., and Mann, R. V.** The Jones' fracture revisited. *J. Bone Joint Surg.,* 1978; 60(A):776–782.

42. **Keating, T. M.** Stress fracture of the sternum in a wrestler. *Am. J. Sports Med.,* 1987; 15:92–93.

43. **Lombardo, S. J. and Benson, D. W.** Stress fractures of the femur in runners. *Am. J. Sports Med.,* 1982; 10:219–227.

44. **Markey, K. L.** Stress fractures. *Clin. Sports Med.,* 1987; 6:405–425.

45. **Matheson, G. O., Clement, D. B., McKenzie, D. C., et al.** Scintigraphic uptake of 99m Tc at non-painful sites in athletes with stress fractures: the concept of bone strain. *Sports Med.,* 1987; 4:65–75.

46. **Matheson, G. O., Clement, D. B., McKenzie, D. C., et al.** Stress fractures in athletes: a study of 320 cases. *Am. J. Sports Med.,* 1987; 15:46–58.

47. **Matin, P.** Basic principles of nuclear medicine techniques for detection and evaluation of trauma and sports medicine injuries. *Sem. Nucl. Med.,* 1988; 18:90–112.

48. **McBryde, A. M.** Stress fractures in runners. *Clin. Sports Med.,* 1985; 4:737–752.

49. **McKeag, D. B. and Dolan, C.** Overuse syndromes of the lower extremity. *Phys. Sportsmed.,* 1989; 17:108–123.

50. **McKenzie, D. C.** Stress fracture of the rib in a elite oarsman. *Int. J. Sports Med.,* 1989; 10:220–222.

51. **Moss, A. and Mowat, A. G.** Ultrasonic assessment of stress fractures. *Br. Med. J.,* 1983; 1479–1480.

52. **Mutch, Y., Mori, T., Suzuki, Y., et al.** Stress fractures of the ulna in athletes. *Am. J. Sports Med.,* 1982; 10:365–367.

53. **Noakes, T. D., Smith, J. A., Lindberg, G., et al.** Pelvic stress fractures in long distance runners. *Am. J. Sports Med.,* 1985; 13:120–123.

54. **Nuber, G. W. and Diment, M. T.** Olecranon stress fractures in throwers. A report of two cases and a review of the literature. *Clin. Orthop.,* 1992; 278:58–61.

55. **Orava, S., Jormakka, E., and Kulkko, A.** Stress fractures in young athletes. *Arch. Orthop. Trauma Surg.,* 1981; 98:271–274.

56. **Orava, S. and Hulkko, A.** Delayed unions and nonunions of stress fractures in athletes. *Am. J. Sports Med.,* 1988; 16:378–382.

57. **Orava, S. and Hulkko, A.** Stress fracture of the mid-tibial shaft. *Acta Orthop. Scand.,* 1984; 55:35–37.

58. **Orava, S., Karpakko, J., Hulkko, A., Vaananen, K., Takala, T., Kallinen, M., and Alen, M.** Diagnosis and treatment of stress fractures located at the mid-tibial shaft in athletes. *Int. J. Sports Med.,* 1991; 12:419–422.

59. **Pavlov, H., Nelsen, T. L., Wararen, R. F., et al.** Stress fractures of the pubic ramus. *J. Bone Joint Surg.,* 1982; 64(A):1020–1025.

60. **Pavlov, M., Torg, J. S., and Freiberger, R. M.** Tarsal navicular stress fractures: radiographic evaluation. *Radiology,* 1983; 48:641–645.

61. **Pećina, M., Bojanić, I., and Ribarić, G.** Stres fraktura baze pete metatarzalne kosti — Jonesov prijelom. *Acta Orthop. Iugosl.,* 1988; 19:118–123.

62. **Pećina, M., Bojanić, I., and Dubravič, S.** Stress fractures in figure skaters. *Am. J. Sports Med.,* 1990; 18:277–279.

63. **Posinkovič, B. and Pavlovič, M.** Prijelom zamora. *Liječ Vjesn.,* 1989; 111:228–231.

64. **Rettig, A. C.** Stress fracture of the ulna in an adolescent tournament tennis player. *Am. J. Sports Med.,* 1983; 11:103–109.

65. **Rettig, A. C. and Beltz, M. F.** Stress fracture in the humerus in an adolescent tennis tournament player. *Am. J. Sports Med.,* 1985; 13:55–58.

66. **Rettig, A. C., Shelbourne, K. D., McCarrol, J. R., et al.** The natural history and treatment of delayed union stress fractures of the anterior cortex of the tibia. *Am. J. Sports Med.,* 1988; 16:250–255.

67. **Rupani, H. D., Holder, L. E., Espinola, D. A., et al.** Three-phase radionuclide bone imaging in sports medicine. *Radiology,* 1985; 156:187–196.

68. **Shelbourne, K. D., Fisher, D. A., Rettig, A. C., et al.** Stress fractures of the medial malleolus. *Am. J. Sports Med.,* 1988; 16:60–63.

69. **Stafford, S. A., Rosenthal, D. I., Gebhardt, M. C., et.** MRI in stress fractures. *AJR,* 1986; 147:553–556.

70. **Stanitski, C. L., McMaster, J. H., and Scranton, P. E.** On the nature of stress fractures. *Am. J. Sports Med.,* 1978; 6:391–396.

71. **Sterling, J. C., Edelstein, D. W., Caho, R. D., and Webb, R., II.** Stress fractures in athletes. Diagnosis and management. *Sports Med.,* 1992; 14:336–346.

72. **Sullivan, D., Warren, R. F., Pavlov, H., et al.** Stress fractures in 51 runners. *Clin. Orthop.,* 1984; 187:188–192.

73. **Torg, J. S. and Moyer, R. A.** Non-union of a stress fracture through the olecranon epiphyseal plate observed in an adolescent baseball pritcher. *J. Bone Joint Surg.,* 1977; 59(A):264–265.

74. **Torg, J. S., and Pavlov, H., Cooley, L. H.** Stress fractures of the tarsal navicular: a retrospective review of twenty-one cases. *J. Bone Joint Surg.,* 1982; 63(A):700–712.

75. **Torg, J. S., Balduini, F. C., Zelko, R. R., et al.** Fractures of the base of the fifth metatarsal distal to the tuberosity: classification and guidelines for non-surgical and surgical management. *J. Bone Joint Surg.*, 1984; 66(A):209–214.

76. **Van Hal, M. E., Keene, J. S., Lange, T. A., et al.** Stress fractures of the great toe sesamoids. *Am. J. Sports Med.*, 1982; 10:122–128.

77. **Volpin, G., Milgrom, C., Goldsher, D., et al.** Stress fracture of the sacrum following strenuous activity. *Clin. Orthop.*, 1989; 243:184–188.

78. **Zogby, R. G. and Baker, B. E.** A review of non-operative treatment of Jones' fracture. *Am. J. Sports Med.*, 1987; 15:304–457.

79. **Zwas, S. T., Elkanovitch, R., and Frank, G.** Interpretation and classification of bone scintigraphic findings in stress fractures. *J. Nucl. Med.*, 1987; 28:452–7.

12

Nerve Entrapment
Syndromes

Long-term repetitive microtrauma can lead to nerve entrapment syndromes, which is why they are included among overuse injuries.

In contemporary medical literature, we can find numerous reports on various nerve entrapment syndromes. Acute trauma and especially long-term repetitive microtrauma have been indicated as possible instigating agents.[6,14,24,46,47,72,89,96] Certain sports or physical activities that have been mentioned lead to specific nerve entrapment syndromes, e.g., cyclist's palsy and bowler's thumb. Nerve entrapment syndromes in athletes are not as rare as they were once considered to be. It is also evident that when athletes have pain, one must always consider the possibility of nerve entrapment syndromes. Diagnosis relies on a detailed history and physical examination with modern diagnostic equipment. In most cases, nonoperative treatment is sufficient, and surgery is therefore seldom recommended. The purpose of this chapter is to present currently available information about nerve entrapment syndromes in athletes.

I. UPPER LIMB

A. Thoracic Outlet Syndrome

The syndrome of upper limb pain, paresthesias, vascular insufficiency, and motor dysfunction secondary to compression of the brachial plexus, subclavian artery, or subclavian vein before their division and separation bears the name *thoracic outlet syndrome*. Thoracic outlet syndrome has been described in athletic population, especially with regard to certain sports such as swimming and other activities within which swing motion of the arm is required (i.e., throwing).[43,50,93] Compression in the outlet may occur at any one of three levels: (1) interscalene triangle, (2) costoclavicular space, and (3) pectoralis minor muscle insertion on the coracoid process. Abnormal structural variations (cervical rib, fibrous band, "abnormal" scalene muscle development) may compress or cause friction of the plexus or vessels at the level of the interscalene triangle. Compression of neurovascular structures through the costoclavicular space is usually caused by dynamic changes, especially in shoulder girdle mechanics, i.e., functional anatomy of the shoulder girdle.[77] The coracoid process and pectoralis minor muscle insertion act as a fulcrum over which the neurovascular structures change direction when the arm is elevated. This site has been implicated as a source of neurovascular compression among athletes who repetitively hyperabduct the arm, i.e., swimmers, tennis players, and pitchers. In swimmers, neurovascular compression in this area may develop as a result of the pectoralis minor muscle hypertrophy.[42] Different patterns of clinical presentations are seen depending on where and which neurovascular structures are compressed. The majority of patients' symptoms are created by neurological compression.[43] Typical symptoms are pain, numbness, or paresthesias. Sensory loss and muscle atrophy are rare but can occur. Vascular symptoms of thoracic outlet syndrome are quite rare. Venous obstruction may cause arm edema, cyanotic discoloration, and venous collaterization across the shoulder and chest wall, whereas arterial obstruction produces symptoms of coolness, numbness, ischemic pain, and external fatigue. A very common symptom pattern in thoracic outlet syndrome is that of "mixed involvement". In mixed symptom pattern, patients have symptoms of both upper and lower trunk compression, along with variable degrees of vascular insufficiency. Thoracic outlet syndrome remains a clinical diagnosis, based almost entirely on the history and physical examination.[43] Therefore, thoracic outlet syndrome should be a diagnosis of exclusion. Initial treatment should be nonoperative, including rest from athletic activities.[43,50,72] Surgical treatment is indicated in patients with significant neurological or vascular involvement that does not respond to nonoperative treatment.[43,50,72]

Compression of the brachial plexus may arise from both intrinsic and extrinsic factors. Both of these mechanisms may occur in association with athletic activity. The most common external agent creating compression of the brachial plexus is a knapsack.[34,49,100] In Hirasawa and Sakakida's series,[34] most of the observed brachial plexus lesions were described as *backpack paralysis*. Brachial plexus compression results when large, heavy backpacks are carried for long periods. The axillary straps create a compression force around the plexus with the clavicle as a firm strut against which compression can occur. The shoulder girdle is pulled posteriorly by the heavy pack, adding a component of traction. Treatment of backpack paralysis consists of avoidance of mechanisms thought to have caused it and participation in physical therapy. Physical therapy restores one's strength, allowing complete recovery.

B. Axillary Nerve

Entrapment of the axillary nerve in the quadrilateral space is rare in athletes.[2] It has been described in baseball pitchers.[81]

C. Suprascapular Nerve

Suprascapular nerve entrapment is an infrequently observed disorder and is often misdiagnosed. The manner of presentation of this syndrome depends on the anatomical site of compression. Entrapment usually occurs at the suprascapular notch (Figure 1). Patients, mostly throwing athletes, suffer from poorly localized

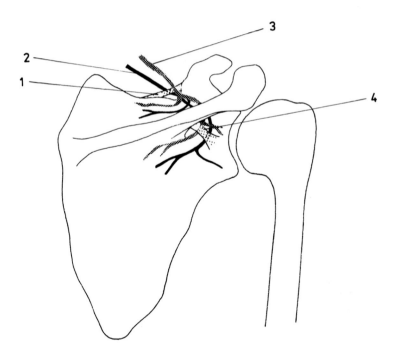

FIGURE 1. Suprascapular notch and pertinent anatomical relationships of the scapula and ligament to the neurovascular bundle. (1) Transverse scapular ligament; (2) suprascapular nerve; (3) suprascapular artery; (4) spinoglenoid ligament.

shoulder pain, intact sensation, weakness of external rotation and abduction, and atrophy of the supraspinatus and infraspinatus muscle.[52,62,76,84] Occasionally, entrapment occurs distally, at the spinoglenoid notch. Patients may be asymptomatic or may describe mild pain and weakness of the shoulder because of denervation of the infraspinatus.[5,8,23,29] Ferretti et al.[23] found 12 top-level volleyball players with an isolated asymptomatic paralysis of the infraspinatus muscle. Ganzhorn et al.[27] described the case of a weight lifter who noted wasting in the region of the dorsal scapula while posing in the mirror. When the entrapment is localized at the suprascapular or spinoglenoid notch, restraint from athletic activities, nonsteroidal anti-inflammatory medication, and local steroid injections may be useful.[62,76] If such nonoperative measures are unsuccessful, surgical exploration is indicated.

D. Musculocutaneous Nerve Entrapment

Musculocutaneous nerve entrapment in the shoulder region do not occur commonly, but several cases have been reported among athletes after heavy physical activity.[7,45,58,74] This syndrome was initially described by Braddom and Wolfe in 1978 who based their experience on two weight lifters.[7] Musculocutaneous nerve compression leads to biceps brachii muscle wasting and weakness (Figure 2). Sensory complaints are referred to the radial aspect of the forearm. Typically, no pain is associated. Neurologic findings include absent biceps reflex, decreased biceps

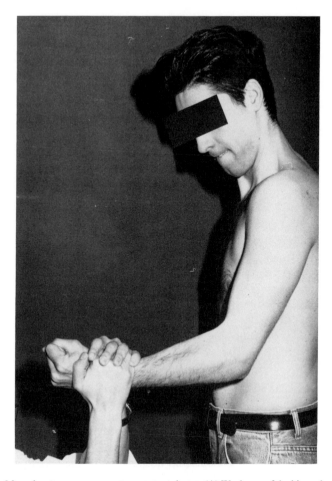

FIGURE 2. Musculocutaneous nerve entrapment syndrome. (A) Weakness of the biceps brachii muscle.

tone, and hypesthesias and paresthesias in the radial aspect of the forearm. This syndrome usually resolves spontaneously with cessation of the strenuous activity.[74] Compression of the musculocutaneous nerve at the elbow, i.e., of the lateral antebrachial cutaneous nerve, may occur when the nerve passes below the tendon of the biceps muscle before piercing the brachial fascia. According to Bassett and Numley,[1] the lateral free margin of the biceps aponeurosis compresses the nerve against the brachial fascia with elbow extension, and pronation further increases nerve compression.

E. Radial Nerve

Entrapment of the radial nerve above the elbow is rare in athletes.[75] The site of compression is in the region of the lateral intermuscular septum, which the radial nerve pierces as it enters the anterior aspect of the arm. It has been reported in weight lifting following strenuous muscular activities.[53] Patients develop a complete radial

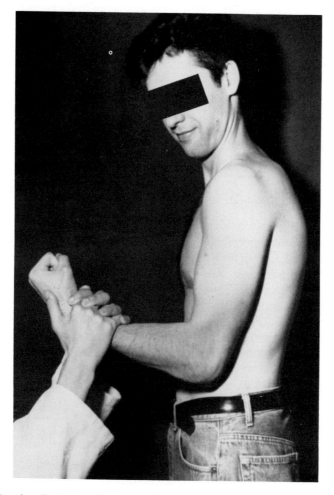

FIGURE 2 (continued). (B) Return of strength and breadth to the biceps muscle 6 weeks after ceasing strenuous physical work.

nerve palsy. Treatment is rest and cessation of all strenuous activities. In most cases, the symptoms will disappear within several weeks. Persistent or progressive symptoms suggest the need for surgical decompression.[53,75]

F. Radial Tunnel Syndrome

In their study of a group of patients with chronic tennis elbow, Roles and Maudsley[86] recognized the compression of the radial nerve within its tunnel and called it *radial tunnel syndrome*. The syndrome differs from a posterior interosseous nerve syndrome in which the problem is localized to compression of the nerve at one particular site, the arcade of Frohse, and results in only a motor deficit.[61,65,82,98] In radial tunnel syndrome, there may be a spectrum of complaints, including pain, paresthesias, and weakness.[66] A motor deficit is not nearly as common as in a posterior interosseous nerve syndrome. There are five potential sites of compression within the radial tunnel: (1) fibrous bands at its proximal portion, (2) fibrous medial edge along the extensor carpi radialis brevis, (3) "fan" of radial recurrent vessels, (4) arcade of Frohse, and (5) fibrous band at the distal edge of the supinator muscle. The radial tunnel syndrome occurs most commonly in tennis players, but may also be seen in rowers and weight lifters.[75] Nonoperative measures should be the first form of treatment. Such measures include rest of the elbow and wrist from repetitive stressful activity and a course of anti-inflammatory medication. Surgical exploration with neurolysis is indicated if nonoperative treatment fails.[75,85]

G. Wartenberg's Disease

Athletes involved in sports requiring repetitive pronation supination ulnar flexion activities may acquire Wartenberg's disease — entrapment of the superficial sensory branch of the radial nerve in the forearm.[15,83] Wearing wrist bands as in racquet sports has also been implicated as a cause of this syndrome; this is also known as *handcuff neuropathy*.[19,57,61] The patient's main complaints are burning pain or numbness and tingling over the dorsoradial aspect of the wrist, thumb, and web space, usually aggravated by wrist movement. If the syndrome occurs from external compression, nonoperative therapy can be successful. It may take several months for the symptoms to resolve. Surgical exploration is necessary if nonoperative therapy fails.[15,83]

H. Ulnar Nerve

Ulnar nerve entrapment at the elbow is most frequently encountered by throwing athletes, such as baseball pitchers, tennis players, and javelin throwers, but is also observed in skiing, weight lifting, and stick-handling sports.[16,26,30,101,104] Because of its position in the cubital tunnel (Figure 3), the ulnar nerve is vulnerable to repetitive "tension" or "traction" stresses in athletes. This may also be compounded by subluxation or instability of the nerve. Childress[10] reported that 16.2% of the population demonstrated recurrent dislocation of the ulnar nerve when the elbow was flexed and extended. Repeated stress and injury may lead to inflammation, adhesions, and progressive compressive neuropathy. The intermittent nature of the athletic endeavors may confuse the presentation of the athlete with entrapment of the ulnar nerve at the elbow. Sometimes, the first symptom will consist of pain along the medial joint line either associated with or exacerbated by overhead activities. As the inflammation of the nerve progresses, pain and paresthesias will be noted down the ulnar aspect of the forearm to the hand. Sensory changes definitely precede motor changes; however, a careful evaluation of the intrinsic musculature of the hand is essential to detect any weakness. Quite often, recalcitrant ulnar nerve entrapment at the elbow requires surgery. However, many transient episodes can be treated nonoperatively.[30] Del Pizzo et al.[16] reported 19 baseball players with ulnar nerve entrapment at the elbow who underwent surgery. The surgery consisted of anterior transfer of the nerve deep into the origin of the flexor muscles.

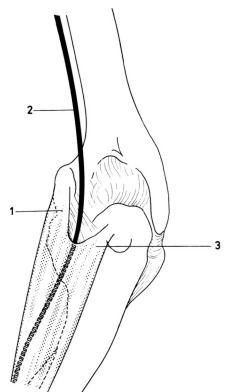

FIGURE 3. Compression of the ulnar nerve, distal to the elbow, by the heads of the flexor carpi ulnaris muscle. (1) Humeral head of the flexor carpi ulnaris muscle; (2) ulnar nerve; (3) ulnar head of the flexor carpi ulnaris muscle.

I. Ulnar Tunnel Syndrome

Entrapment of the ulnar nerve in Guyon's canal (ulnar tunnel syndrome) is seen in cyclists and racquetball players as a result of chronic external compression. The first report of ulnar neuropathy as a complication of long-distance cycling was published in 1896.[17] Several reports have since described this complication, called *cyclist's* or *handlebar palsy*.[9,13,22,25,39,56,91,97] Factors reported in the literature as contributing to the development of neuropathies in cyclists include the use of worn-out gloves, unpadded handlebars, prolonged grasping of dropped handlebars, riding an improperly adjusted bicycle, and vibratory trauma from rough roads. Jackson[39] recently studied 20 cyclists with riding experience of more than 100 miles per week and found that 9 of 20 cyclists complained of either hand or finger numbness during cycling which disappeared after completion of the ride. They reported that their hand numbness or pain was reduced after adjusting their hand position. Conventional treatment for nerve compression syndrome at the wrist consists of changes in cycling technique, including frequently varying hand position, the use of properly padded gloves and handlebars, and changes in the bicycle to ensure a proper fit.[39,56] These changes frequently will relieve symptoms in most cases without need for surgical decompression of the Guyon's canal.

J. Hypothenar Hammer Syndrome

Repetitive trauma to the heel of the palm can cause ulnar artery spasm, thromboses, or aneurysms and thus compromise the ulnar nerve function with a more vascular type of presentation. This condition, known as *hypothenar hammer syndrome*, has been described in conjunction with several sports, including karate, judo, tennis, and lacrosse.[12,35,69,83] Nonunion of the hook of the hamate or of the pisiform, which may be fractured during a tennis, baseball, or golf swing, can also cause entrapment within the ulnar tunnel (Guyon's canal).[61] It is also important to keep in mind the possibility of a double crush injury of the ulnar nerve with coexistence of the syndrome of the flexor carpi ulnaris muscle (cubital tunnel syndrome) and ulnar tunnel syndrome.[36,39]

K. Median Nerve

Entrapment of the median nerve at the elbow is termed *pronator teres syndrome* and may result from repetitive exercises and hypertrophy of the flexor-pronator muscle group.[11,36,99] Patients complain of pain and tenderness in the volar aspect of their forearms over the area of compression, which worsens with exertional activities. Sensory complaints are common, consisting of numbness and paresthesias in part or all of the median nerve distribution of the hand. Pronator teres syndrome is often a difficult diagnosis and must be distinguished from carpal tunnel syndrome. Since the majority of cases are intermittent and mild, nonoperative treatment should be utilized initially.[36,39] Persistent or progressive symptoms suggest the need for surgical intervention.[36,99]

L. Anterior Interosseous Syndrome (Kiloh-Nevin Syndrome)

It has been described in association with repetitive activities such as throwing, racquet sports, or weight lifting.[70,75] It is characterized by a vague feeling of discomfort in the proximal forearm, which may mimic pronator teres syndrome. The classic finding is that the patient loses his ability to pinch between his thumb and index finger. However, this is not always present. Initial treatment should be nonoperative because in many cases spontaneous improvement will occur. However, if there is no improvement after 8 to 12 weeks, a surgical decompression and neurolysis should be performed.[36,72]

M. Carpal Tunnel Syndrome

It is the most described among nerve entrapment syndromes, but its incidence as a sports-related problem is surprisingly low. Carpal tunnel may be seen in sports secondary to gripping, throwing, cycling, repetitive wrist flexion/extension activity, as well as direct trauma.[11,34,36,61,65,72,83,87,97,102] Since carpal tunnel syndrome is so rare in the athlete, unusual causes must be suspected when the diagnosis is entertained.

N. Digital Nerve Entrapment Syndromes

In athletes, the digital nerve entrapment syndromes are less common than those occurring at the wrist level. Digital nerves may be compressed during their course in the distal palm or at the proximal digit level. Bowler's thumb is the most common syndrome, involving the digital nerve in the hand.[11,18,21,37,61,63,65,83,90,97,102] Repetitive compression of the ulnar digital nerve to the thumb secondary to direct pressure on the nerve from the thumb hole of a bowling ball has been implicated as a cause of bowler's thumb. Incidentally, bowler's thumb has been reported in a baseball player.[61] On physical examination, the patients have tenderness over the ulnar volar aspect of the metacarpophalangeal joint of the thumb and a positive Tinel's sign in this area with paresthesias radiating to the ulnar aspect of the tip of the thumb. There is no motor involvement; however, grip strength may be somewhat diminished secondary to pain. Bowler's thumb should be treated nonoperatively with rest, cessation of activity, nonsteroidal anti-inflammatory medication, and modification of equipment and technique.[18,83] In the advanced cases, a molded plastic thumb guard is recommended to prevent trauma. Surgical treatment is indicated for those with persistent significant symptoms.[18,63,83] Surgical options include resection of the neuroma and primary repair of the nerve, neurolysis, and transfer to a new location.

Compression of digital nerves in tennis players has recently been reported.[68,70] Symptoms include numbness along the volar surface of the index finger of the racquet hand and an abnormal sweat pattern, especially in players who have recently started playing or who have recently increased their amount of playing. Physical finding usually include calluses over the second metacarpal head, which implies rubbing of the digital nerve between the fixed bone and the racquet handle. Early recognition, improved technique, better equipment, and protective measures are helpful in treating this problem.[68,70] Surgery is very rarely indicated.

II. LOWER LIMB

A. Piriformis Muscle Syndrome

It is not discussed with specific reference to athletes although athletic activities may cause such changes which significantly contribute to the muscle and sciatic nerve, direct and indirect trauma, muscular hypertrophy, inflammation, and local ischemia.[14,71–73,96] Piriformis muscle syndrome has many similarities with and overlaps symptoms of low back pain, ischialgias, vascular disease, and lower extremity pathologies.[38,72] Pain in the sacral or gluteal region remains the most constant symptom. The pain increases with sitting or walking and decreases with lying supine. Frequently, diagnosis requires eliminating other cause of sciatic pain. Nonoperative treatment includes physiotherapy, nonsteroidal anti-inflammatory medication, and local steroid injection.[14,72] Surgical treatment must be initiated within 6 to 8 months of presentation. Surgical treatment consists of sectioning the piriformis muscle at its tendinous origin and external neurolysis of sciatic nerve.[72,73]

B. Meralgia Paresthetica

It is an entrapment syndrome of the lateral femoral cutaneous nerve as it enters the thigh through or under the superolateral end of the inguinal ligament, causing burning sensations, paresthesias and dysesthesias of the anterior and lateral thigh. This entrapment may be secondary to direct or repetitive traumas. In the athletic population, it has been described in gymnasts.[55] Meralgia paresthetica usually responds to nonoperative treatment, including avoidance of repetitive traumas or pressure sources, nonsteroidal anti-inflammatory medications, and steroid injections.[14,55,96] Resistant cases require surgical intervention, neurolysis, or nerve resection.

C. Entrapment of Saphenous Nerve

In the athletic population, the saphenous nerve may be compressed within the adductor canal (Hunter's or subsartorial canal) or where it exits the fascia (Figure 4) during strong contraction of the surrounding musculature, i.e., with knee extensions or squats.[14,20,103] Hemler et al.[32] reported saphenous nerve entrapment caused by pes anserine

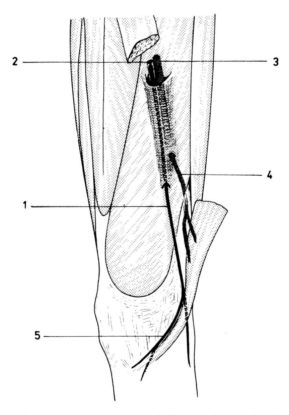

FIGURE 4. Compression of the saphenous nerve typically occurs in the region shown. (1) Saphenous nerve; (2) femoral vein; (3) femoral artery; (4) descending genicular artery; (5) infrapatellar branch of the saphenous nerve.

bursitis. Entrapment of the saphenous nerve causes medial knee pain, dysesthesias, and hypesthesias in the distal distribution of the nerve. Relief is usually obtained with nonoperative measures, but surgical exploration and neurolysis may be necessary.[14,103]

D. Sural Nerve Entrapment

It may occur anywhere along its course. In the athletic population, it is most often described in runners.[14,88,96] Recurrent ankle sprains may lead to fibrosis and subsequent nerve entrapment.[78] The patients complain of shooting pain and paresthesias along the lateral border of the foot, sometimes extending proximally to immediately behind the lateral malleolus and up the posterior lateral aspect of the lower leg. Usually, nonoperative treatment is successful.[14,88] Several cases of sural nerve entrapment have been described in athletes who sustained avulsion fractures of the base of the fifth metatarsal bone.[31] In these cases, due to persisting symptoms and nonunion of the fracture, surgical excision of the nonunited fragment and a neurolysis of the sural nerve were performed.

E. Common Peroneal Nerve Entrapment

There were only a few case reports about common peroneal nerve entrapment in runners.[64,92] Recently, Leach et al.[48] reported eight athletes, seven runners, and one soccer player with common peroneal nerve entrapment. In all reported patients, running induced pain and numbness. Examination after running revealed muscle weakness and a positive Tinel's test where the nerve winds around the fibular neck. Due to failure of various nonoperative treatments, all of the patients were treated surgically by neurolysis of the peroneal nerve as it travels under the sharp fibrous edge of the peroneus longus muscle origin. Leach et al.[48] reported that seven of eight operated athletes returned to their previous level of activity without any further symptoms.

F. Superficial Peroneal Nerve Entrapment

It occurs most commonly in runners, but may also be seen in soccer players, hockey players, tennis players, bodybuilders, and dancers.[44,54,60,94,95] Loss of or disturbances in sensation over the dorsum of the foot during exercise is a common sign of entrapment. Occasionally, patients only complain of pain at the function of the middle and distal third of the leg, with or without the presence of local swelling. The pain is typically worse with any physical activity, including walking, jogging, running, or squatting. Relief by conservative measures is uncommon. Decompression by local fasciectomy and fasciotomy of the lateral compartment have been reported to give good results.[94,95]

G. Deep Peroneal Nerve Entrapment (Anterior Tarsal Tunnel Syndrome)

It has been described in runners, soccer players, skiers, and dancers.[14,88] Patients frequently give a history of recurrent ankle sprains or previous trauma. Tight, high-heeled shoes or ski boots have also been implicated as inciting factors.[28,51] An osteophyte on the dorsum of the talus or of the intermetatarseum at the tarsometatarsal joint can also press on the nerve.[67] Baxter and co-workers[14,67,88] described this entrapment in joggers who put keys under the tongue of their running shoes and in athletes who did sit-ups with their feet hooked under a metal bar. The patients complained of dorsal foot pain, numbness, and paresthesias over the first web space. The pain usually occurs during athletic activities. Most patients will respond well to nonoperative therapy with local steroid injections, alteration of footwear, and orthotic devices.[88,105] Occasionally, when these measures fail, a patient may require surgical decompression.

H. Tarsal Tunnel Syndrome

It is an uncommon condition in the athletic population, although it has been described in runners, ballet dancers, and basketball players.[40,41,59,67,79] The most common etiology is alteration of the normal spacial relationships secondary to space — occupying lesions, such as lipomas, ganglion cysts, neurilemomas, neurofibromas, varicose veins, and enlarged venous plexus (Figure 5). Other causes have included severe pronation of the hindfoot, chronic flexor tenosynovitis, posttraumatic scarring, and inflammatory collagen vascular disease. According to the literature, many of the cases are idiopathic. Athletes usually suffer from burning, sharp pain at the medial malleolus radiating into the sole of the foot, the heel, and sometimes the calf. They may also notice numbness and burning paresthesias on the plantar aspect of the foot and in the toes, which also may radiate up the calf. Initially, symptoms may be intermittent but may become more constant over time. The symptoms are accentuated by prolonged standing, walking, and especially prolonged running. Treatment should be directed toward identifying and correcting the etiology of the syndrome. Nonoperative treatment of the athlete with tarsal tunnel syndrome includes rest, nonsteroidal anti-inflammatory medication, local steroid injection, flexibility exercises, well-fitting shoes, and custom-made foot orthotics to help control abnormal mechanics.[40,41,67,79] Failure of nonoperative treatment necessitates surgical exploration and decompression of the nerve.

I. Entrapment of the First Branch of the Lateral Plantar Nerve

One of the most commonly overlooked causes of chronic heel pain in athletes is entrapment of the first branch of the lateral plantar nerve (nerve to the abductor digiti quinti muscle). Although runners and joggers account for the overwhelming majority of cases, this entrapment has been reported in athletes who participate in soccer, dance, tennis, and other track and fields events.[3,4,33,67] Entrapment occurs between the heavy deep fascia of the abductor hallucis muscle and the medial caudal margin of the medial head of the quadratus plantae muscle. Athletes complain of chronic heel pain intensified by walking and especially by running. Tenderness over the course of the nerve, maximal in the area of entrapment, is a characteristic and pathognomonic finding. Treatment is similar to that of other forms of heel pain: rest,

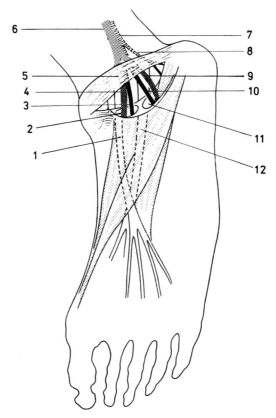

FIGURE 5. This figure reveals the complex anatomy of the tarsal tunnel. (1) Flexor digitorum muscle; (2) upper (medial) tarsal tunnel; (3) medial plantar nerve; (4) medial plantar artery; (5) ligamentum lacinatum; (6) posterior tibial artery; (7) tibial nerve; (8) calcaneal branches of the tibial nerve; (9) lateral plantar artery; (10) lateral plantar nerve; (11) lower (lateral) tarsal tunnel; (12) flexor hallucis longus muscle.

nonsteroidal anti-inflammatory medication, heel cups, stretching programs, and occasionally local steroid injections.[3,33,67] If 6 to 12 months of nonoperative therapy fail to relieve the symptoms and other possible causes of heel pain have been ruled out, then surgical intervention is indicated.

J. Medial Plantar Nerve Entrapment

It is known as jogger's foot and occurs in the region of the Master Knot of Henry.[80] The patients, usually middle-age joggers, complain of aching or shooting pain in the medial aspect of their arch during running. Most characteristically, the onset of pain is associated with the use of a new arch support. Physical examination reveals point tenderness of the plantar aspect of the medial arch in the region of the navicular tuberosity. The pain may be reproduced by everting the heel or having the patient stand on the ball of the foot. Nonoperative treatment is usually sufficient.[80,88]

K. Interdigital Neuromas (Metatarsalgia)

They are not uncommon in athletes, especially in runners.[14,67,72,88] Patients characteristically complain of plantar or forefoot pain associated with sprints or long-distance running. The pain is described as burning or sharp and frequently radiates to the toes. Patients may also notice numbness or tingling in the affected toes. They will often give a history of many shoe changes in an attempt to seek relief. Typically, the pain is relieved by rest, removal of the shoes, and massage of the forefoot. A variety of metatarsal pads and orthotic devices have been suggested, but they are usually uncomfortable and are rejected by athletes. A small percentage of interdigital neuromas respond to local steroid injections. Most of them require surgical excision of the neuroma.[14,67,72,88]

REFERENCES

1. **Bassett, H. F. and Numley, A. J.** Compression of the musculocutaneous nerve at the elbow. *J. Bone Joint Surg.*, 1982; 64A:1050–1052.
2. **Bateman, J. E.** Nerve injuries about the shoulder in sports. *J. Bone Joint Surg.*, 1967; 49A:785–792.
3. **Baxter, D. E., Pfeffer, G. B., and Thigpen, M.** Chronic heel pain: treatment rationale. *Orthop. Clin. N. Am.*, 1989; 20:563–269.
4. **Bazzoli, A. S. and Polina, F. S.** Heel pain in recreational runners. *Phys. Sportsmed.*, 1989; 17:55–61.
5. **Black, K. P. and Lombardo, J. A.** Suprascapular nerve injuries with isolated paralysis of the infraspinatus. *Am. J. Sports Med.*, 1990; 18:225–228.
6. **Bora, F. W. and Osterman, A. L.** Compression neuropathy. *Clin. Orthop.*, 1982; 163:20–32.
7. **Braddom, R. L. and Wolfe, C.** Musculocutaneous nerve injury after heavy exercise. *Arch. Phys. Med. Rehab.*, 1978; 59:290–293.
8. **Bryan, W. J. and Wild, J. J.** Isolated infraspinatus atrophy: a common cause of posterior shoulder pain and weakness in throwing athletes. *Am. J. Sports Med.*, 1989; 17:130–131.
9. **Burke, E. R.** Ulnar neuropathy in bicyclists. *Phys. Sportsmed.*, 1981; 9:53–56.
10. **Childress, H. M.** Recurrent ulnar nerve dislocation at the elbow. *J. Bone Joint Surg.*, 1956; 38A:978–984.
11. **Collins, K., Storey, M., Peterson, K., and Nuttler, P.** Nerve injuries in athletes. *Phys. Sportsmed.*, 1988; 16:92–100.
12. **Conn, J., Bergan, J. J., and Bell, J. L.** Hypothenar hammer syndrome. Posttraumatic digital ischemia. *Surgery*, 1970; 68:1122–1128.
13. **Converse, T. A.** Cyclist palsy (letter). *N. Engl. J. Med.*, 1979; 301:1397–1398.
14. **Deese, J. M., Jr., and Baxter, D. E.** Compressive neuropathies of the lower extremity. *J. Musculoskel. Med.*, 1988; 5:68–91.
15. **Dellon, A. L. and Mackinnon, S. E.** Radial sensory nerve entrapment in the forearm. *J. Hand Surg.*, 1986; 11A:199–205.

16. **Del Pizzo, W., Jobe, F. W., and Norwood, L.** Ulnar nerve entrapment syndrome in baseball players. *Am. J. Sports Med.,* 1977; 5:182–185.
17. **Destot, M.** Paralysie cubitale per l'usage de la bicyclette. *Gaz. Hop. Civ. Mil.,* 1896; 69:1176–1177.
18. **Dobyns, J. H., O'Brien, E. T., and Linscheid, R. L.** Bowler's thumb, diagnosis and treatment: review of 17 cases. *J. Bone Joint Surg.,* 1972; 54A:751–755.
19. **Dorfman, L. J. and Jayoram, A. R.** Handcuff neuropathy. *JAMA,* 1978; 239:957.
20. **Dumitru, D. and Windsor, R. E.** Subsartorial entrapment of the saphenous nerve of a competitive female bodybuilder. *Phys. Sportsmed.,* 1989; 17:116–125.
21. **Dunham, W., Haines, G., and Spring, J. M.** Bowler's thumb. (Ulnovolar neuroma of the thumb). *Clin. Orthop.,* 1972; 83:99–101.
22. **Eckman, P. B., Perlstein, G., and Altrocchi, P. H.** Ulnar neuropathy in bicycle riders. *Arch. Neurol.,* 1975; 32:130–131.
23. **Ferretti, A., Cerullo, G., and Russo, G.** Suprascapular neuropathy in volleyball players. *J. Bone Joint Surg.,* 1987; 69A:260–263.
24. **Fischer, M. A. and Gorelick, P. B.** Entrapment neuropathies: differential diagnosis and management. *Postgrad. Med.,* 1985; 77:160–174.
25. **Frontera, W. R.** Cyclist palsy: clinical and electrodiagnostic findings. *Br. J. Sports Med.,* 1983; 17:91–93.
26. **Fulkerson, J. P.** Transient ulnar neuropathy from Nordic skiing. *Clin. Orthop.,* 1980; 153:230–231.
27. **Ganzhorn, R. W., Hocker, J. T., Horowitz, M., and Switzer, H. E.** Suprascapular nerve entrapment. *J. Bone Joint Surg.,* 1981; 63A:492–494.
28. **Gessini, L., Jandolo, B., and Pietrangeli, A.** The anterior tarsal syndrome: report of four cases. *J. Bone Joint Surg.,* 1984; 66A:786–787.
29. **Glennon, T. P.** Isolated injury of the infraspinatus branch of the suprascapular nerve. *Arch. Phys. Med. Rehab.,* 1992; 73:201–202.
30. **Glousman, R. E.** Ulnar nerve problems in the athlete's elbow. *Clin. Sports Med.,* 1990; 9:365–377.
31. **Gould, N. and Trevino, S.** Sural nerve entrapment by avulsion fracture of the base of the fifth metatarsal. *Foot Ankle,* 1981; 2:153–155.
32. **Hemler, D. E., Ward, W. K., Karstetter, K. W., and Bryant, P. M.** Saphenous nerve entrapment caused by pes anserine bursitis mimicking stress fracture of the tibia. *Arch. Phys. Med. Rehab.,* 1991; 72:336–337.
33. **Henricson, A. S. and Westlin, N. E.** Chronic calcaneal pain in athletes: entrapment of the calcaneal nerve? *Am. J. Sports Med.,* 1984; 12:152–154.
34. **Hirasawa, Y. and Sakakida, K.** Sports and peripheral nerve injury. *Am. J. Sports Med.,* 1983; 11:420–426.
35. **Ho, P. K., Dellon, A. L., and Wilgis, E. F. S.** True aneurysms of the hand resulting from athletic injury. *Am. J. Sports Med.,* 1985; 13:136–138.
36. **Howard, F. M.** Controversies in nerve entrapment syndromes in the forearm and wrist. *Orthop. Clin. N. Am.,* 1986; 17:375–381.
37. **Howell, A. E. and Leach, R. E.** Bowler's thumb: perineural fibrosis of the digital nerve. *J. Bone Joint Surg.,* 1970; 52A:379–381.
38. **Hunter, S. C. and Poole, R. M.** The chronically inflamed tendon. *Clin. Sports Med.,* 1987; 6:371–388.
39. **Jackson, D. L.** Electrodiagnostic studies of median and ulnar nerves in cyclists. *Phys. Sportsmed.,* 1989; 17:137–148.
40. **Jackson, D. L. and Haglund, B.** Tarsal tunnel syndrome in athletes. Case reports and literature review. *Am. J. Sports Med.,* 1991; 19:61–65.

41. **Jackson, D. L. and Haglund, B. L.** Tarsal tunnel syndrome in runners. *Sports Med.,* 1992; 13:146–149.

42. **Johnson, D. C.** The upper extremity in swimming. In: *Symposium on Upper Extremity Injuries in Athletes.* Pettrone, F. A., Ed. St. Louis: C. V. Mosby, 1986:36–46.

43. **Karas, S. E.** Thoracic outlet syndrome. *Clin. Sports Med.,* 1990; 9:297–310.

44. **Kernohan, J., Levack, B., and Wilson, J. N.** Entrapment of the superficial peroneal nerve: three case reports. *J. Bone Joint Surg.,* 1985; 67B:60–61.

45. **Kim, S. M. and Goodrich, J. A.** Isolated proximal musculocutaneous nerve palsy: case report. *Arch. Phys. Med. Rehab.,* 1984; 65:735–736.

46. **Komar, J.** *Alagut — Szindromak.* Budapest: Medicina - Konyvkiado, 1977.

47. **Kopel, H. P. and Thompson, W. A. L.** Peripheral entrapment neuropathies of the lower extremity. *N. Engl. J. Med.,* 1960; 262:55–60.

48. **Leach, R. E., Purnell, M. B., and Saito, A.** Peroneal nerve entrapment in runners. *Am. J. Sports Med.,* 1989; 17:287–291.

49. **Leffert, R. D.** Brachial plexus injuries. *N. Engl. J. Med.,* 1974; 291:1059–1066.

50. **Leffert, R. D.** Thoracic outlet syndrome and the shoulder. *Clin. Sports Med.,* 1983; 2:439–52.

51. **Lindenbaum, B. L.** Ski boot compression syndrome. *Clin. Orthop.,* 1979; 140:19–23.

52. **Liveson, J. A., Bronson, M. J., and Pollack, M. A.** Suprascapular nerve lesions at the spinoglenoid notch: report of three cases and review of the literature. *J. Neurol. Neurosurg. Psych.,* 1991; 54:241–243.

53. **Lotem, M., Fried, A., and Levy, M.** Radial palsy following muscular effort: a nerve compression syndrome possibly related to a fibrous arch of the lateral band of the triceps. *J. Bone Joint Surg.,* 1971; 53B:500–506.

54. **Lowdon, I. M. R.** Superficial peroneal nerve entrapment: a case report. *J. Bone Joint Surg.,* 1985; 67B:58–59.

55. **McGregor, J., Moncur, J. A.** Meralgia paresthetica — a sports lesion in girl gymnasts. *Br. J. Sport Med.,* 1977; 11:16–19.

56. **Maimaris, C. and Zadeh, H. G.** Ulnar nerve compression in the cyclist's hand: two case reports and review of the literature. *Br. J. Sport Med.,* 1990; 24:245–246.

57. **Massey, E. W. and Pleet, A. B.** Handcuffs and cheiralgia paresthetica. *Neurology,* 1978; 28:1312–1313.

58. **Mastiglia, F. L.** Musculocutaneous neuropathy after strenuous physical activity. *Med. J. Aust.,* 1986; 145:153–154.

59. **Mattalino, A. J., Deese, J. M., Jr., and Campbell, E. D., Jr.** Office evaluation and treatment of lower extremity injuries in runners. *Clin. Sports Med.,* 1989; 8:461–475.

60. **McAuliffe, T. B., Fiddian, N. J., and Browett, J. P.** Entrapment neuropathy of the superficial peroneal nerve: a bilateral case. *J. Bone Joint Surg.,* 1985; 67B:62–63.

61. **McCue, F. C., III, and Miller, G. A.** Soft-tissue injuries of the hand. In: *Symposium on Upper Extremity Injuries in Athletes.* Pettrone, F. A., Ed. St. Louis: C. V. Mosby, 1986:79–94.

62. **Mendoza, F. X. and Main, K.** Peripheral nerve injuries of the shoulder in the athlete. *Clin. Sports Med.,* 1990; 9:331–342.

63. **Minkow, F. V. and Basset, F. H. III.** Bowler's thumb. *Clin. Orthop.,* 1972; 83:115–117.

64. **Moller, B. N. and Kadin, S.** Entrapment of the common peroneal nerve. *Am. J. Sports Med.,* 1987; 15:90–91.

65. **Mosher, J. F.** Peripheral nerve injuries and entrapment of the forearm and wrist. In: *Symposium on Upper Extremity Injuries in Athletes.* Pettrone, F. A., Ed. St. Louis: C. V. Mosby, 1986:174–181.

66. **Moss, S. H. and Switzer, H. E.** Radial tunnel syndrome. A spectrum of clinical presentations. *J. Hand Surg.*, 1983; 8:414–420.
67. **Murphy, P. C. and Baxter, D. E.** Nerve entrapment of the foot and ankle in runners. *Clin. Sports Med.*, 1985; 4:753–763.
68. **Naso, S. J.** Compression of the digital nerve: a new entity in tennis players. *Orthop. Rev.*, 1984; 13:47.
69. **Nuber, G. W., McCarthy, W. J., Yao, J. S. T., Schafer, M. F., and Suker, J. R.** Arterial abnormalities of the hand in athletes. *Am. J. Sports Med.*, 1990; 18:520–523.
70. **Osterman, L. A., Moskow, L., and Low, D. W.** Soft-tissue injuries of the hand and wrist in racquet sports. *Clin. Sports Med.*, 1988; 7:329–48.
71. **Pećina, M.** Contribution to the etiological explanation of the piriformis syndrome. *Acta Anat. (Basel)*, 1979; 105:181–187.
72. **Pećina, M., Krmpotić-Nemanić, J., and Markiewitz, A. D.** *Tunnel Syndromes*. Boca Raton: CRC Press, 1991.
73. **Pećina, M., Bojanić, I., and Markiewitz, A. D.** Nerve entrapment syndrome in athletes. *Clin. J. Sport Med.*, 1993; 3:36–43.
74. **Pećina, M. and Bojanić, I.** Nervus musculocutaneous entrapment syndrome in the shoulder region. *Int. Orthop. (SICOT)*, 1993; (in print).
75. **Posner, M. A.** Compressive neuropathies of the median and radial nerves at the elbow. *Clin. Sports Med.*, 1990; 93:34–63.
76. **Post, M. and Mayer, J.** Suprascapular nerve entrapment. *Clin. Orthop.*, 1987; 223:126–136.
77. **Priest, J. D.** A physical phenomenon: shoulder depression in athletes. *Sports Care Fit.*, 1989; 3/4:20–24.
78. **Pringle, R. M., Protheroe, K., and Mukherjee, S. K.** Entrapment neuropathy of the sural nerve. *J. Bone Joint Surg.*, 1974; 56B:465–467.
79. **Radin, E. L.** Tarsal tunnel syndrome. *Clin. Orthop.*, 1983; 181:167–170.
80. **Rask, E. L.** Tarsal plantar neuropraxia (jogger's foot): report of three cases. *Clin. Orthop.*, 1978; 134:193–198.
81. **Redler, M. R., Ruland, L. J., and McCue, F. C., III.** Quadrilateral space syndrome in a throwing athlete. *Am. J. Sports Med.*, 1986; 14:511–513.
82. **Regan, W. D.** Lateral elbow pain in the athlete: a clinical review. *Clin. J. Sport Med.*, 1991; 1:53–58.
83. **Rettig, A. C.** Neurovascular injuries in the wrist and hands of athletes. *Clin. Sports Med.*, 1990; 9:389–417.
84. **Ringel, S. P., Treihaft, M., Carry, M., Fisher, R., and Jacobs, P.** Suprascapular neuropathy in pitchers. *Am. J. Sports Med.*, 1990; 18:80–86.
85. **Ritts, G. D., Wood, M. B., and Linscheid, R. L.** Radial tunnel syndrome: a ten-year surgical experience. *Clin. Orthop.*, 1987; 219:201–205.
86. **Roles, N. C. and Maudsley, R. H.** Radial tunnel syndrome. Resistant tennis elbow as a nerve entrapment. *J. Bone Joint Surg.*, 1972; 54B:499–508.
87. **Ruby, L. K.** Common hand injuries in the athlete. *Orthop. Clin., N. Am.*, 1980; 11:819–839.
88. **Schon, L. C., Baxter, D. E.** Neuropathies of the foot and ankle in athletes. *Clin. Sports Med.*, 1990; 9:489–509.
89. **Sheon, R. P.** Peripheral nerve entrapment, occupation-related syndromes, and sports injuries. *Curr. Opin. Rheumatol.*, 1992; 4:219–225.
90. **Siegel, I. M.** Bowling thumb neuroma (letter). *JAMA*, 1965; 192:263.
91. **Smail, D. F.** Handelbar palsy (letter). *N. Engl. J. Med.*, 1975; 292:322.

92. **Stack, R. E., Bianco, A. J., and MacCarty, C. S.** Compression of the common peroneal nerve by ganglion cysts. *J. Bone Joint Surg.,* 1965; 47A:773–778.

93. **Strukel, R. J. and Garick, J. G.** Thoracic outlet compression in athletes. *Am. J. Sports Med.,* 1978; 6:35–39.

94. **Styf, J.** Entrapment of the superficial peroneal nerve: diagnosis and results of decompression. *J. Bone Joint Surg.,* 1989; 71B:131–135.

95. **Styf, J.** Chronic exercise-induced pain in the anterior aspect of the lower leg: an overview of diagnosis. *Sports Med.,* 1989; 7:331–339.

96. **Tackmann, W., Richter, H. P., and Stohr, M.** *Kompressionssyndrome peripherer Nerven.* Berlin: Springer-Verlag, 1989.

97. **Weinstein, S. M. and Herring, S.** Nerve problems and compartment syndromes in the hand, wrist, and forearm. *Clin. Sports Med.,* 1992; 11:161–188.

98. **Werner, C. O.** Lateral elbow pain and posterior interosseous nerve entrapment. *Acta Orthop. Scand. (Suppl.),* 1979; 174:1–62.

99. **Wilhelm, A.** Unklare Schmmerzzustande an der oberen Extremitat. *Orthopadie,* 1987; 16:458–464.

100. **White, H. H.** Pack palsy: a neurological complication of scouting. *Pediatrics,* 1968; 41:1001–1003.

101. **Wojtys, E. M., Smith, P. A., and Hankin, F. M.** A cause of ulnar neuropathy in a baseball pitcher: a case report. *Am. J. Sports Med.,* 1986; 14:522–524.

102. **Wood, M. B. and Dobyns, J. H.** Sports-related extraarticular wrist syndromes. *Clin. Orthop.,* 1986; 202:93–102.

103. **Worth, R. M., Kettelkamp, D. B., Defalque, R. J., and Duane, K. V.** Saphenous nerve entrapment. A case of medial knee pain. *Am. J. Sports Med.,* 1984; 12:80–81.

104. **Yocum, L. A.** The diagnosis and nonoperative treatment of elbow problems in the athlete. *Clin. Sports Med.,* 1989; 8:39–51.

105. **Zongzhao, L., Jiansheng, Z., and Li, Z.** Anterior tarsal tunnel syndrome. *J. Bone Joint Surg.,* 1991; 73B:470–473.

Chapter
13

Overuse Injuries in the Young Athletes

I. OVERVIEW OF YOUNG ATHLETE INJURIES

During the past few decades, there has been a dramatic increase of top world-ranking results accomplished by young athletes, most notably in swimming and gymnastics. Other athletic activities are also following this trend with serious training and organized competition beginning at increasingly earlier ages. Heavy sports participation coupled with ongoing growth creates unique problems which often result in athletic injuries belonging to the overuse injuries group.[2,3,5,7,10,12]

In the U.S. one half of males and one fourth of females between 8 to 16 years of age are engaged in some type of competitive, organized sports activity during the school year. An additional 20% of the children in this age range are involved in community sports programs. Three fourths of U.S. junior and middle schools have significant competitive sports programs. The growing involvement of children in organized sports and fitness activities has been paralleled by an increased number of new types of injuries in children.[1,2,3,9,12,13] When impact or macrotrauma injuries are compared, there is certainly no clear evidence that organized sports are in any way more dangerous, or more safe, than free play. However, there is a whole new genre of injuries occurring in children engaged in organized sports, which rarely occur in the free play situation. These injuries are overuse injuries, such as tendinitis, stress fractures, patellofemoral stress syndrome of the knee, bursitis, etc. Although the child subjected to repetitive training now appears to be susceptible to many of the same overuse injuries as adults, there are several overuse injuries unique to the growing child. These unique overuse injuries are associated with the presence of growth cartilage in the child, and additionally, with the growth process itself. Among the risk factors for overuse injuries, training errors, musculotendinous imbalance, anatomic malalignment of the lower extremities, inadequate footwear, playing surface, and growth (in particular, the growth spurt) must be added when assessing the occurrence of overuse injuries in the young athlete. The growth cartilage, particularly the growing articular cartilage, is less resistant to repetitive microtraumas than adult cartilage. Growth cartilage is located at three sites in the child: the epiphyseal plate, the joint surface, and the apophyseal insertions of major muscle-tendon units. Each of these sites may be injured and may have a particular susceptibility to repetitive microtraumas.[9] Overuse injuries, the result of repetitive microtraumas, have rarely been identified at the epiphysis (Freiberg's disease, Kohler-Mouchet's disease or even Legg-Calve-Perthes' disease, growth plate Scheuermann's diseases, Blount's diseases), but are seen with increasing frequency at the joint surface (osteochondritis dissecans, chondromalacia and apophysitis, Osgood-Schlatter's disease, Sever's disease). Injuries to the growth plate from repetitive trauma caused by athletic activities has been suggested as an etiologic factor in the onset of adult arthritis of the hip, presumably as a result of minimal capital femoral epiphyseal displacement from this repetitive microtrauma. Chantraine[9] reported that a long-term follow-up of soccer players suggested that they had a bilaterally increased incidence of genu varum and osteoarthritis at the knee when compared to the general population. *Little League shoulder* is a term applied to nondisplaced but symptomatic microfractures at the growth plate of the proximal humerus; this is often found in children and adolescent baseball pitchers after they have repetitive trauma of throwing a ball. There is increasing evidence that the child's articulare surface is more susceptible to shear than adult cartilage, particularly at the elbow, knee, and ankle.[4] Repetitive trauma's are responsible for many cases of osteochondritis dissecans, e.g., at the elbow of a child pitcher, with an increased incidence of osteochondritis of the capitellum, with or without associated loose bodies in the joint, injury and premature closure of the proximal radial epiphysis, overgrowth of the radial head, and irritation of the medial epicondyle. The mechanism of injury is the repetitive valgus strain applied to the elbow when throwing, with compression medially and traction laterally. Little League elbow is the general label applied to this overuse injury sustained by some young throwers. It is obvious that some of the overuse injuries in young athletes can be labeled as "overgrowth" injuries. Traction apophysitises are the most common overuse and overgrowth injuries in young athletes. Traction apophyses are sites of active growth in the child, consisting of columns of growth cartilage uniting tendon with bone. Injuries at the traction apophyses may result from repetitive microtraumas. The resultant pain, swelling, and on occasion, bony and cartilaginous overgrowth are referred to as apophysitis. The inflammation may be a component of the body's response to repetitive tiny avulsions. Being a secondary process, subsequent healing occurs at the involved apophysis. Thus, labeling these injuries "apophysitis" tends to obscure the primary traumatic nature of the injury. Until now, we have discussed overuse injuries of the cartilage, especially the growing cartilage, but all of the structural components of the musculoskeletal system, i.e., the muscle-tendon units, ligaments, tendons, bursae, and muscles, are potential sites of overuse injuries. Perhaps the most obvious "new" overuse injuries in children are stress fractures. These fractures were not known in children prior to the advent of organized sports training in the early 1950s. They appear to be most frequently associated with improper training and to be highly preventable if proper attention is paid to the rate and intensity of training.[8] Tendinitis can certainly occur in the young athletes, although much less frequently than in the adult. Usually, the site of tendon insertion, the apophysis, becomes symptomatic before the tendon itself, although both may become painful and inflamed.[6,7,10,11] Overuse injuries of the joint capsule or ligament are frequently diagnosed as bursitis. A bursa, of course, becomes swollen or inflamed when adjacent tissues, such as tendon or ligament, sustain irritation or injury. As with

TABLE 1
The Most Common Overuse Injuries in Young Athletes

Site	Overuse injury
Shoulder	"Little League shoulder"
	Impingement syndromes (primary and secondary; instability)
Elbow	"Little League elbow"
	Medial epicondylitis
Hand	Closure of the distal radial epiphysis
Spine	Scheuermann's disease
	Spondylolysis
Hip and pelvis	Iliac apophysitis
	Rectus femoris apophysitis
	Sartorius apophysitis
	Iliopsoas apophysitis
	Apophysis of greater trochanter (Mandl)
Knee	Osgood-Schlatter's disease
	Sinding-Larson-Johansson's disease
	Patellofemoral stress syndrome
Ankle and foot	Sever's disease
	Accessory navicular syndrome
	Iselin's disease
	(Apophysitis at the base of the fifth metatarsal)
	Medial malleolus apophysitis
Variety of localization	Bursitis
Variety of localization	Stress fractures

tendinitis, bursitis in the young athletes usually responds quite rapidly to relative rest or conservative treatment.

The aim of this short chapter about overuse injuries in young athletes is not to describe all of the potential overuse syndromes, but only to indicate the presence of this "new chapter" in sports medicine. The most common overuse injuries in childhood and adolescents are shown in Table 1.

In conclusion, we would like to cite the opinion of Micheli[9], "Certainly, the role of maltraining, usually too much over too short a period of time, appears to be common to most overuse injuries, including children's injuries in sports. It now appears that the 'weekend warrior' syndrome may even affect the very young child, and so aging, though perhaps still a factor in susceptibility to overuse injury, is probably less important than once thought."

REFERENCES

1. **Benezis, C., Simeray, J., and Simon, L.** *Muscles, Tendon et Sport.* Paris: Masson, 1990; 187–197.
2. **Clain, M. R. and Hershman, E. B.** Overuse injuries in children and adolescents. *Phys. Sportsmed.,* 1989; 17:111–123.

3. **Dalton, S. E.,** Overuse injuries in adolescent athletes. *Sports Med.,* 1992; 13:58–70.
4. **Dupuis, J. M.** Croissance et sport. *Actual. Sport Med.,* 1992; 18:10–16.
5. **Katz, J. F.** Nonarticular osteochondroses. *Clin. Orthop.,* 1981; 158:70–76.
6. **Lehman, R. C., Gregg, J. R., and Torg, E.** Iselin's disease. *Am. J. Sports Med.,* 1986; 14:494–496.
7. **Longis, B., Surzur, P., and Moulies, D.** Apophysites de croissance. *Actual. Sport Med.,* 1992; 19:9–10.
8. **Maffulli, N.** Intensive training in young athletes. The orthopaedic surgeon's viewpoint. *Sports Med.,* 1990; 9:229–243.
9. **Micheli, L. J.** Overuse injuries in children's sports: the growth factor. *Orthop. Clin. N. Am.,* 1983; 14:337–359.
10. **Micheli, L. J.** The traction apophysitis. *Clin. Sports Med.,* 1987; 6:389–404.
11. **Micheli, L. J. and Ireland, M. L.** Prevention and management of calcaneal apophysitis in children: an overuse syndrome. *J. Pediatr. Orthop.,* 1987; 7:34–38.
12. **O'Neill, D. B. and Micheli, L. J.** Overuse injuries in the young athlete. *Clin. Sports Med.,* 1988; 7:591–610.
13. **Stanitski, C. L.** Management of sports injuries in children and adolescents. *Orthop. Clin. N. Am.,* 1988; 19:689–697.

Subject Index

Subject Index

Author Index

Author Index

Reference numbers are in parentheses and indicate that the author's work is referred to in text. Numbers in italics show the page on which the complete reference is given.

A

Aalto, K., 49(89), *54*
Aalto, T., 180(110), 181(110), *213, 216*
Abel, M. S., 292(1), *305*
Abelin, T., 195(166), *218*
Abrahamsson, P., 134(6), *155*
Abrams, J. S., 42(25), *51*
Adeleine, P., 175(16), *212*
Agins, H. J., 49(74), *53*
Aglietti, P., *211*
Aho, H., 229(8), *246*
Ahovuo, J., 46(5), *50*
Ahstrom, J. P., 255(1), 256(1), 257(1), 258(1), *266*
Ain, B. R., 65(31), *72*
Aldam, C. H., 241(31), *246*
Aldridge, M. J., 291(10), *305*
Alen, M., 297(58), *307*
Allander, E., 56, *70*
Allen, M. E., 290(2), *305*
Allen, W. C., 143(61), 144(61), 145(61), 147(61), *158*
Alroham, E., 65(20), 66(20), 67(20), *71*
Alten, S. R., 179(78), *215*
Alter, M. J., 22(1), *25*
Altrocchi, P. H., 315(22), *323*
Amato, F., 241(67), *248*, 279(21), 280(21), *282*
Amis, J., 251(2), 253(2), *266*
Amit, S., 287(28), 292(28), *306*
Ammann, W., 125(10), 129(10), 135(10), 137(10), *155*
Anderson, A. H., 175(15), *212*
Anderson, B., 22(2), *25*
Anderson, D. L., 235(32), 238(32), *247*
Anderson, R. B., 264(53), *268*

Andrews, J. R., 19(3), *25*, 67(58), 68(58), 69(59, 63), *73*, 199(152), *218*
Andrish, J. T., 229(1), *245*
Anticevic´, D., 203(185), 205(185), *219*
Apple, D. F., Jr., 189, 190, *214*
Arons, M. S., 75(1), *85*
Asai, H., 146, 147(47), *157*
Ashewer, J., 41(31), *52*

B

Bajraktarevic, T., 40(17), *51*, 175(2, 50), *211, 213*
Baker, B. E., 302(78), *308*
Balduini, F. C., *308*
Balint, B. J., 241(51), *247*
Bandi, W., 177(3), *211*
Baratta, R., *158*
Barber, F. A., 195(181), 197(181), 199(181), *219*
Barnes, D. A., 69(60), *73*
Barnett, P. R., 166, *212*
Barrow, G. W., 284, *305*
Basmaijam, J. V., 107(1), *118*
Basset, F. H., III, 151(65), *158*, 179(81), *215, 207(194), 219*, 312(1), *322*, 317(63), *324*
Bateman, J. E., 38(1), *50*, 310(2), *322*
Bates, B. T., 222(7), 230(48), 231(48), 236(48), *246, 247*
Batt, M. E., 75(2), *85*
Baumgard, S. H., 65(2), 66(2), 67, *71*
Baxter, D. E., 261(51), *268*, 309(14), 317(14), 318(14), 319(14, 88), 320, 321(3, 67, 88), 322(14, 67, 88), *322, 325*
Bazzoli, A. S., 320(4), *322*
Beagley, M. J., 175(66), *214*, 276(20), *282*